DECISION MAKING IN

Psychiatric and Psychosocial Nursing

Decision Making in Clinical Nursing™ Series

Baird:
Decision Making in Oncology Nursing

Baumann, Johnston, Antai-Otong:
Decision Making in Psychiatric and Psychosocial Nursing

Drain:
Decision Making in Postanesthesia Nursing

Gorzeman, Bowdoin:
Decision Making in Medical-Surgical Nursing

Knor:
Decision Making in Obstetrical Nursing

Mancini:
Decision Making in Emergency Nursing

Murphy:
Decision Making in Pediatric Nursing

Wells:
Decision Making in Perioperative Nursing

Williams:
Decision Making in Critical Care Nursing

DECISION MAKING IN

Psychiatric and Psychosocial Nursing

Andrea Baumann, RN, BScN, MScN, PhD

Associate Professor
School of Nursing
Faculty of Health Sciences
McMaster University
Hamilton, Ontario, Canada

Nancy E. Johnston, RN, MHSc

Assistant Professor
School of Nursing
Faculty of Health Sciences
University of Ottawa
Ottawa, Ontario, Canada

Deborah Antai-Otong, MS, RNCS, ANP

Psychiatric Clinical Specialist
Dallas Veterans Administration Medical Center
Dallas, Texas

1990 B.C. Decker Inc. • Toronto • Philadelphia

Publisher

B.C. Decker Inc
3228 South Service Road
Burlington, Ontario L7N 3H8

B.C. Decker Inc
320 Walnut Street
Suite 400
Philadelphia, Pennsylvania 19106

Sales and Distribution

United States and Puerto Rico
The C.V. Mosby Company
11830 Westline Industrial Drive
Saint Louis, Missouri 63146

Canada
McAinsh & Co. Ltd.
2760 Old Leslie Street
Willowdale, Ontario M2K 2X5

Australia
McGraw-Hill Book Company Australia Pty. Ltd.
4 Barcoo Street
Roseville East 2069
New South Wales, Australia

Brazil
Editora McGraw-Hill do Brasil, Ltda.
rua Tabapua, 1.105, Itaim-Bibi
Sao Paulo, S.P. Brasil

Colombia
Interamericana/McGraw-Hill de Colombia, S.A.
Apartado Aereo 81078
Bogota, D.E. Colombia

Europe
McGraw-Hill Book Company GmbH
Lademannbogen 136
D-2000 Hamburg 63
West Germany

France
MEDSI/McGraw-Hill
6, avenue Daniel Lesueur
75007 Paris, France

Hong Kong and China
McGraw-Hill Book Company
Suite 618, Ocean Centre
5 Canton Road
Tsimshatsui, Kowloon
Hong Kong

India
Tata McGraw-Hill Publishing Company, Ltd.
12/4 Asaf Ali Road, 3rd Floor
New Delhi 110002, India

Indonesia
P.O. Box 122/JAT
Jakarta, 1300 Indonesia

Italy
McGraw-Hill Libri Italia, s.r.l.
Piazza Emilia, 5
I-20129 Milano MI
Italy

Japan
Igaku-Shoin Ltd.
Tokyo International P.O. Box 5063
1-28-36 Hongo, Bunkyo-ku,
Tokyo 113, Japan

Korea
C.P.O. Box 10583
Seoul, Korea

Malaysia
No. 8 Jalan SS 7/6B
Kelana Jaya
47301 Petaling Jaya
Selangor, Malaysia

Mexico
Interamericana/McGraw-Hill de Mexico, S.A. de C.V.
Cedro 512, Colonia Atlampa
(Apartado Postal 26370)
06450 Mexico, D.F., Mexico

New Zealand
McGraw-Hill Book Co. New Zealand Ltd.
5 Joval Place, Wiri
Manukau City, New Zealand

Panama
Editorial McGraw-Hill Latinoamericana, S.A.
Apartado Postal 2036
Zona Libre de Colon
Colon, Republica de Panama

Portugal
Editora McGraw-Hill de Portugal, Ltda.
Rua Rosa Damasceno 11A–B
1900 Lisboa, Portugal

South Africa
Libriger Book Distributors
Warehouse Number 8
"Die Ou Looiery"
Tannery Road
Hamilton, Bloemfontein 9300

Southeast Asia
McGraw-Hill Book Co.
348 Jalan Boon Lay
Jurong, Singapore 2261

Spain
McGraw-Hill/Interamericana de Espana, S.A.
Manuel Ferrero, 13
28020 Madrid, Spain

Taiwan
P.O. Box 87–601
Taipei, Taiwan

Thailand
632/5 Phaholyothin Road
Sapan Kwai
Bangkok 10400
Thailand

United Kingdom, Middle East and Africa
McGraw-Hill Book Company (U.K.) Ltd.
Shoppenhangers Road
Maidenhead, Berkshire
SL6 2QL England

Venezuela
McGraw-Hill/Interamericana, C.A.
2da. calle Bello Monte
(entre avenida Casanova y Sabana Grande)
Apartado Aereo 50785
Caracas 1050, Venezuela

NOTICE

The authors and publisher have made every effort to ensure that the patient care recommended herein, including choice of drugs and drug dosages, is in accord with the accepted standards and practice at the time of publication. However, since research and regulation constantly change clinical standards, the reader is urged to check the product information sheet included in the package of each drug, which includes recommended doses, warnings, and contraindications. This is particularly important with new or infrequently used drugs.

Decision Making in Psychiatric and Psychosocial Nursing

ISBN 1–55664–158–3

Library of Congress catalog card number: 89–50927

10 9 8 7 6 5 4 3 2 1

CONTRIBUTORS

DEBORAH ANTAI-OTONG, MS, RNCS, ANP

Psychiatric Clinical Specialist, Psychiatric (Opt) Triage Unit, Dallas Veterans Administration Medical Center, Dallas, Texas

ANDREA BAUMANN, RN, BScN, MScN, PhD

Associate Professor, School of Nursing, Faculty of Health Sciences, McMaster University, Hamilton, Ontario, Canada

ANN C. BECKINGHAM, RN, PhD

Associate Professor, School of Nursing; Joint Appointee, Educational Centre for Aging and Health, McMaster University, Hamilton, Ontario, Canada

ROSA BELGARD, RN, MS

Director of Nursing, The Haven, DeSoto, Texas

MAGDA BISHAI, RN, MEd

Clinical Educator, School of Nursing, Faculty of Health Sciences, University of Ottawa; Clinical Educator, School of Nursing, Algonguin College, Ottawa, Ontario, Canada

SHERYL L. BOBLIN, BScN, MEd

Assistant Professor, Faculty of Health Sciences, McMaster University, Hamilton, Ontario, Canada

DIANE T. BRISSON, RN, BSN, MSc

Assistant Professor, School of Nursing, Faculty of Health Sciences, University of Ottawa, Ottawa, Ontario, Canada

BARBARA BROWN, BA, BScN, MScN

Associate Professor, School of Nursing, Faculty of Health Sciences, McMaster University; Public Health Associate, Bereavement Team, Hamilton-Wentworth Department of Public Health Services, Hamilton, Ontario, Canada

KAY BURKE, BS, MS, RN, LPC

Psychiatric and Mental Health Clinical Nurse Specialist, Mental Hygiene Clinic, Department of Veterans Affairs, Dallas Veterans Administration Medical Center, Dallas, Texas

HOWARD KARL BUTCHER, RN, BS, BSN, MScN

Clinical Nurse Specialist—Mental Health, Psychiatric Institute of Washington, D.C., Washington, D.C.

M.T. MILDRED CARSWELL, RN, BScNEd, MSN, CNM

Associate Professor, School of Nursing, Faculty of Health Sciences, University of Ottawa, Ottawa, Ontario, Canada

DONNA CILISKA, RN, PhD

Associate Professor, Faculty of Health Sciences, McMaster University; Clinical Nurse Consultant, Teaching Health Unit, Hamilton-Wentworth Department of Public Health Services, Hamilton, Ontario, Canada

LYNN COCHRANE, RN, BScN

Manager, Ottawa Salus Corporation, Ottawa, Ontario, Canada

MARILYN E. DEWIS, RN, BScN, MEd

Assistant Professor, School of Nursing, University of British Columbia, Vancouver, British Columbia, Canada

VIOLA DUFF, RN, MEd

Lecturer, School of Nursing, Faculty of Health Sciences, University of Ottawa, Ottawa, Ontario, Canada

PATRICIA ELLIS, RN, BS, MS

Associate Professor, School of Nursing, Faculty of Health Sciences, McMaster University; Clinical Associate, McMaster University Medical Center, Hamilton, Ontario, Canada

NONA FLYE, RN, MSN

Psychiatric Nurse, The Day Hospital, Dallas Veterans Administration Medical Center, Dallas, Texas

CHERYL FORCHUK, RN, BA, BScN, MScN

Doctoral Student, College of Nursing, Wayne State University, Detroit, Michigan; Clinical Nurse Specialist, Hamilton Psychiatric Hospital, Hamilton, Ontario, Canada

FRANCES FOTHERGILL-BOURBONNAIS, RN, BScN, MN

Associate Professor, School of Nursing, Faculty of Health Sciences, University of Ottawa, Ottawa, Ontario, Canada

PATRICIA A. GERVAIZE, PhD, CPsych

Adjunct Professor, School of Psychology, Department of Obstetrics and Gynecology, School of Medicine, Faculty of Health Sciences, University of Ottawa; Clinical Research Psychologist, Ottawa Civic Hospital, Ottawa, Ontario, Canada

IRENE L. GOLDSTONE, RN, BN, MSc

Adjunct Professor, School of Nursing, University of British Columbia; Director, Medical Nursing, St. Paul's Hospital, Vancouver, British Columbia, Canada

BRENDA INGRAM, RN, MS

Head Nurse, Acute Psychiatry, Dallas Veterans Administration Medical Center, Dallas, Texas

GULROSEBEGUM N. JIWANI, RN, MN

Clinical Nurse Specialist, Brockville Psychiatric Hospital, Brockville, Ontario, Canada

NANCY E. JOHNSTON, RN, MHSc

Assistant Professor, School of Nursing, Faculty of Health Sciences, University of Ottawa, Ottawa, Ontario, Canada

HELEN KIRKPATRICK, RN, BScN, MScN

Clinical Lecturer, School of Nursing, Faculty of Health Sciences, McMaster University; Clinical Nurse Specialist, Hamilton Psychiatric Hospital, Hamilton, Ontario, Canada

ALISON C. LEE, BScN, BA

PhD Student, Department of Psychology, University of Ottawa, Ottawa, Ontario, Canada

MARY-LOU MARTIN, RN, BScN, MScN

Assistant Clinical Professor, School of Nursing, Faculty of Health Sciences, McMaster University; Clinical Nurse Specialist, Hamilton Psychiatric Hospital, Hamilton, Ontario, Canada

ELIZABETH McCAY, RN, BNSc, MScN

Clinical Associate, University of Toronto; Research Associate, Sunnybrook Medical Centre, Toronto, Ontario, Canada

ERLINDA T. MORALES-MANN, RN, MA

Assistant Professor, School of Nursing, Faculty of Health Sciences, University of Ottawa, Ottawa, Ontario, Canada

ANNETTE M. O'CONNOR, RN, PhD

Associate Professor, School of Nursing, Faculty of Health Sciences, University of Ottawa, Ottawa, Ontario, Canada

KAREN PERKINS, RN, MSN

Clinical Nurse Specialist, Outpatient Psychiatry Manager, Outpatient Clinic, Parkland Memorial Hospital, Dallas, Texas

ELIZABETH PODNIEKS, RN, MES

Professor, School of Nursing, Ryerson Polytechnical Institute, Toronto, Ontario, Canada

ROSEMARIE RIDDELL, RN, BSN

Instructor, Medical Nursing, St. Paul's Hospital, Vancouver, British Columbia, Canada

ROBERTA RONAYNE, RN, MSc(A)

Assistant Professor, School of Nursing, Faculty of Health Sciences, University of Ottawa, Ottawa, Ontario, Canada

S. TAYLOR STEPHENS, MSN, RN

Nurse Manager, Willow Creek Adolescent Center, Residential Treatment Center, Arlington, Texas

B. HELEN THOMAS, RN, MSc

Assistant Professor, School of Nursing, Faculty of Health Sciences, McMaster University; Public Health Associate, Hamilton-Wentworth Department of Public Health Services, Hamilton, Ontario, Canada

JAN WESTWELL, RN, BScN, MScN

Assistant Clinical Professor, Faculty of Health Sciences, McMaster University; Clinical Nurse Specialist, Hamilton Psychiatric Hospital, Hamilton, Ontario, Canada

M. ANNE WYNESS, RN, MN

Assistant Professor, School of Nursing, University of British Columbia; Faculty Associate, Division of Nursing, Vancouver General Hospital, Vancouver, British Columbia, Canada

PREFACE

Nursing, like many other disciplines, is in a state of evolution. The rapid expansion of knowledge and increase in decision-making responsibilities have increased demands on the nurse to provide informed, comprehensive care. Critical thinking and informed decision making are imperative.

The prototypes chosen for this book are the most common psychiatric and psychosocial problems seen in nursing practice. With each chapter, there is the clinical algorithm and text with a recent bibliography. The format is designed to provide a succinct overview of the problems and demonstrates the expanded role of the nurse. The algorithmic format outlines both the theoretical framework and the decisions necessary in each prototype.

The nursing models and the psychosocial concepts chapters provide a theoretical overview of major concepts with an algorithm that highlights those concepts. As with other texts in the Decision Making series, this volume "outlines the facts and integrates a number of ideas at a glance" (Dubrovsky). This format is useful for both nurse educators and clinicians who need an overall approach to what are sometimes complex clinical phenomena. The authors of the clinical prototypes are nurse clinicians who have broad ranges of experience in psychiatric and psychosocial nursing as well as clinical decision making.

Andrea Baumann
Nancy E. Johnston
Deborah Antai-Otong

CONTENTS

I TRENDS AND CONCEPTS IN NURSING

Mental Health
Culturally Relevant Care in Mental Health Nursing
Assessing the Environment

Decision Making

Crisis State
Decision Making During a Crisis State
Dealing with Clients' Decisional Conflict

Nursing Models and Theories

Selecting or Developing a Model for Use in Clinical Practice: A Process-Oriented Approach
The Neuman Systems Model
Orem's Self-Care Model
Orlando's Need-Oriented Theory
Peplau's Interpersonal Theory
Roy's Adaptation Model
Rogers' Science of Unitary Human Beings Model

MENTAL HEALTH

Ann C. Beckingham
Andrea Baumann

A. The traditional definition of health includes physical health, mental health, and social well-being. The recent trend examines societal effects on an individual's mental health. Health and Welfare Canada defines mental health as the capacity of the individual, the group, and the environment to interact with one another in ways that promote subjective well-being, the optimal development and use of mental abilities (cognitive, affective, and relational), the achievement of individual and collective goals consistent with justice, and the attainment and preservation of conditions of fundamental equality.

B. As nurses, we must agree upon a concept of mental health that accentuates the importance of mental and social well-being within the context of society as a whole. In the continuum, one must differentiate between a mental health problem and a mental disorder. A mental health disorder is a psychopathologic problem, whereas a mental health problem may indicate external environmental factors. These factors may include the inability to cope with routine societal problems, such as stress or lack of adequate day care. Initiatives in the community must be aimed at encouraging approaches in which health promotion activities take their place along with rehabilitative efforts. Nurses and other health professionals can respond to mental health issues in many ways, play an integral and informed part in decision making in the delivery of mental health services, and work to reduce structural and attitudinal impediments to this process.

C. Societal factors that affect the mental health continuum are such factors as the stressors of poverty, which not only affect a person's capacity to alter the environment but also contribute to mental health problems. The mental health of individuals is enhanced by adequate shelter and income, a nurturing, accepting setting that promotes personal growth and development, and opportunities to have meaningful social roles (see "Assessing the Environment," p 6). Many features of modern society feed into mental health problems, as evidenced by family breakdown, substance abuse, and increased crime. In some cases, it is the environment and not the individual that needs change. Mental health becomes more than just the absence of diseases; it becomes a quality-of-life issue.

D. The mental health continuum fluctuates between a balance of equilibrium and disequilibrium. In general terms, a mental health problem can be described as a stressful imbalance among the respective demands and resources of the individual and family within that environment. The disequilibrium results in ineffective, dysphoric, or destructive patterns of thought, mood, and behavior not conducive to a healthy environment.

E. The goals are to support and maintain mental and physical health, prevent disability, and ensure that prevention receives adequate recognition as part of primary health care. Health promotion and disease prevention include proper nutrition, housing, and community resources. Implementation strategies include fostering public participation, strengthening community services and increasing their accessibility, and coordinating public policy with the overall objective of promoting mental health.

References

Beck C, Rawlins R, Williams G. Mental health and psychiatric nursing. St. Louis: CV Mosby, 1988.

Health and Welfare Canada. Mental health for Canadians: striking a balance. Ottawa: Ministry of Supply and Services, 1989.

Johnson B. Psychiatric and mental health nursing. Adaptation and growth. Philadelphia: JB Lippincott, 1986.

Pasquali EA, Arnold HM, DeBasio N, Alesi EG. Mental health nursing: a holistic approach. St. Louis: CV Mosby, 1985.

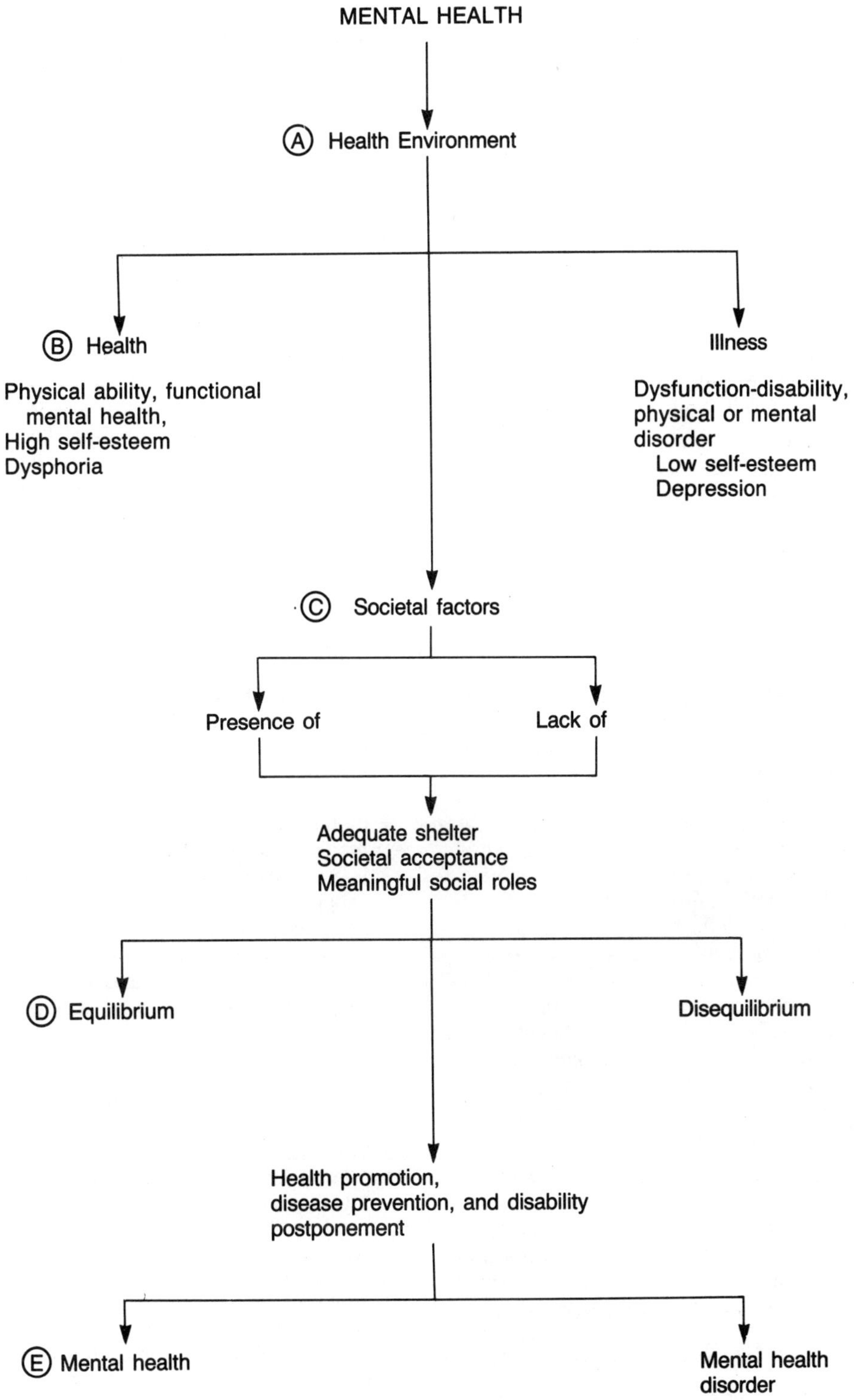
MENTAL HEALTH
(A) Health Environment
(B) Health
Physical ability, functional mental health,
High self-esteem
Dysphoria
Illness
Dysfunction-disability, physical or mental disorder
Low self-esteem
Depression
(C) Societal factors
Presence of
Lack of
Adequate shelter
Societal acceptance
Meaningful social roles
(D) Equilibrium
Disequilibrium
Health promotion, disease prevention, and disability postponement
(E) Mental health
Mental health disorder

CULTURALLY RELEVANT CARE IN MENTAL HEALTH NURSING

Nancy E. Johnston

A. Cultural differences between the nurse and client may lead to misunderstandings and disappointments and can prevent the development of a therapeutic relationship. It therefore becomes essential to assess the likelihood of cultural congruence at the beginning of the relationship. The nurse with knowledge of and comfort with cultures other than her own is an invaluable asset in providing culturally sensitive and relevant care.

B. In situations of significant cultural difference, it becomes necessary for the nurse to acknowledge her limitations and actively seek out resources that will help to bridge the gap. These resources may include the help of a colleague from the same culture as or one similar to the client's, the assistance of an interpreter, or consultation with a nurse specialist possessing advanced training in transcultural issues.

C. The client and nurse may come to the health-care setting with very different belief systems about the causation of mental illness. Whereas the nurse may believe that mental illness is caused by such factors as genetic predispositions, biochemical and hormonal imbalances, and adverse social conditions, the client may attribute spirit possession, the evil eye, or yin-yang imbalances as the cause of mental illness. Illnesses that are attributed to nonscientific causation fit into two broad categories: personalistic and naturalistic illnesses. Personalistic illnesses are believed to result from aggression or punishment directed toward the individual. Beliefs in voodoo and the evil eye are common expressions of this belief. Naturalistic illnesses are believed to be caused by impersonal factors and are frequently based on the equilibrium model. Examples of the most prevalent are the yin-yang model of Chinese culture, the American Navajo model of balance and harmony with nature, and the hot and cold model of Hispanic cultures.

D. Since positive client outcomes have been demonstrated to relate significantly to the client's belief in the efficacy of care, it is essential to facilitate the use of culturally salient health-care practices where they are practical and feasible. In many situations, the comfort that is derived by attributing a cause to an otherwise perplexing phenomenon and carrying out the prescribed interventions to deal with it results in appreciable relief of symptoms.

E. In some situations, however, the individual continues to decompensate, and it is at this point that a collaborative approach using both scientific and indigenous models of treatment is likely to be most effective.

F. Symptoms of mental illness are found in every culture, and although aspects of the expression of the mental illness vary across cultures, certain core symptoms seem to be universal. Those core symptoms frequently observed with schizophrenic patients include flatness of affect, delusions, hallucinations, and social withdrawal. Core symptoms of psychotic depression frequently include insomnia, early morning awakening, diurnal mood variation, and social withdrawal. Frequently, indigenous cultural groups are well aware that the symptoms a member exhibits are in the "serious" category and warrant western, scientific treatment approaches.

G. Secondary symptoms of the disorders mentioned above are, by contrast, culturally specific. The content of delusions and hallucinations is related directly to the individual's experience and preoccupations with the culture to which he or she belongs.

H. Western scientific models of treatment for psychotic illnesses predictably include the administration of psychotropic medication and perhaps even electroconvulsive therapy. Traditional or indigenous models would approach the illness in a different but potentially complementary manner. According to traditional Chinese medicine, for example, emotional disturbances are closely associated with dysfunction of internal organs. Relevant prescriptions might include acupuncture, massage, special diet, herbs, and exercise. Provided there are no contraindications for combining scientific and indigenous treatment strategies, a collaborative approach may prove to potentiate the therapeutic effects of both models.

References

Ben-Tovim DI. Development psychiatry: mental health and primary health care in Botswana. London and New York: Tavistock Publications, 1987.

Flaskerud JH. A proposed protocol for culturally relevant psychotherapy. Clin Nurse Spec 1987; 1:150–157.

Leininger M. Transcultural nursing: an overview. Nurs Outlook, 32(92):72–73.

Orque MS, Bloch B, Ahumada Monrroy LS, eds. Ethnic nursing care: a multi-cultural approach. Toronto: CV Mosby, 1983.

Tripp-Reimer T. Cultural diversity in therapy. In: Beck CM, Rawlins RP, Williams SR, eds. Mental health-psychiatric nursing. Toronto: CV Mosby, 1984: 381–398.

Xu JM. Some issues in the diagnosis of depression in China. Can J Psychiatry 1987; 32:368–370.

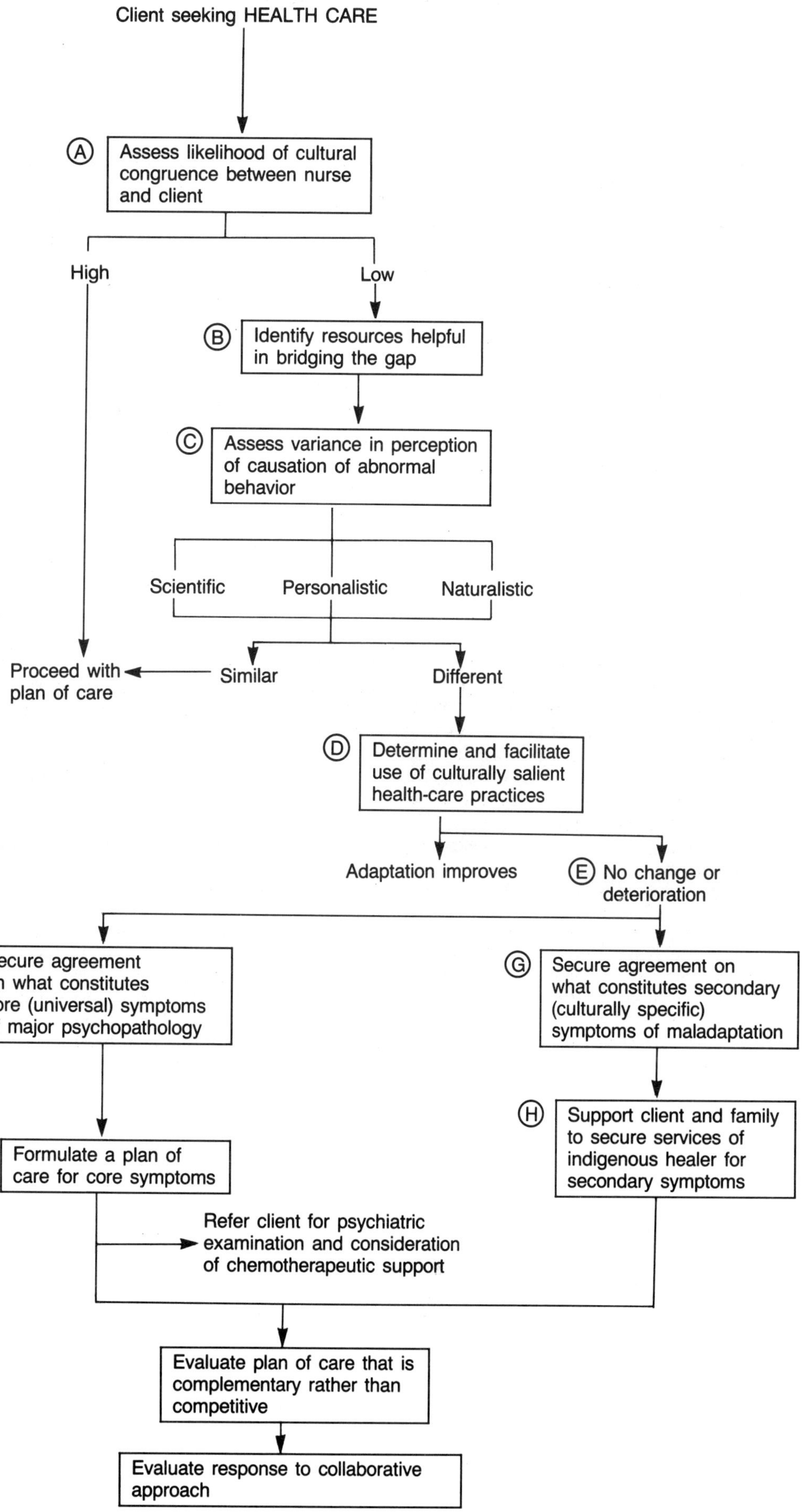
Client seeking HEALTH CARE
Ⓐ Assess likelihood of cultural congruence between nurse and client
High
Low
Ⓑ Identify resources helpful in bridging the gap
Ⓒ Assess variance in perception of causation of abnormal behavior
Scientific
Personalistic
Naturalistic
Proceed with plan of care
Similar
Different
Ⓓ Determine and facilitate use of culturally salient health-care practices
Adaptation improves
Ⓔ No change or deterioration
Ⓕ Secure agreement on what constitutes core (universal) symptoms of major psychopathology
Ⓖ Secure agreement on what constitutes secondary (culturally specific) symptoms of maladaptation
Ⓗ Support client and family to secure services of indigenous healer for secondary symptoms
Formulate a plan of care for core symptoms
Refer client for psychiatric examination and consideration of chemotherapeutic support
Evaluate plan of care that is complementary rather than competitive
Evaluate response to collaborative approach

ASSESSING THE ENVIRONMENT

Cheryl Forchuk

Environment is a broad term that encompasses not only the physical surroundings, but also the constellation of attitudes, beliefs, opportunities, responsibilities, and expectations. It encompasses the past, present, and future. The environment can maintain illness or promote health.

A. The initial assessment ensures that the client's basic needs are attended to adequately. Meeting basic human needs as well as mandated legal requirements are required to meet minimum standards.

B. If all minimum standards are not adequately maintained, immediate corrective action is essential.

C. Once minimum standards are assured, evaluating the therapeutic nature of the environment can begin. The current setting must be examined in context of the past and probable future settings to determine if it is supportive or nonsupportive.

D. To identify areas of disparity or congruence it may be helpful to think of the similarity and differences between activities that occur on a daily basis. Consider activities and expectations, such as when or how a person rises; expectations about bedmaking, meal preparation and organization, and hygiene activities; attendance at work, school, or programs; transportation arrangements; leisure activities; opportunities for privacy; medication responsibilities; financial resources; activities that occur in weekly, monthly, or annual patterns (e.g., opportunities and responsibilities for laundry, input into decisions, seasonal activities, and handling of birthdays and holidays). Reflect on the differences in expectations and attitudes of others within the system and opportunities for autonomy and recognition of the individual.

E. Areas of congruence support growth if they promote autonomy and respect for the individual. Strengths and competencies are maintained through areas of congruence. Areas of congruence do not support growth if they threaten the autonomy or respect for the individual or restrict the increasing capacities and competencies of the individual.

F. Disparities between past and present settings support growth if the change reflects changing capacities and competencies of the individual.

G. Determine the direction of disparities within the current setting and the probable future setting.

H. If the disparities reflect a decrease in opportunities, autonomy, responsibilities, or expectations, is this a reflection of decreasing competencies or capabilities of the individual?

I. If so, such disparities are reasonable.

J. If the changing opportunities and responsibilities do not reflect changing abilities of the individual, are the current agencies' opportunities and responsibilities unrealistic, or are the future settings inappropriate?

K. Disparities reflecting an increase in opportunities, autonomy, responsibilities or expectations reflect increasing competencies or capacities of the individual.

L. If so, such disparities are reasonable and signal a need for health teaching or experiences to facilitate the transition (e.g., if the new setting involves new responsibilities for meal preparation, necessary prerequisites are meal planning and nutrition knowledge).

References

Chambers L, Forchuk C, Munroe-Blum H, et al. The development of guidelines to promote a therapeutic environment in lodging homes. Can Ment Health 1988; Dec:14–15.

Chopoorian TJ. Reconceptualizing the environment. In: Moccia P, ed. New approaches to theory development. New York: National League for Nursing, 1986.

Frills S. Characteristics of a good ward atmosphere. Acta Psychiatr Scand 1986; 74:469–473.

Gutheil TG. The therapeutic milieu: changing themes and theories. Hosp Commun Psychiat 1985; 36:1279–1285.

Schafer SC. Modifying the environment. Geriatr Nurs 1985; 3:157–159.

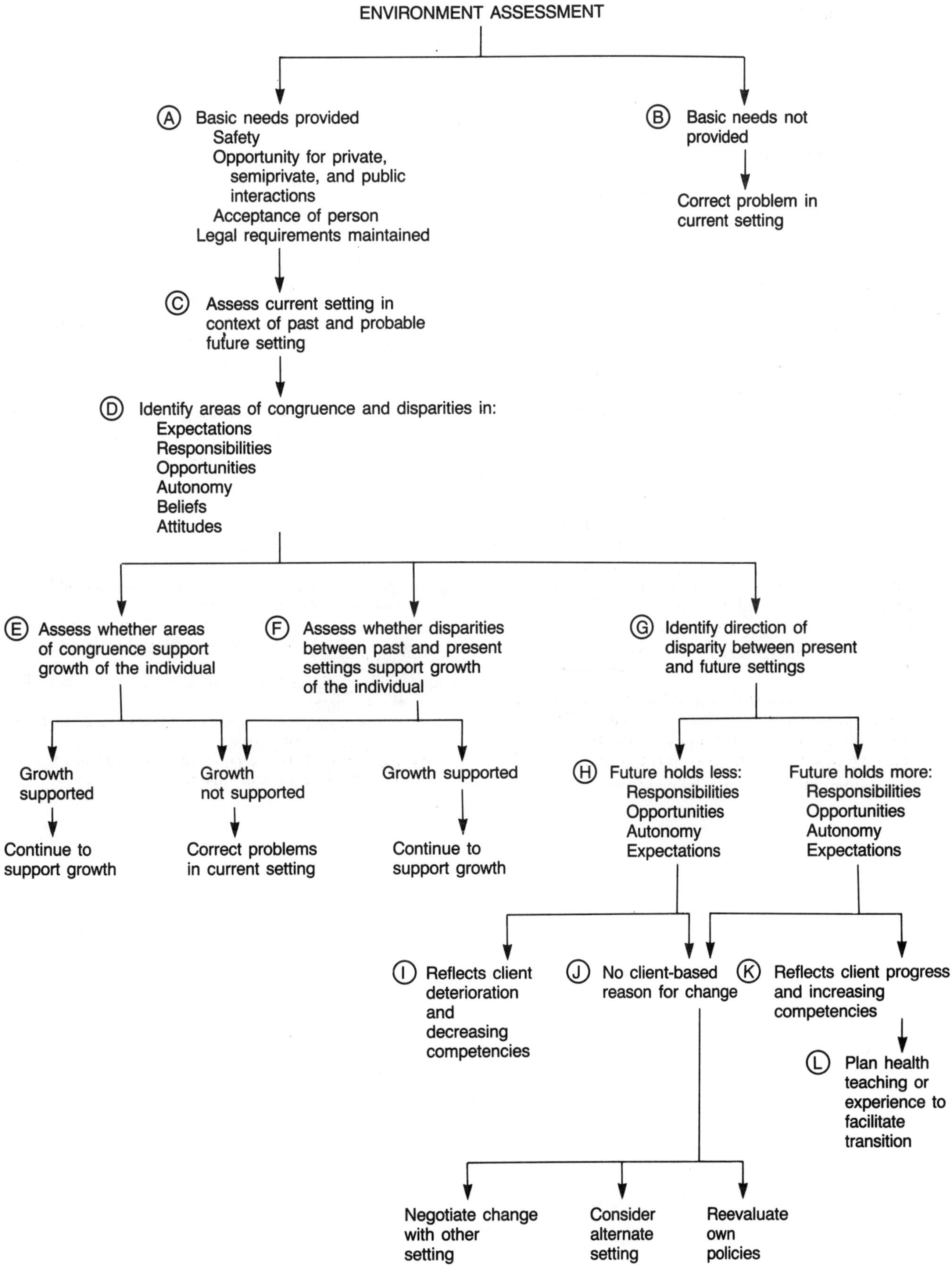
ENVIRONMENT ASSESSMENT
(A) Basic needs provided
Safety
Opportunity for private, semiprivate, and public interactions
Acceptance of person
Legal requirements maintained
(B) Basic needs not provided
Correct problem in current setting
(C) Assess current setting in context of past and probable future setting
(D) Identify areas of congruence and disparities in:
Expectations
Responsibilities
Opportunities
Autonomy
Beliefs
Attitudes
(E) Assess whether areas of congruence support growth of the individual
(F) Assess whether disparities between past and present settings support growth of the individual
(G) Identify direction of disparity between present and future settings
Growth supported
Continue to support growth
Growth not supported
Correct problems in current setting
Growth supported
Continue to support growth
(H) Future holds less:
Responsibilities
Opportunities
Autonomy
Expectations
Future holds more:
Responsibilities
Opportunities
Autonomy
Expectations
(I) Reflects client deterioration and decreasing competencies
(J) No client-based reason for change
(K) Reflects client progress and increasing competencies
(L) Plan health teaching or experience to facilitate transition
Negotiate change with other setting
Consider alternate setting
Reevaluate own policies

CRISIS STATE

Andrea Baumann

A crisis state is defined as a temporary situation characterized by change or loss that poses a threat to the steady state of an individual and/or family. This threat to the integrity provokes a behavioral, emotional, and physiological reaction.

A. Nursing history and assessment include assessing the person's reaction to the crisis and defining the characteristics of the crisis. The client's perception and definition of the problem is very important. Ascertain how the person has coped with problems in the past and the availability of support systems. Coexisting stressors and how the client perceives the present crisis affect a person's inherent ability to handle stress. Observe both the psychological and physical effects of the crisis on the client. Symptoms such as extreme anxiety, shortness of breath, or poor judgment demonstrate difficulty in coping. During the acute crisis state, determining the potential for harm to self or others is important.

B. Crises have been defined as situational or maturational. A situational crisis is a sudden, unanticipated event, such as a death of a family member. A maturational crisis is one that occurs through the life cycle, such as retirement or the empty nest syndrome when a child leaves home. Crises may be compounded by the development of more than one problem, which may result in ineffective coping.

C. If the client has a realistic perception of the problem and has adequate adaptive mechanisms, there will be a rapid resolution of the problem and a return to the precrisis state. However, if the crisis is not resolved, a period of disequilibrium ensues, and the need for crisis intervention is apparent. Crisis intervention is a concept originating in 1964 with Caplan and expanded by nursing authors such as Aguilera and Messick, Hoff, and Infante. It is short-term therapy where the objective is the resolution of the present problem and restoration of precrisis functioning. Interventions focus on assisting the client to understand the crisis and promoting effective decision making (see "Decision Making During a Crisis State," p 10). Supportive counseling and understanding of behavior under crisis assist the client to make decisions to reach a successful resolution of the crisis.

D. If the person is unable to identify the problem and does not have support or strong coping mechanisms, there will be a further increase in the crisis state, further disequilibrium, and need for more intensive therapy (see "Short-Term Psychotherapy," p 112).

References

Aguilera D, Messick J. Crisis intervention: theory and methodology. St. Louis: CV Mosby, 1986.

Barbato L. Crisis intervention. In: Mancini M, ed. Decision making in emergency nursing. Toronto: BC Decker, 1987:198–199.

Caplan G. Principles of preventative psychiatry. New York: Basic Books, 1964.

Hoff L. People in crisis understanding and helping. Menlo Park, CA: Addison Wesley, 1978.

Infante MS. Crisis theory: a framework for nursing practice. Reston, VA: Prentice-Hall, 1982.

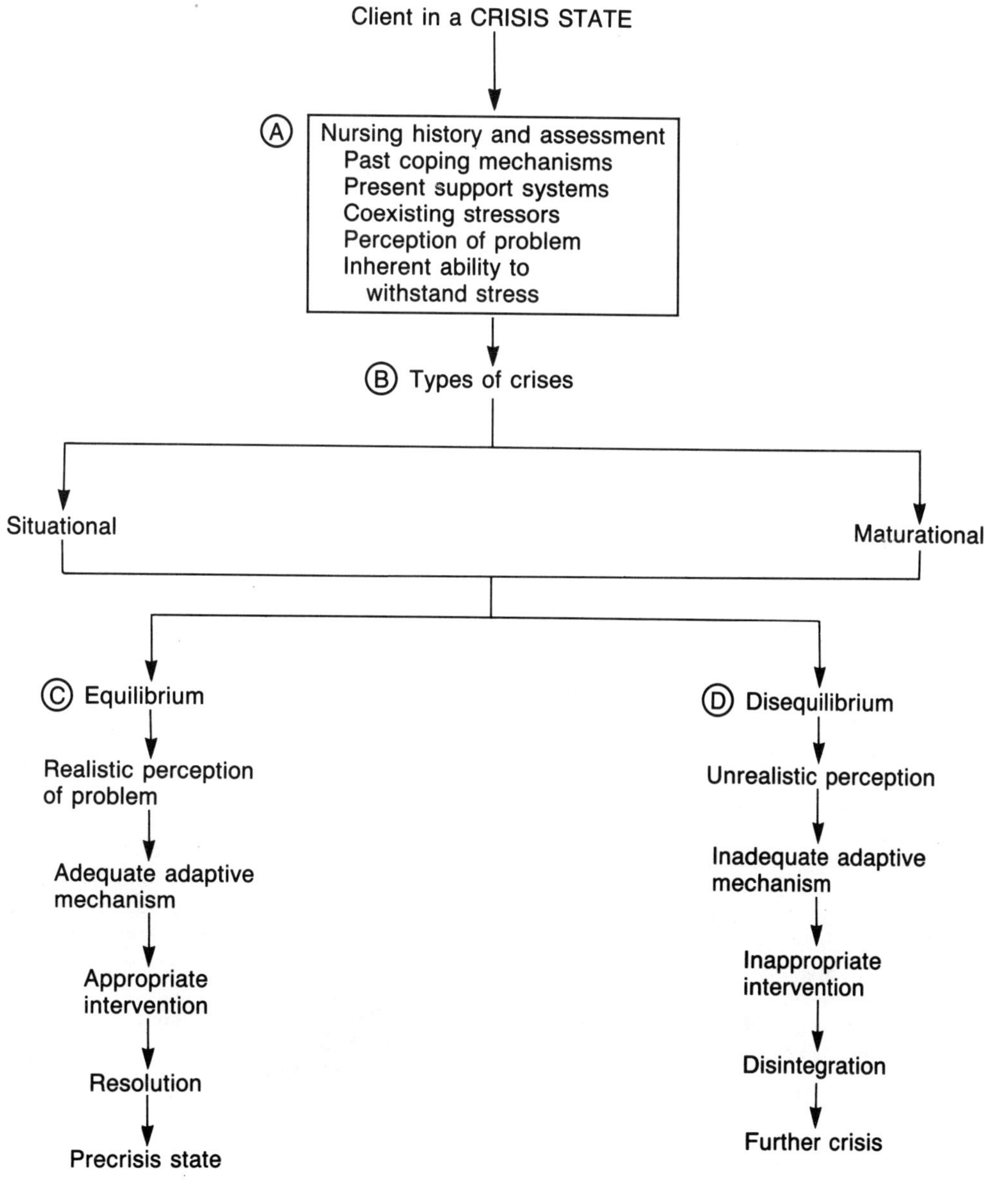
Client in a CRISIS STATE
A
Nursing history and assessment
Past coping mechanisms
Present support systems
Coexisting stressors
Perception of problem
Inherent ability to withstand stress
B
Types of crises
Situational
Maturational
C
Equilibrium
Realistic perception of problem
Adequate adaptive mechanism
Appropriate intervention
Resolution
Precrisis state
D
Disequilibrium
Unrealistic perception
Inadequate adaptive mechanism
Inappropriate intervention
Disintegration
Further crisis

DECISION MAKING DURING A CRISIS STATE

Andrea Baumann

A. Decision making during a crisis state is characterized by high risk to the individual and short decision making time. In times of crisis, a client and/or family are called upon to make decisions within a limited time frame using limited resources. As a result, all necessary factors are not considered, nor is the time taken to come to an informed decision. When there is more time, comprehensive resources can be tapped, people can be consulted, and optimal decision making can proceed.

B. The nurse must assess the decision-making behavior of clients and family. It is important to assist the client and/or family to identify the problem, potential alternatives, and resources available to solve the problem.

C. It is important to recognize that during crisis, inappropriate decision-making behavior may be manifested, primarily because of the stress of the situation. Anxiety due to the uncertainty of the situation persists beyond identification of the problem, even though decision-making behavior may proceed. There may be initial denial, disorganization, and uncertainty about which action to take. (See "Dealing with Clients' Decisional Conflict," p 12.) The nurse may observe a decrease in attention span, increased reliance on past experience, and decreased sensitivity to another's perspective. The stress of the situation can cause regressive behavior, manifested by anger and child-like behavior. There is usually an inability to integrate a lot of information as the client and/or family attends to only a few cues in the environment. Clients may display cognitive rigidity and have difficulty reviewing all aspects of the situation. The desire to find a quick solution may result in premature closure and lack of consideration of all possible alternatives.

D. In order to try to understand the problem (the first step in the decision-making process), clients search for past experiences or similar experiences which they feel represent the problem. This reliance on past experience as a basis for making decisions has been documented by Kahneman, Slovic, and Tversky. Clients use simple but misleading processing strategies (heuristics) to reduce the complexity of decision making. Heuristics such as "availability" (ease of recall of past occurrences) lead people to apply past information to present situations when it may not be applicable. Although the use of heuristics in crisis situations has not been demonstrated experimentally, it can be observed in families as they try to relate a situation to a neighbors' experience or one that happened in the past to their own family. Once such behavior is recognized by a nurse, families can be assisted to see what it is about this situation that is unique and what may have possible parallels with the past. Encouragement can be given to exclude erroneous information and retain only the most relevant information for the purpose of making a decision.

E. Once the ineffective decision-making behavior is identified, the nurse can assist the family in reducing anxiety. Reliance on past experience and behavior may not be applicable in this situation; the client must be encouraged to look at all aspects of the present situation, at the same time recognizing past successful coping mechanisms. Anger and hostility can be diffused by a warm, nonjudgmental approach. Clearly defining the problem and focusing the client and/or family on the problem are essential. Denial may be reduced by identifying immediate problems and the possible alternatives. Since the client's attention span is reduced, discussions should be clear and simple. The use of repetition is helpful since the client may have difficulty attending to the information. In the early stages of crisis, a more direct approach may be appropriate because the client and family may not have mobilized the necessary resources and information. Once support, reassurance, and information are given and the immediate crisis has passed, the client and family can be assisted to review all potential problems and feasible alternatives (see "Dealing with Client's Decisional Conflict, p 10, and "Problem Solving," p 106). Again, a calm, reassuring approach can assist the client in using a more comprehensive decision-making approach in a crisis.

References

Baumann A, Fothergill-Bourbonnais F. Rapid decision making in crisis situations: a case study approach for nurses. Toronto: McGraw-Hill Ryerson, 1984.

Holsti OR. Limitations of cognitive abilities in the face of crisis. In: Smart C, Standbury W, eds. Studies in crisis management. Toronto: Butterworth, 1978:53–67.

Kahneman D, Slovic P, Tversky A. Judgment under uncertainty: heuristics and biases. Cambridge: Cambridge University Press, 1982.

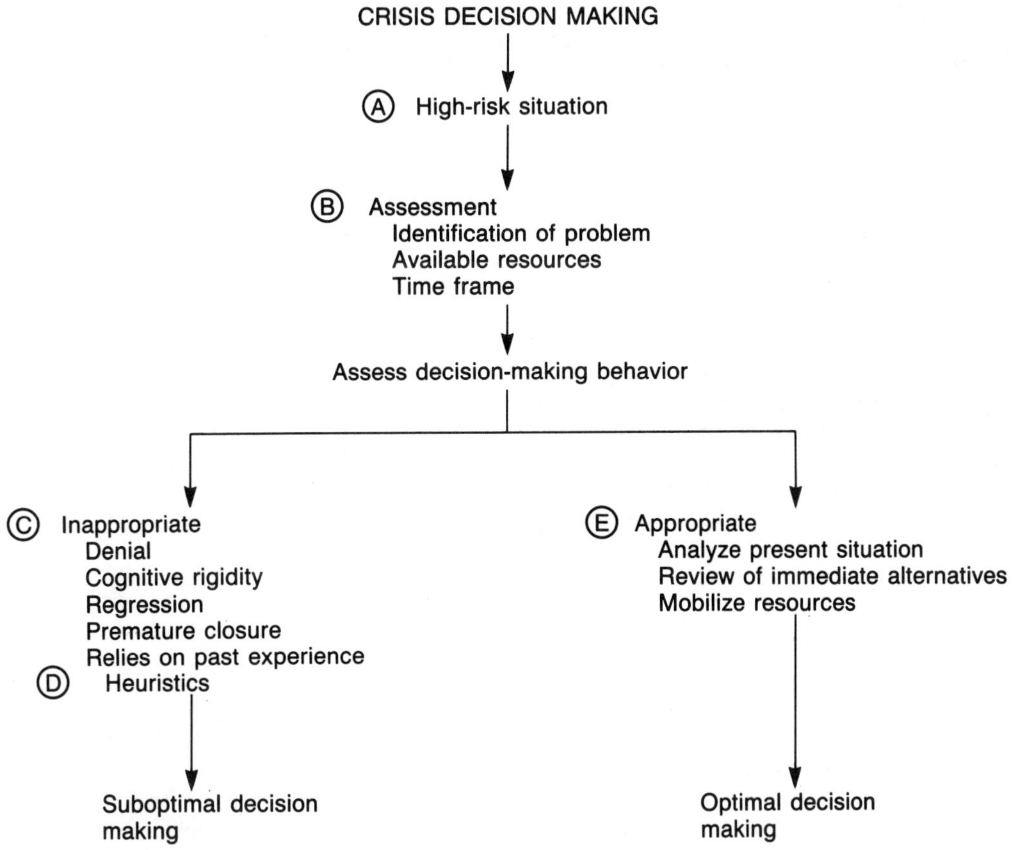

CRISIS DECISION MAKING
(A) High-risk situation
(B) Assessment
Identification of problem
Available resources
Time frame
Assess decision-making behavior
(C) Inappropriate
Denial
Cognitive rigidity
Regression
Premature closure
Relies on past experience
(D) Heuristics
Suboptimal decision making
(E) Appropriate
Analyze present situation
Review of immediate alternatives
Mobilize resources
Optimal decision making

DEALING WITH CLIENTS' DECISIONAL CONFLICT

Annette M. O'Connor

Decisional conflict is a state of uncertainty about a course of action to be taken when choice among competing actions involves risk, loss, regret, or challenge to personal life values. Conflicts can arise when making choices regarding health, family relationships, career, finances, or other life events. Major defining characteristics include: (1) verbalized feelings of distress related to uncertainty about choices, (2) verbalization of undesired consequences of the alternative actions being considered, (3) vacillation between alternative choices, (4) delayed decision making, and (5) questioning personal values and beliefs while attempting decision making. Minor defining characteristics include self-focusing and physical signs of distress or tension such as increased muscle tension, restlessness, and increased heart rate. Factors contributing to decisional conflict include: (1) unclear or unrealistic goals and alternatives, (2) unclear or unrealistic expectations of the outcomes of alternatives, (3) unclear values, (4) knowledge or skill deficit in making or implementing a decision, (5) impaired cognitive functioning from underlying illness, drugs, or anxiety, and (6) interference from significant others or health professionals who are imposing their views.

A. Assessment involves asking clients to explain in their own words what makes the decision difficult and validating your impressions. Personal goals and perceived alternatives are elicited. Expectations are assessed by asking clients to indicate what outcomes of each alternative are possible and how likely they are to occur. Values are elicited by asking clients how desirable or undesirable the outcomes of each alternative are and their priority of importance. Resources are assessed by identifying the perceived difficulties in implementing the decision and the client's knowledge, skill, motivation, and other resources to implement the decision.

B. The expected outcome of decisional conflict is that the patient will make an effective decision. Effective decisions are informed, consistent with personal values, and congruent with behavior (i.e., behaviorally implemented). The criteria for judging these outcomes are that the client: (1) identifies viable alternatives, (2) expresses realistic expectations, (3) identifies the source of conflict that makes the decision difficult, (4) prioritizes outcomes of decision alternatives, (5) is clear about which alternative is likely to achieve the most important outcomes, (6) expresses satisfaction at having made the best possible decision at the time, and (7) uses or acquires self-help skills to implement the decision and deal with the consequences.

C. Decision therapy is the process of assisting individuals to make effective decisions. Approaches may range from unstructured counseling to the use of structured decision aids. Part of this process begins in the assessment phase; data generated from the assessment represent a first approximation of the patient goals, alternatives, expectations, and values. It is subsequently revised by two-way interaction where clinician and clients fill gaps, clarify, and share expertise. The specific interventions used in decision therapy depend on the data provided by the client in the first approximation of the decision problem and the clinician's and client's judgment about how clear, complete, salient, accurate, and parsimonious the first approximation is. Goals, alternatives, or outcomes that are too narrow or incomplete are expanded. Options or outcomes that are too numerous are reduced to viable alternatives and salient outcomes. For areas in which information is lacking, the clinician or client provides the data or searches for an appropriate source. Unrealistic expectations are realigned with research data or conventional wisdom. Values are clarified to identify the trade-offs implicit in the decision and the priority of outcomes. Once clients have identified the viable alternatives, realistic expectations, and value trade-offs, they are in a better position to make an informed decision consistent with value trade-offs. Following selection, the client needs to plan strategies for dealing with the consequences of the decision and then act on the decision. Decisional conflict is a recent addition to the taxonomy of nursing diagnoses and requires further scientific investigation to better understand the prevalence of the problem, the factors that explain and predict the problem, and the efficacy of interventions designed to promote effective decision making.

References

Janis IL, Mann L. Decision making. New York: Free Press, 1977.

O'Connor A, D'Amico M. Decisional conflict. In: McFarland GK, Thomas MD, eds. Psychiatric mental health nursing: nursing diagnosis and intervention. Toronto: JB Lippincott, 1989.

Rothert ML, Talarczyk GJ. Patient compliance and the decision-making process of clinicians and patients. J Compliance Health Care 1987; 1:55–71.

Slimmer LW, Brown RT. Parents' decision-making process in medication administration for control of hyperactivity. J School Health 1985; 55:221–225.

Wilberding JZ. Values clarification. In: Bulechek GM, McCloskey JC, eds. Nursing interventions: treatments for nursing diagnoses. Philadelphia: WB Saunders, 1985:173–184.

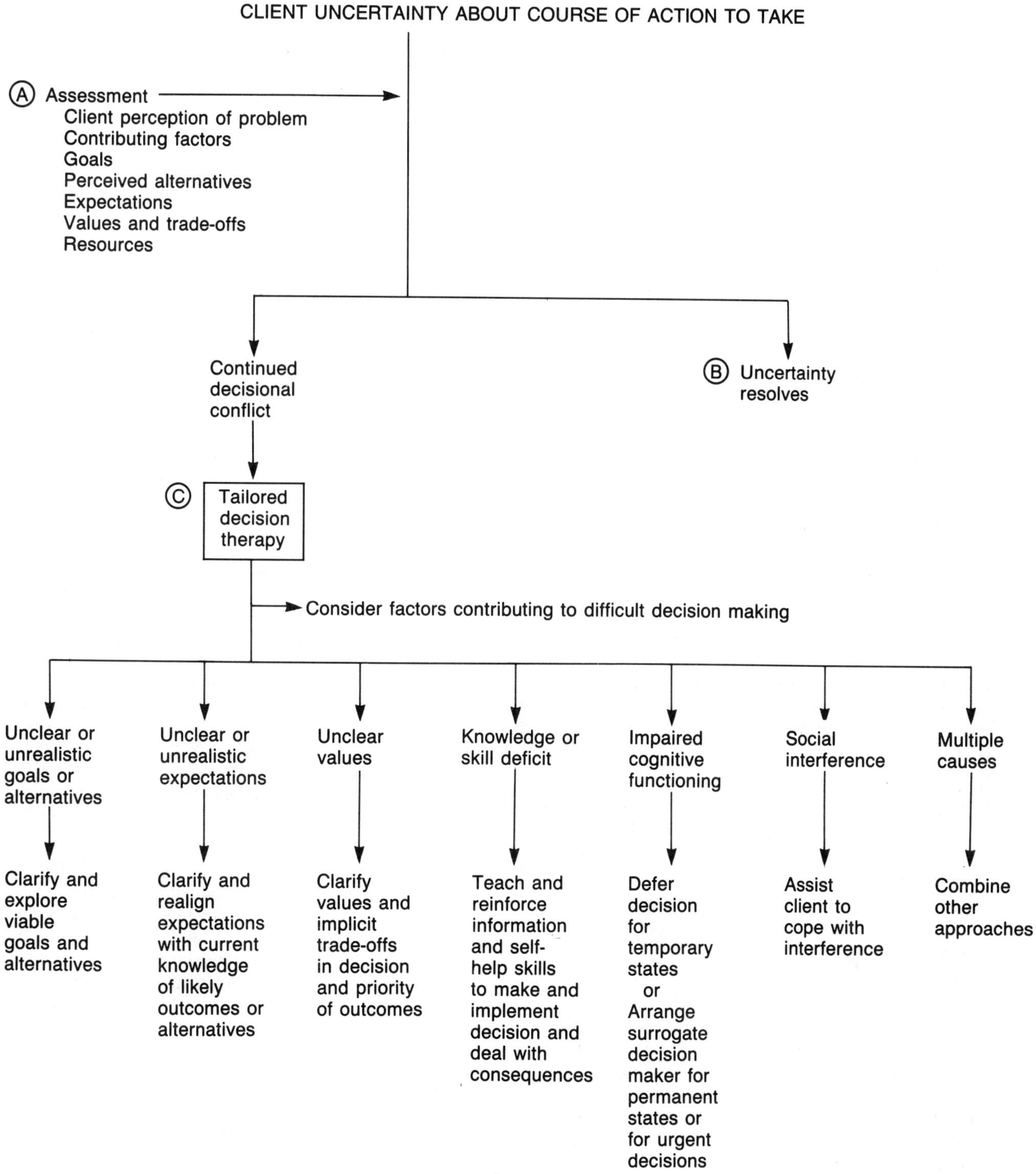
CLIENT UNCERTAINTY ABOUT COURSE OF ACTION TO TAKE
(A) Assessment
Client perception of problem
Contributing factors
Goals
Perceived alternatives
Expectations
Values and trade-offs
Resources
Continued decisional conflict
(B) Uncertainty resolves
(C) Tailored decision therapy
Consider factors contributing to difficult decision making
Unclear or unrealistic goals or alternatives
Unclear or unrealistic expectations
Unclear values
Knowledge or skill deficit
Impaired cognitive functioning
Social interference
Multiple causes
Clarify and explore viable goals and alternatives
Clarify and realign expectations with current knowledge of likely outcomes or alternatives
Clarify values and implicit trade-offs in decision and priority of outcomes
Teach and reinforce information and self-help skills to make and implement decision and deal with consequences
Defer decision for temporary states or Arrange surrogate decision maker for permanent states or for urgent decisions
Assist client to cope with interference
Combine other approaches

SELECTING OR DEVELOPING A NURSING MODEL FOR USE IN CLINICAL PRACTICE: A PROCESS-ORIENTED APPROACH

Nancy E. Johnston
Andrea Baumann

Within the last 30 years much interest has been evinced in the development of nursing as a profession. For nursing to establish credibility as a profession in its own right, it has been necessary to articulate a set of theories that describe, explain, and predict the realm of nursing education, practice, and research.

A. Although nursing practice models have the capacity to describe and explain the nature of nursing, they have not as yet achieved their full stature as theories, since they lack specificity and accuracy to predict outcomes. Nevertheless they have enabled nurses to perform systematic assessments and have provided direction and guidance for nursing interventions. They allow nurses to be clear about what they do, why they do it, and how their practice is distinct from that of other health professionals. The disadvantages of adopting a nursing model are few and relate mainly to the barriers to implementation that can occur such as unavailability of time, effort, and the commitment necessary to conduct a careful analysis of particular practice needs and possibilities. When support for adoption of a model does not exist because of lowered resources, limited interest, or other pressing priorities, postpone implementation until a more conducive atmosphere can be created.

B. To select an appropriate nursing practice model the nurse must articulate, simply and in her own words, her beliefs and assumptions about the person, health, environment, and nursing, since these are the critical components contained in most nursing theories.

C. A summary of the characteristics of clients served, the particular sets of client problems, and the priorities for care related to these clients, enables the nurse to judge the relevance of current nursing practice models and their applicability to the particular client population.

D. It is important to examine, articulate, and document interventions that have been successful or have a high likelihood of being effective. Many of these approaches are recognized as common nursing interventions. Some interventions used in a clinical setting are prescribed and implemented by other disciplines (such as psychopharmacologic approaches, electroconvulsive therapy, and psychological testing). The largest group of interventions are those that are shared among disciplines, with each discipline achieving its own characteristic mix and balance of interventions.

E. Reflecting on the whole spectrum of interventions allows the nurse to synthesize her beliefs and knowledge about the person, health, environment, and nursing. If interventions are effective, it may be reasonable to assume that some truth about man's physical, psychological, social, and/or spiritual essence has been understood, appreciated, and acted upon. Compare the conclusions reached following this analytical process to the nurse's more intuitive, spontaneous ideas (see C). Thoughts that are congruent are further elaborated; conclusions that are incongruent require further analysis, integration, and reformulation.

F. Once the beliefs and assumptions about the person, health, environment, and nursing are articulated, taking into consideration truths attained through clinical experiences, evaluate the ability of existing nursing practice models to deliver a framework that complements what is viewed to be true (congruent), is useful in guiding practice (relevant), is compatible with other non-nursing models (complementary), and is understandable (comprehensible). Choosing a particular nursing practice model involves a process of deciding to what extent and under what conditions complementarity with other health disciplines is desirable. If the nurse works closely with other disciplines and shares common strategies with them, the nursing model must complement the models of the other professionals. However, if the nurse is the only professional therapeutic contact for the client, complementarity with other disciplines is of minimal concern or interest.

G. When the criteria described above are successfully met, an existing nursing practice model can be selected for testing on a trial basis. If existing practice models are felt to be lacking one or more critical ingredients, refine the existing model or develop a nursing practice model that will more adequately meet the particular practice needs.

References

Chinn PL, Jacobs MK. Theory and nursing: a systematic approach. Toronto: CV Mosby, 1983.

Duldt BW, Giffin K. Theoretical perspectives for nursing. Toronto: Little, Brown, 1985.

Fitzpatrick J, Whall A, Johnston R, Floyd J. Nursing models and their psychiatric mental health applications. Bowie, MD: Robert J. Brady, 1982.

Meleis AI. Theoretical nursing: development and progress. Philadelphia: JB Lippincott, 1985.

McGee M, ed. Theoretical pluralism in nursing science. Ottawa: University of Ottawa Press, 1984.

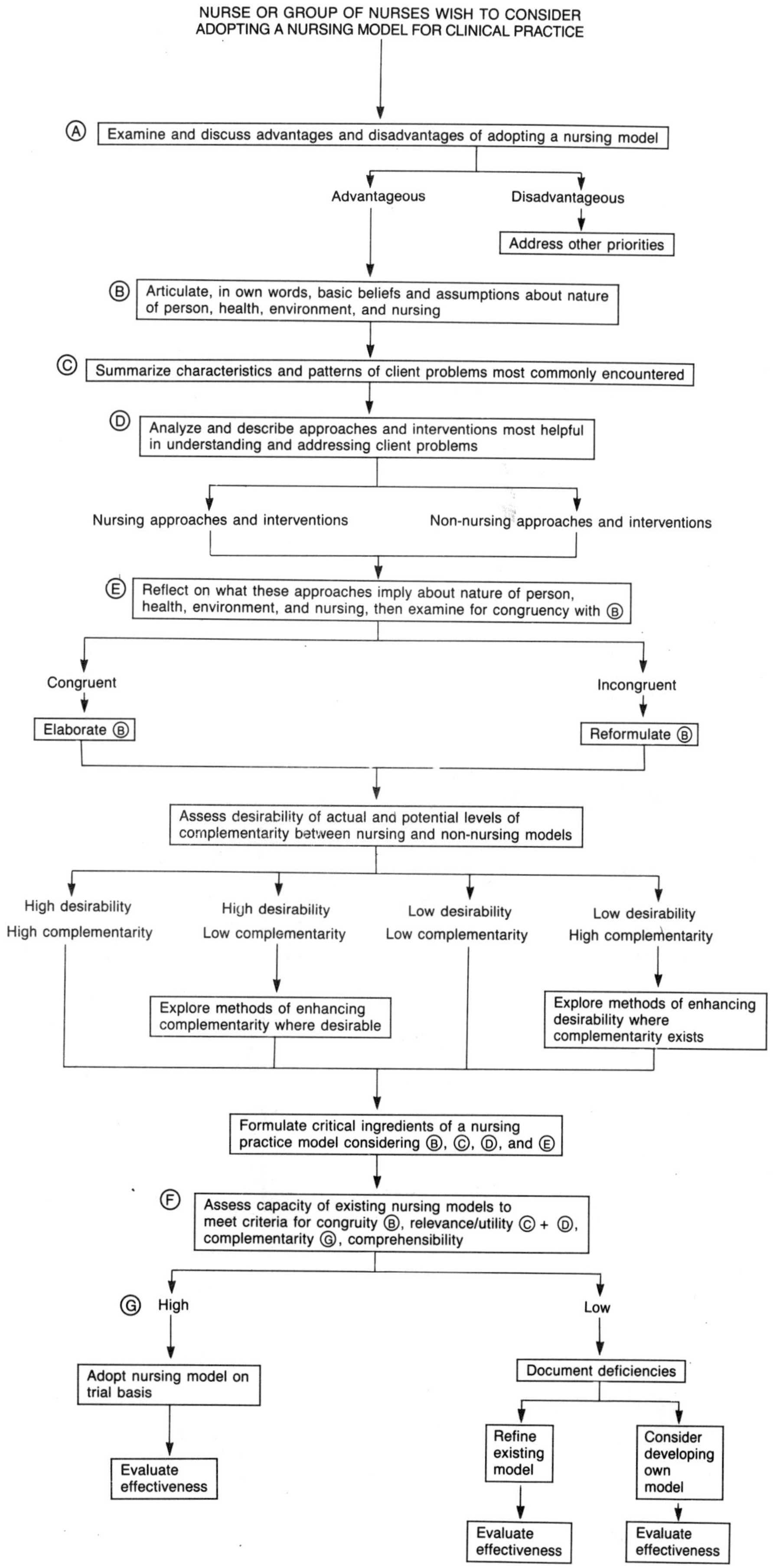
NURSE OR GROUP OF NURSES WISH TO CONSIDER ADOPTING A NURSING MODEL FOR CLINICAL PRACTICE
Ⓐ Examine and discuss advantages and disadvantages of adopting a nursing model
Advantageous
Disadvantageous
Address other priorities
Ⓑ Articulate, in own words, basic beliefs and assumptions about nature of person, health, environment, and nursing
Ⓒ Summarize characteristics and patterns of client problems most commonly encountered
Ⓓ Analyze and describe approaches and interventions most helpful in understanding and addressing client problems
Nursing approaches and interventions
Non-nursing approaches and interventions
Ⓔ Reflect on what these approaches imply about nature of person, health, environment, and nursing, then examine for congruency with Ⓑ
Congruent
Incongruent
Elaborate Ⓑ
Reformulate Ⓑ
Assess desirability of actual and potential levels of complementarity between nursing and non-nursing models
High desirability High complementarity
High desirability Low complementarity
Low desirability Low complementarity
Low desirability High complementarity
Explore methods of enhancing complementarity where desirable
Explore methods of enhancing desirability where complementarity exists
Formulate critical ingredients of a nursing practice model considering Ⓑ, Ⓒ, Ⓓ, and Ⓔ
Ⓕ Assess capacity of existing nursing models to meet criteria for congruity Ⓑ, relevance/utility Ⓒ + Ⓓ, complementarity Ⓖ, comprehensibility
Ⓖ High
Low
Adopt nursing model on trial basis
Evaluate effectiveness
Document deficiencies
Refine existing model
Consider developing own model
Evaluate effectiveness
Evaluate effectiveness

THE NEUMAN SYSTEMS MODEL

Andrea Baumann
Ann C. Beckingham

Betty Neuman has devised a holistic model. It is based on an open systems theory, along with two underlying concepts of stress: the person's reaction to stress and reconstitution. Each stressor is different in its potential to disturb a person's equilibrium. For a complete review of Neuman's model, the reader is referred to Neuman (1989).

A. The individual is viewed as unique and a composite of biological, psychological, sociocultural, spiritual, and developmental factors, which are considered simultaneously.

B. Stressors are described within the context of the intrapersonal, interpersonal, and extrapersonal forces. The intrapersonal forces are forces within an individual such as attitudes, values, and expectations. Interpersonal forces are those occurring between one or more individuals, such as the nurse and the client or relationships with family and friends. Extrapersonal forces occur outside the system of the individual such as financial circumstances or employment. The impact of the stressors is perceived in a unique way by every individual.

C. The model is depicted as a series of concentric circles. The outer circles are the flexible and normal lines of defense. The flexible lines of defense are a protective buffer to prevent breaking through to the normal line of defense. It is important to focus on strengthening the flexible line of defense against various stressors. The next concentric ring surrounding the core structure is the normal line of defense. The normal line of defense is composed of the biological, sociocultural, psychological, and developmental aspects of the person that define the state of wellness or equilibrium. The inner circle is the line of resistance and the person's last line of defense. An example may be the immune system. Assessment of the degree of reaction to stressors is needed to facilitate treatment or intervention.

D. Central to the author's model is primary, secondary, and tertiary prevention. Nursing intervention can begin at any point at which a stressor is either suspected or identified. Primary prevention is focused on risk assessment, reduction of the stressors, and assisting in retaining stability of the system. Secondary prevention begins when

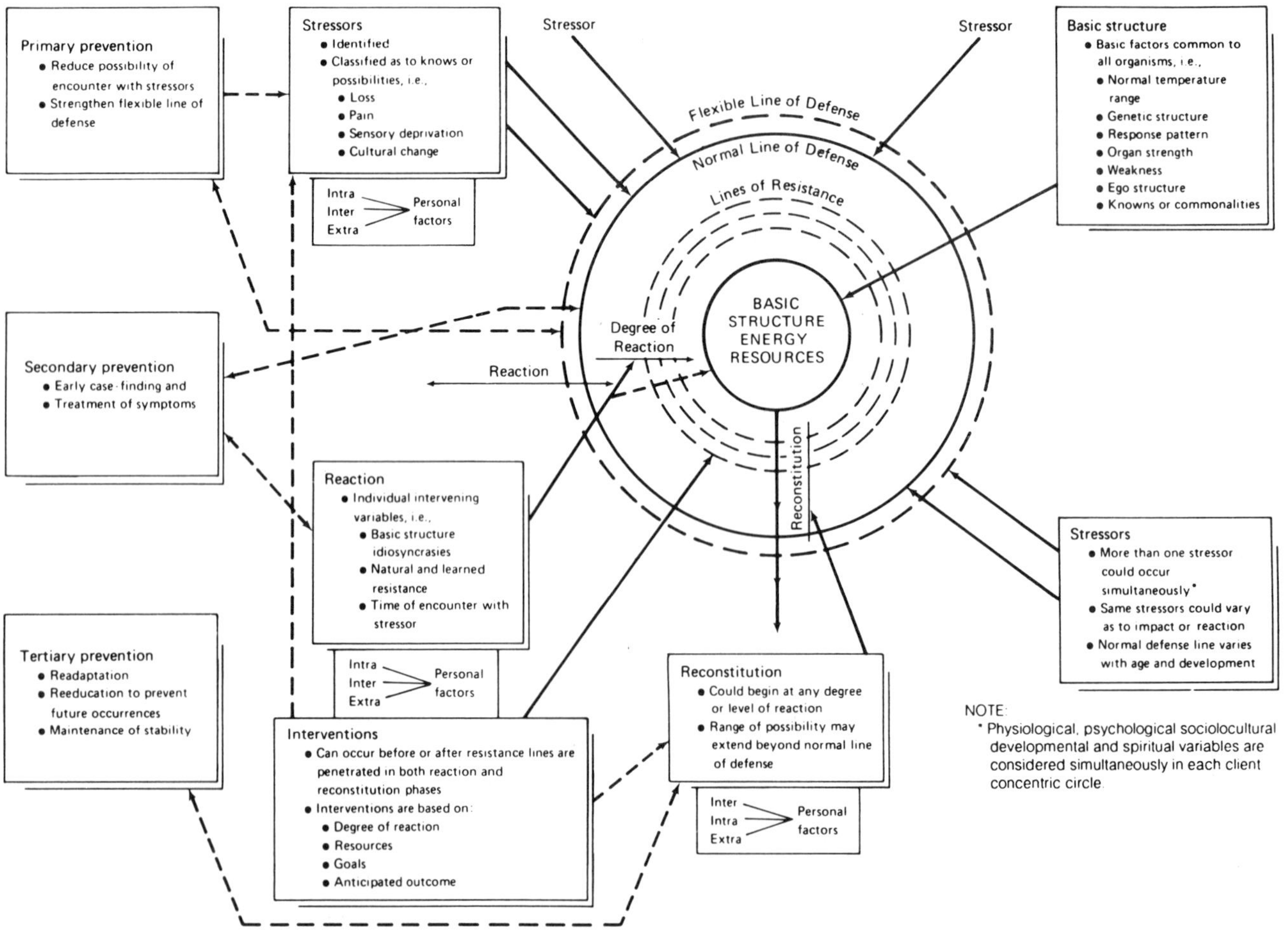

Figure 1 The Neuman Systems Model. (Original diagram ©1970 by Betty Neuman. Reprinted with permission.)

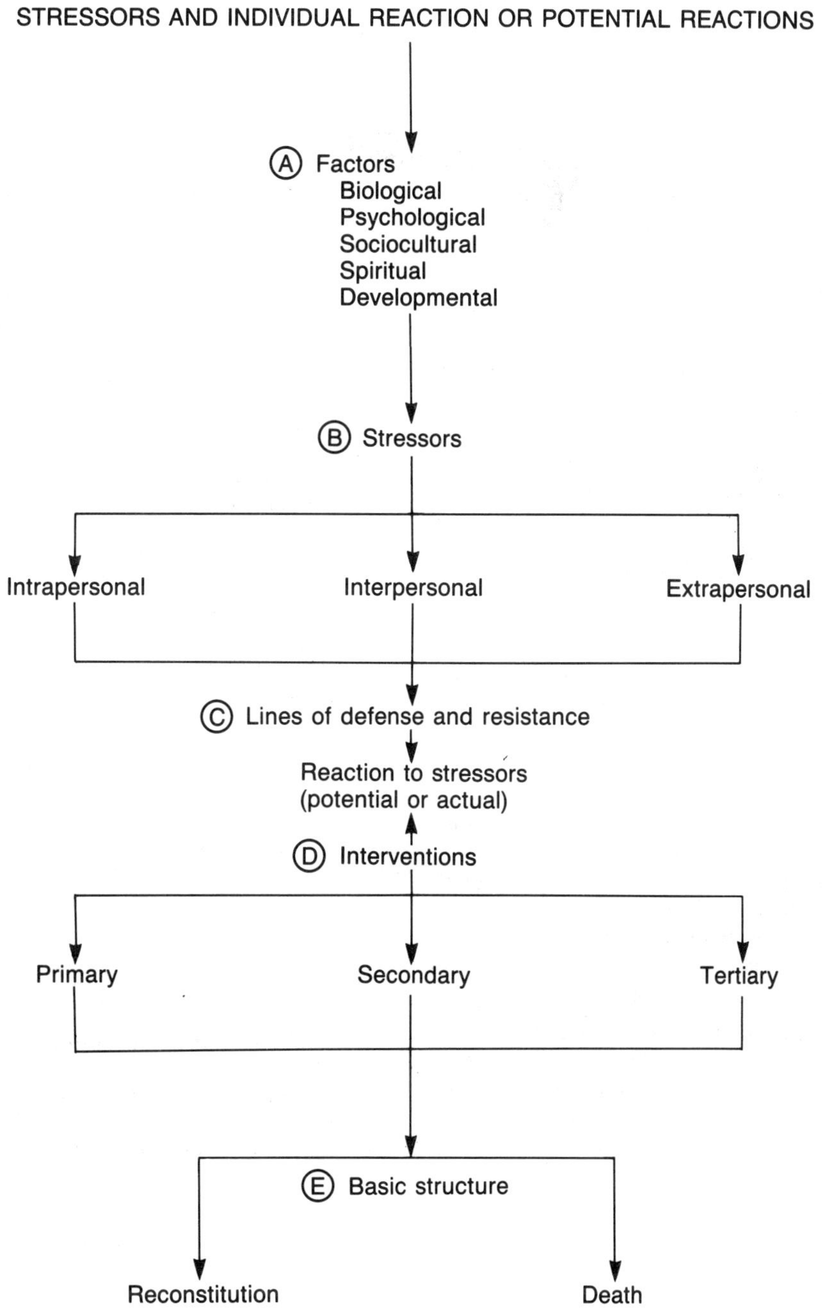

a stressor breaks through the normal line of defense. It involves early detection, and treatment of symptoms during the illness phase to attain stability of the system. Tertiary prevention is focused on adaptation and rehabilitation, leading to maintaining stability of the system.

E. The core is the energy resource or basic structure of the model. Reconstitution can be thought of as beginning at any point following interventions related to the degree of reaction. If the individual fails to reconstitute, death occurs as a result of the failure of the basic core structure to support the intervention.

References

Fawcett J. Analysis and evaluation of conceptual models of nursing. 2nd ed. Philadelphia: FA Davis, 1989.

Lancaster D, Whall A. The Neuman system model. In: Fitzpatrick J, Whall A, eds. Conceptual models of nursing. 2nd ed. Norwalk, CT: Appleton & Lange, 1989: 255–284.

Neuman B. The Neuman systems model: application to nursing education and practice. Norwalk, CT: Appleton & Lange, 1989.

Ross M, Helmer H. A comparative analysis of Neuman's model using the individual and family as units of care. Pub Health Nurs 1988; 5:30–36.

Torres G. Theoretical foundations of nursing. Norwalk, CT: Appleton-Century-Crofts, 1989.

OREM'S SELF-CARE MODEL

Viola Duff

A. The focus of health for individuals is to maintain for themselves and their families a state of wellness. The nurse, in the nursing history, assesses the abilities of the individual or its members to exercise self-care. Self-care is the practice of activities initiated and directed by the person to maintain life, health, and well-being. This may be a simple task of brushing one's teeth or the complex task of noting, assessing, and acting to alleviate a potential medical problem such as an asthmatic attack.

B. Universal requisites (those actions required by everyone) to meet the common requisites must be assessed. The requisites of air, food, and water are needed by everyone. Activity and rest need to be in balance. The requirement of both solitude and social interaction is evident in each person.

C. Developmental requisites (those associated with developmental processes) need to be assessed. A person at any age may show failure to grow along expected organic, psychological, or intellectual dimensions. Much more needs to be known about the developmental requisites of the elderly.

D. Health deviation self-care requisites are those demands that arise as a result of illness, injury, or a life-cycle event. Regular and repeated self-medication may be required whether the client feels well or not. This would be a health deviation self-care requisite. Also, the ability to recognize symptoms that are potentials for problems and the capacity to act on this information is necessary.

E. Self-care agency is the ability of an individual to initiate and perform health-care activities for himself or herself to maintain life, health, and well-being. If this can be done, no nursing intervention is needed. If the individual lacks the knowledge, motivation, or skill to perform self-care, a deficit occurs.

F. A self-care deficit occurs when the actions needed cannot be performed by the individual. Then, and only then, should the nurse give health care to the client.

G. When a self-care deficit exists, the nurse must decide the type of nursing system that is appropriate for the situation. The client must always be given the freedom to do as much self-care as he or she is capable of doing.

H. If the person cannot perform self-care actions because of physical or psychological inabilities, the nurse compensates for this and does these for the client. Washing and dressing the client may need to be done by the nurse.

I. The partially compensatory nursing system is one in which the client and nurse share the self-care measures. The client or the nurse may have the major role in the performance of care measures, depending on the client's abilities, knowledge, and motivation.

J. If the client can and should perform the self-care measures but requires support or teaching, the supportive-educative nursing system is used. Teaching the elderly client the knowledge of which medications must be taken regularly and the skill to be able to do this would be supportive-educative nursing.

References

Joseph L. Self-care and the nursing process. Nurs Clin North Am 1980; 15:131–143.

Orem D. Nursing concepts of practice. New York: McGraw-Hill, 1985.

Underwood P. Facilitating self-care. In: Ethier C, ed. Psychiatric nursing. Boston: Little, Brown, 1980:115–144.

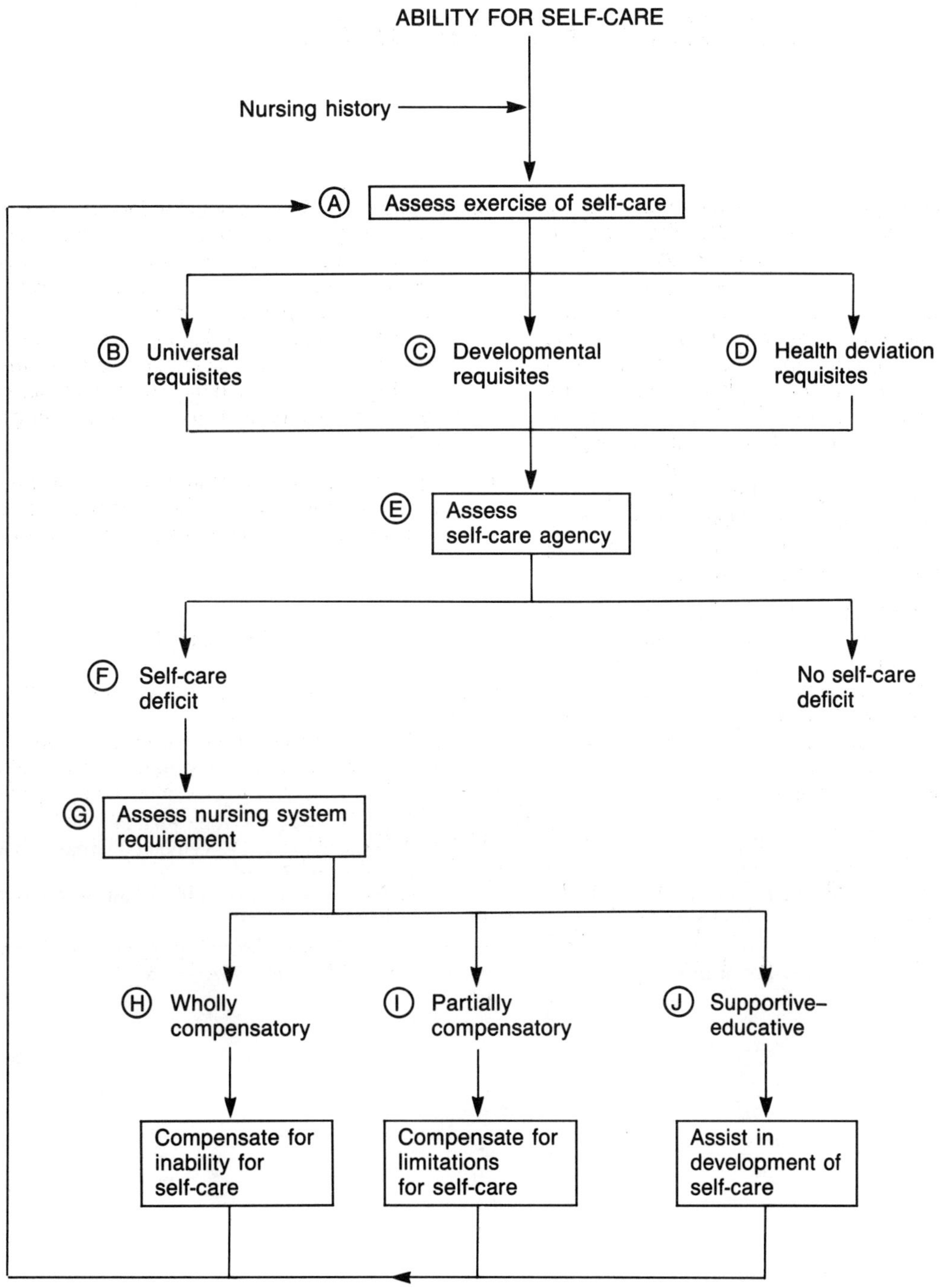
ABILITY FOR SELF-CARE
Nursing history
Ⓐ Assess exercise of self-care
Ⓑ Universal requisites
Ⓒ Developmental requisites
Ⓓ Health deviation requisites
Ⓔ Assess self-care agency
Ⓕ Self-care deficit
No self-care deficit
Ⓖ Assess nursing system requirement
Ⓗ Wholly compensatory
Ⓘ Partially compensatory
Ⓙ Supportive–educative
Compensate for inability for self-care
Compensate for limitations for self-care
Assist in development of self-care

ORLANDO'S NEED-ORIENTED THEORY

Cheryl Forchuk

A. Orlando has developed a need-oriented model focusing on the process of validation. She describes a deliberative nursing process involving self-reflection and validation. She contrasts this with an automatic style of nursing where the nurse acts on her own feelings and assumptions without examining these, trying to understand the meaning of patient behavior and validating assumptions with the patient. In Orlando's 1971 book, she used the phrase "nursing process discipline" to describe the deliberative nursing process. Orlando describes her model as revolving around five major interrelated concepts: (1) the function of professional nursing, (2) the presenting behavior of the client, (3) the immediate reaction or internal response of the nurse, (4) the nursing process discipline, and (5) improvement.

B. The function of professional nursing is the organizing principle around which the other concepts revolve. Simply stated, Orlando sees the function of nursing as identifying and meeting the client's immediate needs for help. She defines a need as "a requirement of the patient which, if supplied, relieves or diminishes his immediate distress or improves his immediate sense of adequacy or well being" (Orlando, 1961).

C. The presenting behavior of the patient is any observable verbal or nonverbal behavior. The nurse's and the client's immediate reactions include their individual perceptions, thoughts, and feelings. For example, the nurse may see the patient pacing, think he or she is bothered about something, and be concerned about this.

D. The nursing process discipline includes the nurse communicating to the client his or her own immediate reaction (i.e., perception, thought, and feeling), clearly identifying that the item expressed belongs to the nurse (i.e., "I see you pacing" rather than "You are pacing"), and then asking for validation or correction. For example, "I notice you are pacing up and down the hall this morning. I'm concerned that something may be bothering you that you haven't shared. Is something bothering you?"

E. Improvement is a resolution or improvement of the presenting behavior, i.e, the patient shares concerns, therefore has immediate needs met, and stops pacing.

References

Lego S. The one-to-one nurse patient relationship. Perspect Psychiatr Care 1980; 18:67–89.

Orlando IJ. The dynamic nurse-patient relationship: function, process and principles. New York: Putnam, 1961.

Orlando IJ. The discipline and teaching of nursing process (An evaluative study). New York: Putnam, 1972.

Orlando IJ. Nursing in the 21st century: alternative paths. J Adv Nurs 1987; 12:405–412.

Schmieding NJ. Putting Orlando's theory into practice. Am J Nurs 1984; 84:759–761.

Schmieding NJ. Analyzing managerial responses in face-to-face contacts. J Adv Nurs 1987; 12:357–365.

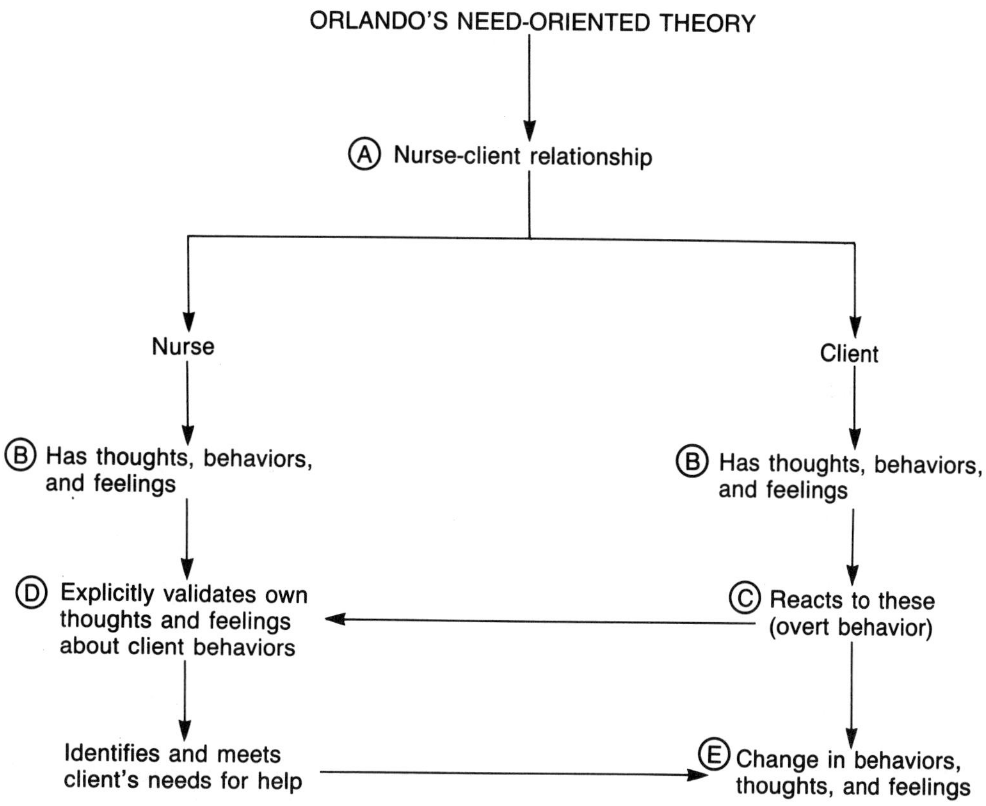
ORLANDO'S NEED-ORIENTED THEORY
(A) Nurse-client relationship
Nurse
Client
(B) Has thoughts, behaviors, and feelings
(B) Has thoughts, behaviors, and feelings
(D) Explicitly validates own thoughts and feelings about client behaviors
(C) Reacts to these (overt behavior)
Identifies and meets client's needs for help
(E) Change in behaviors, thoughts, and feelings

PEPLAU'S INTERPERSONAL THEORY

Cheryl Forchuk

A. The core concept of Peplau's model is the interpersonal process within the nurse-client relationship. The role of the nurse in the therapeutic process is to assist the client to solve problems through new learning and positive change.

B. The goal of the interpersonal process is to increase interpersonal and problem-solving competencies.

C. The increasing competencies lead to the forward movement of the personality that Peplau defines as health.

D. Major concepts include phases of the nurse-client relationship, anxiety, and learning.

E. The relationship always begins in the orientation phase, which is where the purpose and parameters of the relationship are given and tested. The relationship then grows into the working phase, consisting of problem identification and exploitation. In this phase problems are identified and then worked through. The resolution phase of the relationship is the final stage and involves the termination of the relationship.

F. Nursing roles change as the nurse and client work through the relationship. The nurse in the orientation phase always begins in the role of stranger, and all phases include the counselor role. However, the ways and degrees to which the other roles are used vary with each nurse-client dyad. The counseling role is essential for psychodynamic nursing—nursing that promotes forward movement of the personality. If the counseling role does not become the focus (e.g., the mother surrogate role predominates) the nurse's role may become that of a "glorified custodian or super clerk" (Peplau, 1964).

G. Anxiety is a central concept in Peplau's model. It results from any threat to the security of the individual. Unless experiencing euphoria, both the nurse and the patient will experience some anxiety. Peplau's levels of anxiety are mild, moderate, severe, and panic. At each increasing step the individual's focal attention is decreased and behaviors associated with anxiety increase (such as pacing, avoiding eye contact, or wringing hands).

H. Increased levels of anxiety can be an impediment to new learning and growth. Therefore, helping the individual identify anxiety, as well as learning to cope effectively with it, are common nursing goals.

I. Peplau's concept of learning allows the nurse an understanding of eight levels of problem-solving competencies: observe, describe, analyze, formulate, validate, test, integrate, and utilize. Each level is a prerequisite for the next. Increasing anxiety reduces the individual's current level.

J. Peplau focused on learning in an interpersonal context. She believed the nurse and patient would develop both interpersonal and problem-solving competencies through the developing nurse-patient relationship.

K. The process involves the nurse directing the process (through open statements and questions that facilitate elaboration and clarification) while the client directs the content (by choosing the topics to be discussed).

L. Therapeutic use of self includes self reflection and awareness as well as professional closeness (openness to the client, while maintaining professional rather than personal relationship).

M. Peplau described how thoughts cannot be directly observed or changed, but can be inferred indirectly through language. Correction of language through modeling and seeking clarification is therefore seen as a way to impact on cognition.

References

Forchuk C, Brown B. Establishing a nurse-client relationship. J Psychosoc Nurs 1989; 27(2):30–34.

Lego S. The one-to-one nurse-patient relationship. Perspect Psychiatr Care 1980; 18:67–89.

Peplau HE. Basic principles of patient counseling. Philadelphia: Smith, Kline and French, 1964.

Peplau HE. Anxiety. In: Burd SF, Marshall MA, eds. Some clinical approaches to psychiatric nursing. London: MacMillan, 1971.

Peplau HE. Interpersonal relations in nursing. New York: Putnam, 1952.

Peplau HE. Process and concept of learning. In: Burd SF, Marshall MA, eds. Some clinical approaches to psychiatric nursing. London: MacMillan, 1971.

Peplau HE. The art and science of nursing: similarities, differences and relations. Nurs Sci Q 1988; 1:8–15.

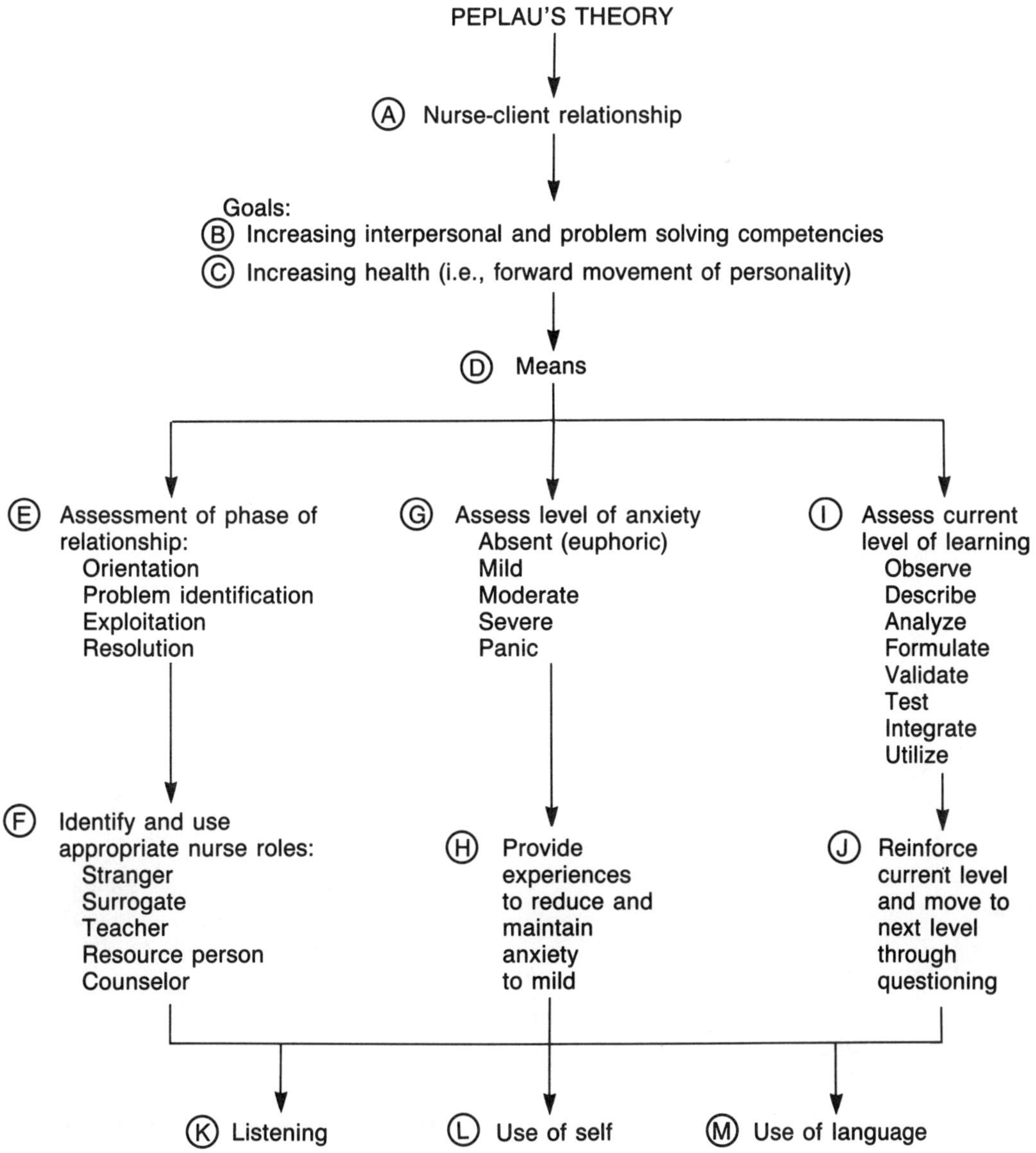
PEPLAU'S THEORY
(A) Nurse-client relationship
Goals:
(B) Increasing interpersonal and problem solving competencies
(C) Increasing health (i.e., forward movement of personality)
(D) Means
(E) Assessment of phase of relationship:
Orientation
Problem identification
Exploitation
Resolution
(G) Assess level of anxiety
Absent (euphoric)
Mild
Moderate
Severe
Panic
(I) Assess current level of learning
Observe
Describe
Analyze
Formulate
Validate
Test
Integrate
Utilize
(F) Identify and use appropriate nurse roles:
Stranger
Surrogate
Teacher
Resource person
Counselor
(H) Provide experiences to reduce and maintain anxiety to mild
(J) Reinforce current level and move to next level through questioning
(K) Listening
(L) Use of self
(M) Use of language

ROY'S ADAPTATION MODEL

Nancy E. Johnston

According to the Roy Adaptation Model, the person as an individual and as a member of a group is described as an adaptive system.

A. The person's adaptive mechanisms can be broadly categorized as regulator mechanisms or cognator mechanisms. Regulator mechanisms are those that respond automatically through neural, chemical, and endocrine activity. Cognator mechanisms are those that respond through four cognitive-emotive channels: perceptual/information processing, learning, judgment, and emotion.

B. Nursing assessment is initially directed toward the assessment of behavior by which regulator and cognator activities are manifested. This is referred to as level I assessment. Observations about behavior are categorized into four modes: the physiologic mode, the self-concept mode, the role-function mode, and the interdependence mode. Within all the adaptive modes are subcomponents that provide useful ways of refining observations about adaptive response. Within the physiologic mode data may be collected pertaining to oxygenation, nutrition, elimination, activity and rest, protection, the senses, fluids and electrolytes, neurologic function, and endocrine function. The examination of two subareas in the self-concept mode, the physical self and the personal self, provides further pertinent information regarding body sensation, body image, self-consistency, self-ideal, and the moral-ethical-spiritual self. A classification of primary, secondary, and tertiary roles and an analysis of instrumental and expressive behaviors within these roles provide further valuable data about the individual's social adequacy within the role-function mode. Affectional adequacy within the interdependence role may be assessed by attention to the individual's capacity for giving and receiving love. Information about the client's support system and the extent to which he or she is able to engage in receptive and contributive behavior is considered.

C. The behavioral outcomes within the four adaptive modes will either be adaptive (i.e., they will support the individual's capacity to adjust effectively to a constantly changing and increasingly complex environment) or they will be ineffective (i.e., they will restrict the individual's range of adaptive response). If ineffective responses continue over a long period of time, they may threaten mastery, growth, or even survival.

D. Further assessment, referred to as level II assessment, is directed toward the factors that influence and produce the behaviors described above. These stimuli are organized into three categories: (1) focal stimuli are those which most immediately confront the individual, (2) contextual stimuli include all other stimuli present in the situation that contribute to the effect of the focal stimuli, and (3) residual stimuli are factors that may affect the individual but cannot be conclusively validated. In this respect they can be understood to be strong possibilities, hypotheses, or educated guesses.

E. Interventions, according to Roy, are directed toward maintaining the stimuli that operate to produce adaptive response or modifying the stimuli that produce ineffective response. In manipulating stimuli it may be possible or necessary to consider increasing stimuli that are deficient, decreasing stimuli that are overwhelming, or removing stimuli that present insurmountable barriers to adaptation.

F. The effectiveness of the nursing interventions may be judged in relation to whether they strengthened adaptive behavior or decreased the strength of ineffective behaviors and whether they contributed to the enhancement of the interaction of the person with his or her environment.

References

Andrews HA, Roy C. Essentials of the Roy adaptation model. Norwalk, CT: Appleton-Century-Crofts, 1986.

Fitzpatrick J, Whall A, Johnston R, Floyd J. Nursing models and their psychiatric mental health applications. Bowie, MD: Robert J. Brady, 1982.

Rambo BJ. Adaptation nursing: assessment and interventions. Philadelphia: WB Saunders, 1984.

Randell B, Tedrow MP, Van Landringham J. Adaptation nursing: the Roy conceptual model applied. St. Louis: CV Mosby, 1982.

Roy C. Introduction to nursing: an adaptation model. Englewood Cliffs, NJ: Prentice-Hall, 1984.

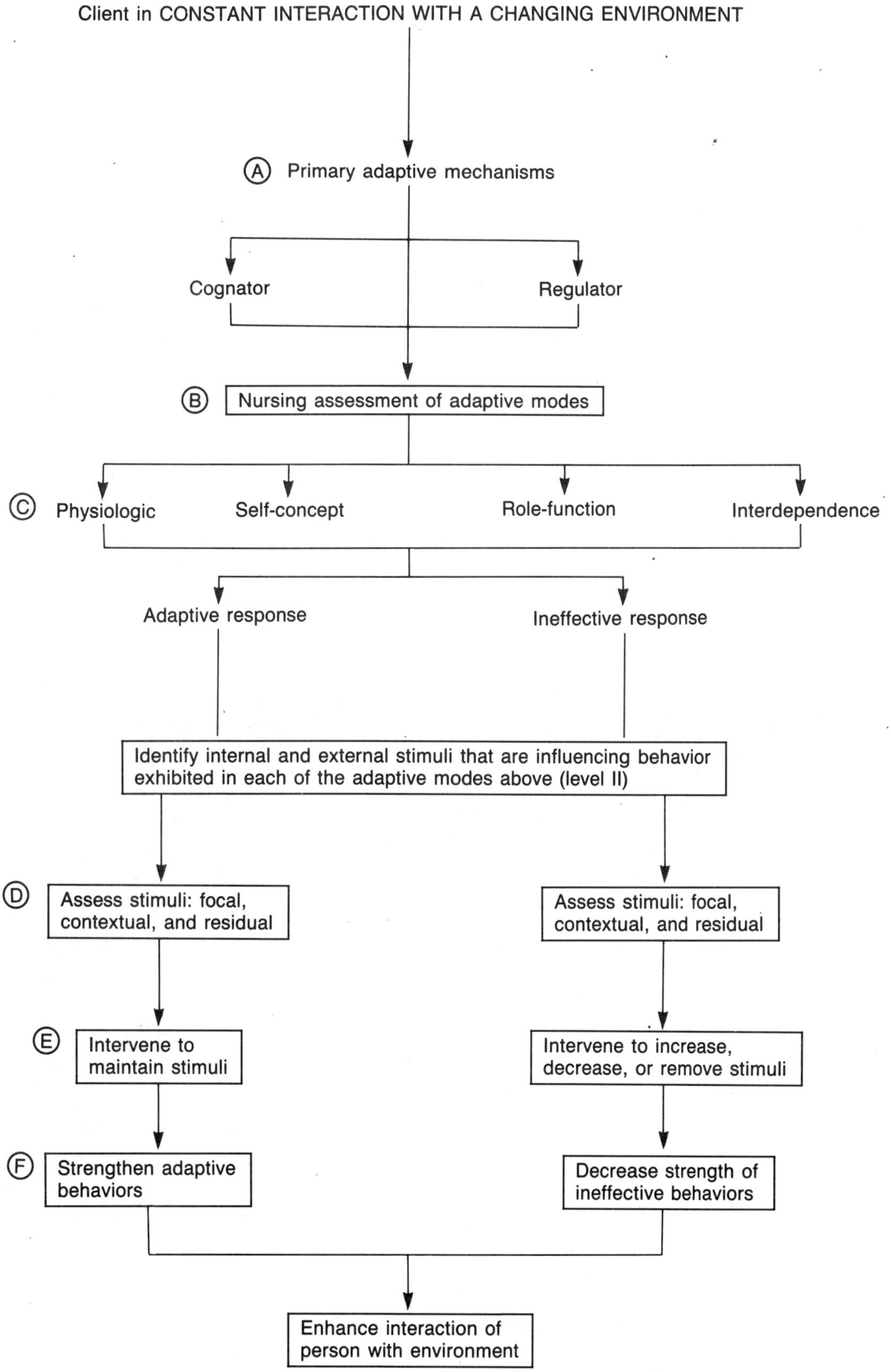
Client in CONSTANT INTERACTION WITH A CHANGING ENVIRONMENT
(A) Primary adaptive mechanisms
Cognator
Regulator
(B) Nursing assessment of adaptive modes
(C) Physiologic
Self-concept
Role-function
Interdependence
Adaptive response
Ineffective response
Identify internal and external stimuli that are influencing behavior exhibited in each of the adaptive modes above (level II)
(D) Assess stimuli: focal, contextual, and residual
Assess stimuli: focal, contextual, and residual
(E) Intervene to maintain stimuli
Intervene to increase, decrease, or remove stimuli
(F) Strengthen adaptive behaviors
Decrease strength of ineffective behaviors
Enhance interaction of person with environment

ROGERS' SCIENCE OF UNITARY HUMAN BEINGS MODEL

Howard Karl Butcher

Practicing nursing from a Rogerian nursing science perspective requires a conceptual shift toward a new world view, a new synthesis, a creative leap toward a new understanding of the nature of the universe (Rogers, 1970, 1988, 1989). See Table 1. Rogers identifies four building blocks as central to her conceptual system: energy fields, a universe of open systems, pattern, and four-dimensionality.

A. Energy field is the fundamental unit of the living and the inanimate. By definition, the energy field is continuously open and dynamic. There is a human energy field and an environmental energy field, which are integral to one another and engaged in a mutual process that is characterized by evolving diversity and creativity.

B. Energy field is characterized by pattern. Pattern evolves from the human-environmental field mutual process. Pattern gives identity to the human and environmental fields. Pattern is an abstraction and cannot be seen directly. Rather, we see manifestations of patterning, and these become the focus of nursing assessment in the Rogerian conceptual system.

C. Four-dimensionality is defined as a nonlinear domain without spatial or temporal attributes. All reality is postulated to be four-dimensional. This concept is helpful in nursing because it emphasizes the relative nature of change. We are our past, present, and future all at once—living in the infinite now. Human experiences of timelessness, precognition, telepathy, reincarnation, and "beyond-waking experiences" can be explained by the postulate of four-dimensionality.

TABLE 1 Prevailing Versus Rogers' World View*

Prevailing View	*Rogers' View*
Cell theory	Field theory
Mechanistic	Organistic
Closed system: feedback	Open system: innovation
Man: homeostatic	Human being: homeodynamic
Man: bio-psycho-social-spiritual parts	Human being: unitary patterns
Causality: single, multiple	Mutual process: pattern
Reductionism	Synthesis
Parts	Wholeness: unitary
Relationships	Interconnectiveness
Man-environment: dichotomous	Human being-environment: integral
Being	Becoming, unfolding
Dynamic equilibrium	Continuous evolving diversity
Assessment	Pattern appraisal
Nursing diagnosis	Health pattern description
Nursing intervention	Mutual patterning
Disease	Well-being, meaning
Deficits	Strengths, actualizing potentials
Structure	Rhythm
Adaptation	Transcendence

* Adapted from Malinski (1986).

D. Three principles are derived from a synthesis of the four building blocks. Rogers refers to the three principles as the "principles of homeodynamics." The term *homeodynamic* signifies the dynamic nature of life and the universe. The *principle of resonancy* is the continuous change from lower- to higher-frequency wave patterns in the human and environmental field. Resonancy describes Rogers' view of the life process of human beings as a symphony of rhythmic vibrations oscillating at various frequencies. The principle of resonancy describes the direction of change as evolving toward a "higher frequency." Higher frequency connotes the accelerating rate of change that is occurring. The *principle of integrality* is the continuous, mutual human field and environmental field process. It emphasizes the inseparability of humans and their environment. They must be viewed as a unity. The principle of integrality identifies the nurse's focus as being the overall pattern and its manifestations. Mechanistic and deterministic explanations of events are not valid in a universe of open systems. Human and the environment are in "mutual process" and therefore change together noncausally. The *principle of helicy* postulates that evolution is a process of continuous, innovative, probabilistic, increasing diversity of human and environmental field patterns characterized by nonrepeating rhythmicities. The nurse values and recognizes patterns of increasing diversity. All change is positive. Diversity is the norm.

E. The focus of nursing practice is on patterning. The Rogerian practice methodology evolves from the three principles of homeodynamics and has two phases: (1) pattern manifestation appraisal and (2) deliberative mutual patterning. Barrett (1988) states that the client is integral to both the appraisal and the patterning phases, which are nonlinear and not necessarily sequential.

F. The first phase, pattern manifestation appraisal, is defined as the continuous process of identifying manifestations of the human-environmental field mutual process that relate to current health events (Barrett, 1988). Manifestations of patterning evolve from the principles of homeodynamics and guide the nurse to focus on the appraisal of the following: the experience of time; sleep-wake and beyond-waking patterns; sense of rhythm; frequencies of light, color, and sound; indicators of increasing diversity, faster rhythms, and creativity; multiple manifestations; near-death experiences; pain-comfort; power; human field motion; pragmatic, visionary approaches to knowing participation in change; personal myth; sense of connectedness to the environment; and one's sense of integrity (Barrett, 1989; Hanchett, 1988; Ference, 1989; and Madrid and Winstead-Fry, 1986).

G. Therapeutic touch and guided imagery are useful unitary pattern appraisal methods within this conceptual system. In addition, the Ference Human Field Motion Tool (1979); Barrett's Power and Knowing Participation in

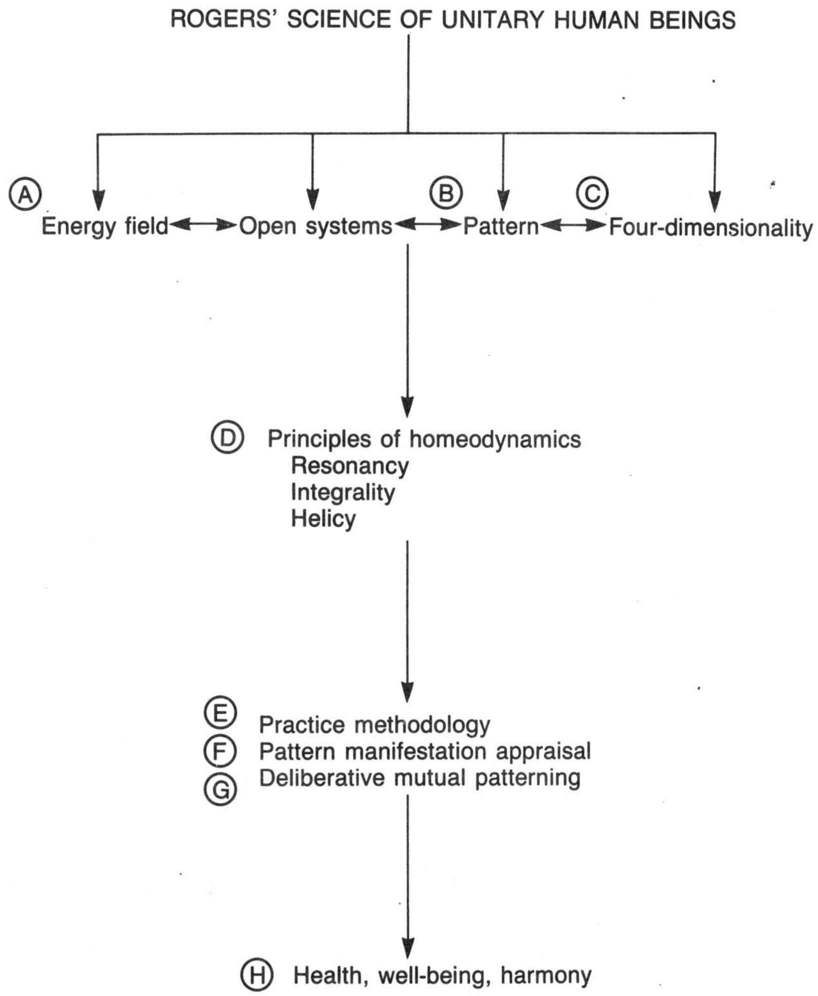

Change Test (1989); and Paletta's Temporal Experience Scales (1987) are pattern appraisal tools developed within Rogers' Science of Unitary Human Beings.

H. Barrett (1988) describes the second phase of the Rogerian practice methodology as deliberative mutual patterning, which is the continuous process whereby the nurse, with the client, patterns the environmental field to promote harmony related to health events. Malinski (1986) states that the nurse patterns the environmental field by using such modalities as sound and music; humor and play; imagery; relaxation and meditative experiences; dialogue; different frequencies of color and light; and touch. Nurses act as facilitators, educators, coordinators, and collaborators by participating actively with clients toward empowering the actualization of their health potentials. Mobilizing health potentials promotes human health and well-being.

References

Barrett EAM. An empirical investigation of Martha E. Rogers' principle of helicy: The relationship of human field motion and power. Ann Arbor, MI: Dissertation Abstracts International, 1984; 45:2, 8406278.

Barrett EAM. Using Rogers' science of unitary human beings in nursing practice. Nurs Sci Quart 1988; 1:50–51.

Barrett EAM. A nursing theory of power for nursing practice: Derivation from Rogers' paradigm. In: Riehl-Sisca JP ed. Conceptual models for nursing practice. 3rd ed. Norwalk, CT: Appleton & Lange, 1989:207–217.

Ference HM. The relationship of time experience, creativity traits, differentiation, and human field motion. Ann Arbor; MI: Dissertation Abstracts International, 1979; 40, 8010281.

Ference HM. Nursing science theories and administration. In: Henry B, Arndt C, DiVincenti M, Marriner-Tomay A, eds. Dimensions of nursing administration: theory, research, education, practice. Boston: Blackwell Scientific Publications, 1989:121–131.

Hanchett ES. Community assessment: Rogers' world view. In: Hanchett ES, ed. Nursing frameworks and community as client: bridging the gap. Norwalk, CT: Appleton & Lange, 1988:137–150.

Madrid M, Winstead-Fry P. Rogers' conceptual model. In: Winstead-Fry P, ed. Case studies in nursing theory. New York: National League for Nursing, 1986:73–102.

Malinski V. Explorations on Martha Rogers' science of unitary human beings. Norwalk, CT: Appleton-Century-Crofts, 1986.

Paletta JL. The relationship of temporal experience to human time. New York: New York University, 1987.

Rogers ME. An introduction to the theoretical basis of nursing. Philadelphia: FA Davis, 1970.

Rogers ME. Nursing science and art: A prospective. Nurs Sci Quart 1988; 1:99–102.

Rogers ME. Nursing: a science of unitary human beings. In: Riehl-Sisca JP, ed. Conceptual models for nursing practice. 3rd ed. Norwalk, CT: Appleton & Lange, 1989:181–188.

II PSYCHIATRIC DISORDERS

ALCOHOL ABUSE

Deborah Antai-Otong

Alcoholism represents a serious public problem in this country. It is estimated that 12 percent of the population use alcohol regularly and 10 million are alcoholics. Alcohol is the most accessible and abused drug in this country.

A. Refer to "Major Depressive Episodes" (p 46) for nursing assessment. In addition, include medical and psychosocial data during the initial assessment. A complete physical examination is imperative and should include complete laboratory work (i.e., complete blood count, chemistries, and toxicology screens). The nurse must assess the client's gait, speech, skin turgor, odor of breath, and nutritional status. The client with chronic alcoholism often has numerous medical problems and reports a history of gastrointestinal disturbances (i.e., gastritis, bleeding, peptic ulcer disease), easy bruising (as a result of cirrhosis or alcohol hepatitis), peripheral neuropathy (i.e., tingling and numbness in extremities), malnutrition, and vitamin deficiencies. A complete history of alcohol and/or drug use must include type, duration of use, frequency, past or present treatment, family history, and support system. The nurse must obtain information from significant others, since these individuals tend to deny or minimize alcohol-related problems. The nurse should also document a history of legal problems related to substance abuse, blackouts, withdrawal seizures, hallucinosis, and delirium tremens (DTs). The client's current social and occupational function must be assessed to determine the extent of use and the effects of alcohol on life-style.

B. Toxicology screens assist in determining the ethanol level, degree of intoxication, and presence of other substances, including illicit and prescribed drugs. Other laboratory tests are useful in assessing the client's nutritional status; often these clients have fluid and electrolyte imbalances, anemia, and liver damage. Poor nutritional status increases the incidence of alcohol withdrawal syndrome and other complications often seen in these individuals such as dementias (i.e., Wernicke's and Korsakoff's syndromes).

C. Alcohol intoxication is manifested by central nervous system depression, euphoria, suicidal ideations, slurred speech, unsteady gait, alcohol on breath, labile mood, and impaired judgment and social and occupational functioning. Most states consider a blood alcohol level of 0.10 percent legal intoxication.

D. Alcohol toxicity is usually manifested by profound central nervous system depression, hyperglycemia, convulsions, cardiovascular collapse, dehydration, and gastrointestinal disturbances.

E. Withdrawal symptoms, which may range from mild to severe, can be seen within hours of the last drink and include weakness, diaphoresis, hyperreflexia, nausea and vomiting, tremulousness, agitation, and shakiness. These symptoms may worsen over 24 to 48 hours and lead to visual and auditory hallucinations, hyperthermia, tachycardia, and hypertension. There is an increased incidence of seizures during this period and up to a week after the last drink or reduced consumption. Alcohol hallucinosis may occur within 48 hours after cessation and is often manifested by persistent or recurrent hallucinations, which usually begin by "seeing things." Most withdrawal syndromes are self-limiting and, if the client survives, dissipate within 5 to 7 days. Approximately 4 to 8 percent of alcoholics may develop DTs within this period. This syndrome constitutes a medical emergency and has a staggering 15 percent mortality rate. Symptoms of this syndrome include vivid persecutory hallucinations, confusion, disorientation, agitation, and resulting autonomic hyperactivity (i.e., hyperthermia, tachycardia, hypertension, cardiovascular collapse, and death).

F. Intravenous fluids must be started upon arrival to replace electrolytes and vitamins and decrease the incidence of severe alcohol withdrawal. Maintaining fluid and electrolyte balance is essential.

G. Benzodiazepines are administered to prevent withdrawal seizures and to decrease the incidence of alcohol withdrawal syndrome. Librium (chlordiazepoxide) is the drug of choice for the treatment of alcohol withdrawal.

References

Jaffe JH. Drug addiction and drug abuse. In: Gilman AG, Goodman LS, Rall TW, Murad F, eds. Goodman and Gilman's the pharmacological basis of therapeutics. 7th ed. New York: Macmillan, 1985:532–581.

Mendelson JH, Mello NK. Biologic concomitants of alcoholism. N Engl J Med 1979; 301:912–921.

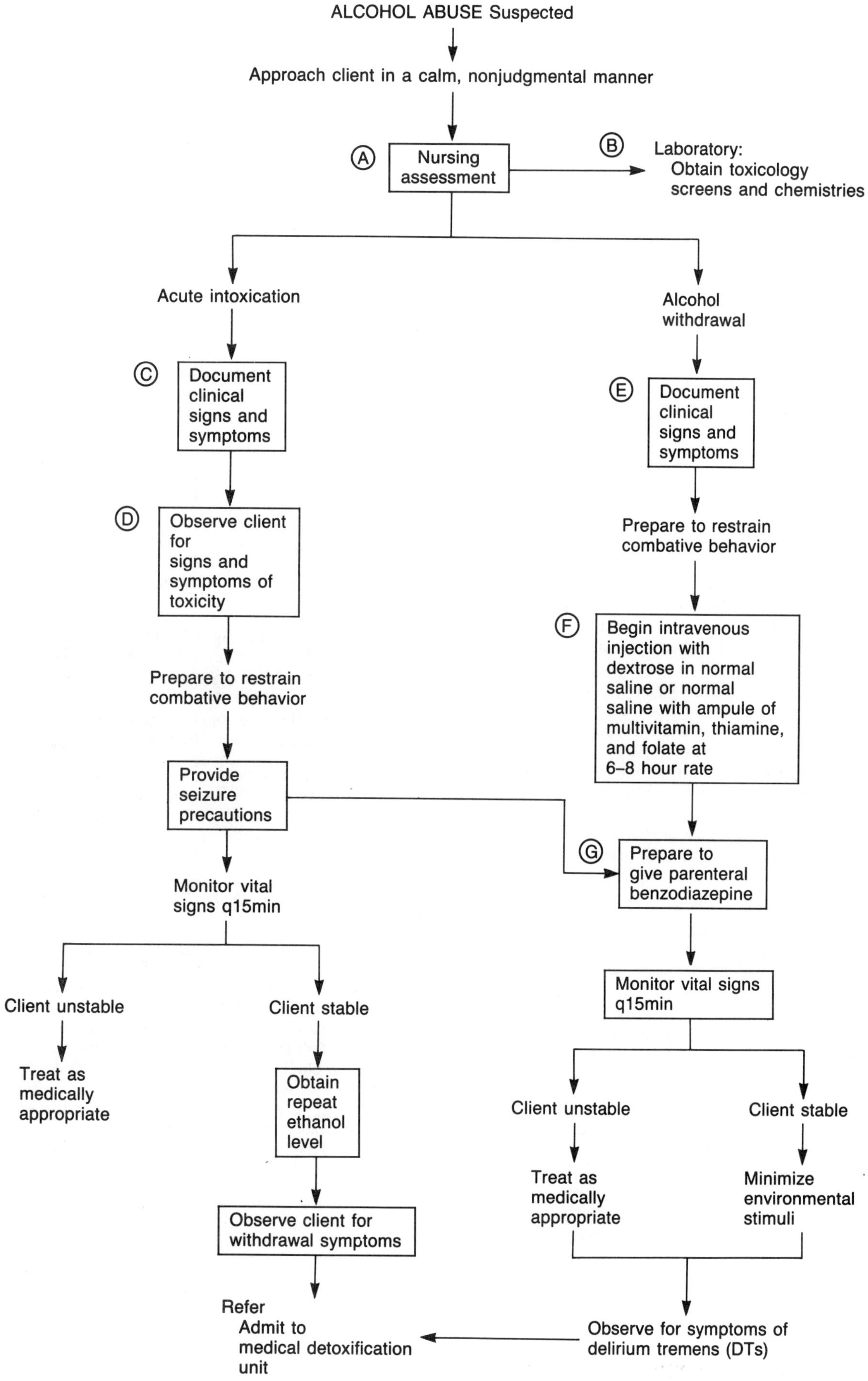
ALCOHOL ABUSE Suspected
Approach client in a calm, nonjudgmental manner
Ⓐ Nursing assessment
Ⓑ Laboratory: Obtain toxicology screens and chemistries
Acute intoxication
Ⓒ Document clinical signs and symptoms
Ⓓ Observe client for signs and symptoms of toxicity
Prepare to restrain combative behavior
Provide seizure precautions
Monitor vital signs q15min
Client unstable
Treat as medically appropriate
Client stable
Obtain repeat ethanol level
Observe client for withdrawal symptoms
Refer
Admit to medical detoxification unit
Alcohol withdrawal
Ⓔ Document clinical signs and symptoms
Prepare to restrain combative behavior
Ⓕ Begin intravenous injection with dextrose in normal saline or normal saline with ampule of multivitamin, thiamine, and folate at 6–8 hour rate
Ⓖ Prepare to give parenteral benzodiazepine
Monitor vital signs q15min
Client unstable
Treat as medically appropriate
Client stable
Minimize environmental stimuli
Observe for symptoms of delirium tremens (DTs)

NARCOTIC ABUSE

Deborah Antai-Otong

A. The history must include asking the client the name of the narcotic, frequency of use, duration, route, the last time used, and present and past chemical abuse treatment. When obtaining histories from these individuals, it is important to remember that the information in some cases may not be reliable. Confirmation of the information by a friend or family member may prove to be invaluable. Documentation of the use of other non-narcotic agents and/or alcohol is also essential. Past and present psychiatric treatment and suicide attempts need to be included in the history. Suicide history must include reasons for the attempt, the method, and whether or not the client was using drugs or alcohol (see "Suicide Attempt," p. 42). Laboratory tests must include toxicology screens (blood and urine), chemistries, physical examination, and a test for human immunodeficiency virus (HIV), especially if intravenous drug abuse is identified. Informed consents must be obtained before a test for HIV is done.

B. The initial nursing assessment should include the client's physical and mental status. Vital signs and neurologic signs include the depth, rate, and quality of respirations. The presence or absence of needle tracks should be noted, and the condition of the tracks must be documented. There is an increased incidence of abscesses in these areas. Individuals with histories of intravenous drug abuse, especially chronic users, have a higher incidence of febrile conditions resulting from bacterial infections. They run a higher risk of developing bacterial endocarditis than the general population. Symptoms indicative of this condition include fever, chills, splenomegaly, and petechiae. The mental status must be documented and must include the presence or absence of hallucinations (tactile, auditory, and visual) and delusions. Clients with histories of chemical abuse must be continuously assessed for changes in their physical and mental status.

C. Narcotic intoxication is manifested by slurred speech, ataxia, constricted pupils, and impairment of memory and judgment. Most narcotic abusers are not seen in hospital settings unless there is a medical problem or the client fears an overdose. Intoxication results from taking the narcotic agent orally, injecting it intravenously, or smoking it. The client may exhibit euphoria and apathy.

D. It is imperative to continuously monitor the intoxicated client and observe for symptoms of overdose, i.e., pinpoint pupils, changes in level of consciousness, depressed respirations, or respiratory arrest. When narcotic overdose is identified, it must be treated as a medical emergency. Assessment of whether or not the overdose was a suicide attempt is essential. This information can be obtained from the client if conscious or from a significant other. If it is a suicide attempt, suicide precautions ("Suicide Attempt," p. 42) must be initiated. Narcotic overdose can be rapidly reversed by an intravenous narcotic antagonist such as Narcan.

E. Narcotic withdrawal, which usually occurs after abrupt cessation of the narcotic agent, rarely constitutes a medical emergency unless other medical problems, such as cardiac disease, exist. Symptoms may range from mild to severe depending on the drug and duration of use. Narcotic withdrawal is manifested by muscle and joint pain, rhinorrhea, tearing, diaphoresis, nausea and vomiting, and diarrhea. Other symptoms include increased blood pressure and pulse, "goose bumps," and irritability. Mild withdrawal rarely requires intervention. Moderate-to-severe withdrawal can be minimized by methadone and clonidine. The client must be assessed for side effects and appropriate response to the medication.

F. The client's support systems must be assessed, and disposition should be determined by available resources. A referral to a local drug treatment program for narcotic abuse or dependence is essential for follow-up and/or detoxification. The local Narcotics Anonymous group will also provide support for the client's significant others.

G. Continuous observation should include assessing the client for symptoms of acute withdrawal, which can occur within 10 minutes of administration of Narcan.

References

Brewer C, Rezae H, Bailey C. Opioid withdrawal and naltrexone induction in 48–72 hours with minimal drop-out, using a modification of the naltrexone-clonidine technique. Br J Psychiatry 1988; 153:340–343.

Jaffe JH. Drug addiction and drug abuse. In: Gilman AG, Goodman LS, Rall TW, Murad F, eds. Goodman and Gilman's the pharmacological basis of therapeutics. 7th ed. New York: Macmillan, 1985:532–581.

Rounsaville BJ, Kosten T, Kleber H. Success and failure at outpatient opioid detoxification, evaluating the process of clonidine and methadone assisted withdrawal. J Nerv Ment Dis 1985; 173:103–110.

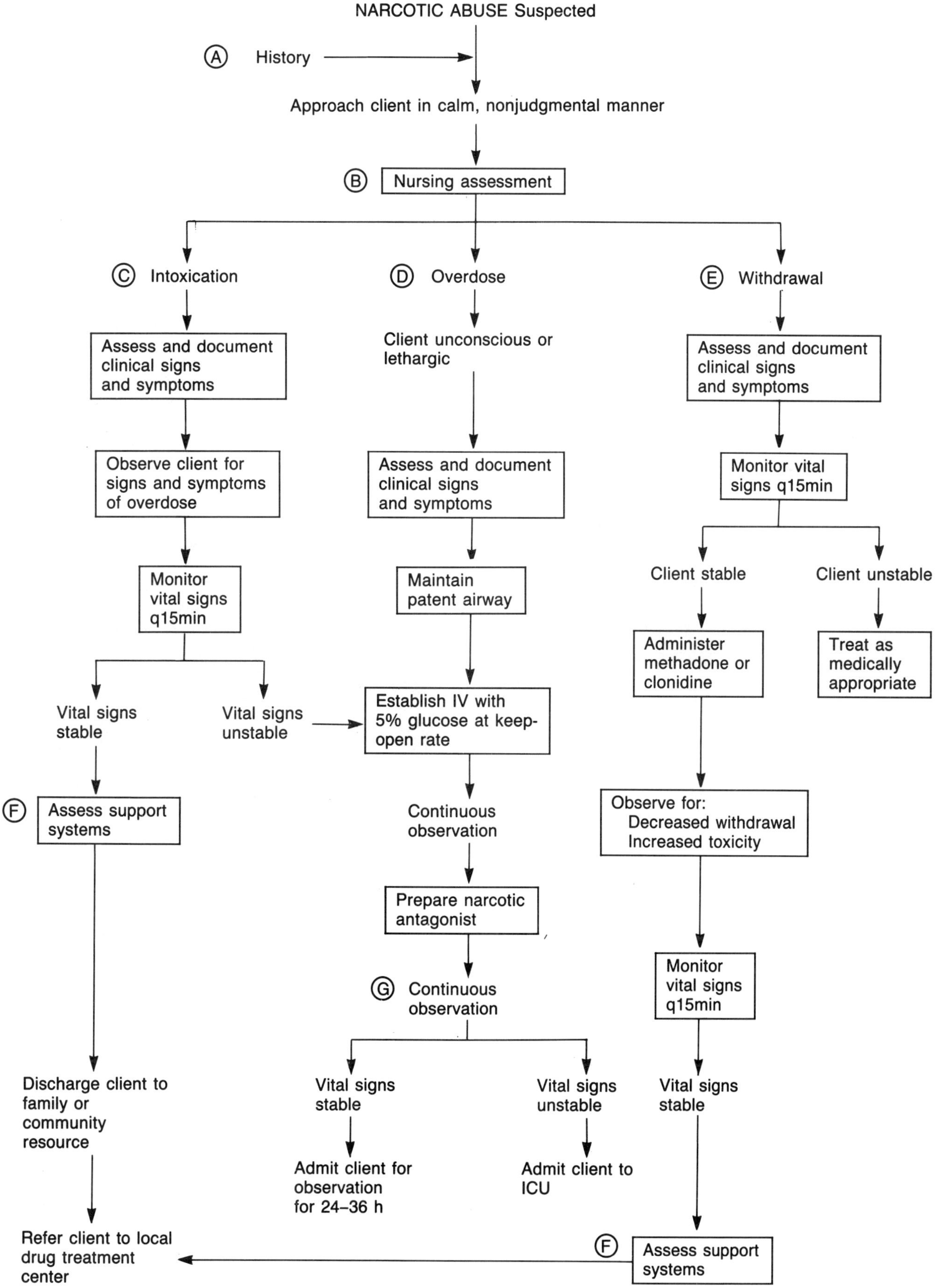
NARCOTIC ABUSE Suspected
(A) History
Approach client in calm, nonjudgmental manner
(B) Nursing assessment
(C) Intoxication
Assess and document clinical signs and symptoms
Observe client for signs and symptoms of overdose
Monitor vital signs q15min
Vital signs stable
Vital signs unstable
(F) Assess support systems
Discharge client to family or community resource
Refer client to local drug treatment center
(D) Overdose
Client unconscious or lethargic
Assess and document clinical signs and symptoms
Maintain patent airway
Establish IV with 5% glucose at keep-open rate
Continuous observation
Prepare narcotic antagonist
(G) Continuous observation
Vital signs stable
Admit client for observation for 24–36 h
Vital signs unstable
Admit client to ICU
(E) Withdrawal
Assess and document clinical signs and symptoms
Monitor vital signs q15min
Client stable
Administer methadone or clonidine
Observe for: Decreased withdrawal Increased toxicity
Monitor vital signs q15min
Vital signs stable
(F) Assess support systems
Client unstable
Treat as medically appropriate

AMPHETAMINE ABUSE

Deborah Antai-Otong

A. Amphetamines are synthetic compounds derived from ephedrine (a potent central nervous system stimulant). Slang terms for amphetamine include crystal, speed, meth, and crank. Other forms of this drug include over-the-counter diet pills and appetite depressants. These agents can be taken orally or intravenously or may be "snorted." The chronic amphetamine user's history sometimes reveals psychotic episodes, significant weight loss, sleeplessness, and irritability. Amphetamine use can precipitate latent schizophrenia or schizophrenia in remission. For further history-taking information see "Alcohol Abuse" (p 30).

B. Refer to "Narcotic Abuse" (p 32) for nursing assessment.

C. Amphetamine intoxication is characterized by agitation, irritability, tachycardia, increased blood pressure, dilated pupils, diaphoresis, chills, confusion, talkativeness, dizziness, and fatigue. Amphetamine intoxication can lead to overdose toxicity, a medical emergency, which is characterized by cardiac arrhythmias, hyperthermia, severe hypertension, and weight loss.

D. Other complications of amphetamine intoxication include delirium and delusional disorder. The client must be continuously observed and monitored for these conditions. Normally, delirium develops within 24 hours after intake of amphetamines, and symptoms include visual, tactile, and auditory hallucinations and paranoid delusions. Precautions must be taken to protect the client and others from injury. The nurse must prepare to restrain the client if violent and aggressive behavior develops. This psychotic reaction frequently responds to antipsychotic (neuroleptic) agents. If the client develops these symptoms, the nurse must attempt to decrease the resulting agitation by decreasing environmental stimuli and avoiding arguments with the client.

E. Withdrawal from amphetamines can be precipitated by cessation of heavy and chronic use. Manifestations of withdrawal symptoms may occur after several days. Clinical signs and symptoms include irritability, restlessness, frustration, fatigue, agitation, and sleeplessness. Other complications include severe depression (p 46) and an increased risk for suicide (p 42). Suicide precautions must be initiated, and environmental stimuli must be minimized with all forms of amphetamine abuse.

References

Antai-Otong DJ. Psychopharmacology. In: Johnson BS, ed. Psychiatric nursing: adaptation and growth. 2nd ed. Philadelphia: JB Lippincott, 1989:268–294.

Jaffe JH. Drug addiction and drug abuse. In: Gilman AG, Goodman LS, Rall TW, Murad F, eds. Goodman and Gilman's the pharmacological basis of therapeutics. 7th ed. New York: Macmillan, 1985:532–581.

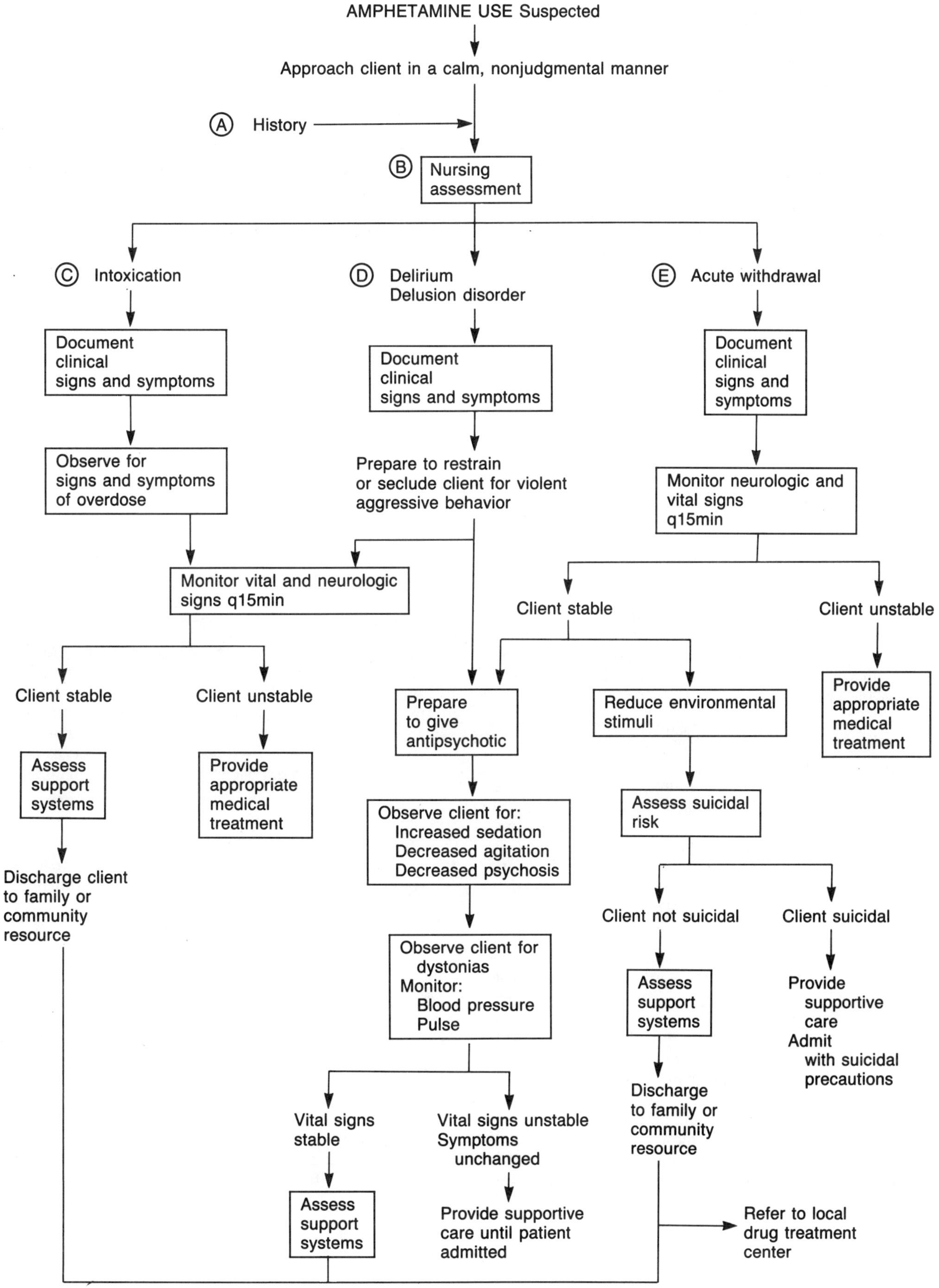
AMPHETAMINE USE Suspected
Approach client in a calm, nonjudgmental manner
Ⓐ History
Ⓑ Nursing assessment
Ⓒ Intoxication
Document clinical signs and symptoms
Observe for signs and symptoms of overdose
Monitor vital and neurologic signs q15min
Client stable
Assess support systems
Discharge client to family or community resource
Client unstable
Provide appropriate medical treatment
Ⓓ Delirium
Delusion disorder
Document clinical signs and symptoms
Prepare to restrain or seclude client for violent aggressive behavior
Prepare to give antipsychotic
Observe client for:
Increased sedation
Decreased agitation
Decreased psychosis
Observe client for dystonias
Monitor:
Blood pressure
Pulse
Vital signs stable
Assess support systems
Vital signs unstable
Symptoms unchanged
Provide supportive care until patient admitted
Ⓔ Acute withdrawal
Document clinical signs and symptoms
Monitor neurologic and vital signs q15min
Client stable
Reduce environmental stimuli
Assess suicidal risk
Client not suicidal
Assess support systems
Discharge to family or community resource
Client suicidal
Provide supportive care
Admit with suicidal precautions
Client unstable
Provide appropriate medical treatment
Refer to local drug treatment center

HALLUCINOGEN ABUSE

Deborah Antai-Otong

The use of hallucinogenic agents reached its peak in the late 1960s. By the late 1970s an estimated 20 percent of the population between 18 and 25 years of age in the United States had used hallucinogens at some time during their lives. With the advent of cocaine and other central nervous system stimulants, the use of hallucinogenic agents has declined drastically in the last 20 years.

Hallucinogens such as LSD and mescaline ("acid," "mushrooms," and "white crosses") are usually taken orally to produce tolerance behavioral effects, which increase with frequent use. They produce "psychedelic" states manifested by induced altered states of feelings and thoughts. They cause heightened euphoria, sensory awareness, and diminished capacity to distinguish boundaries between self, environment, and others. These agents affect areas of the central nervous system ranging from the cortex to the spinal cord. LSD also produces sympathetic stimulation manifested by dilatation of pupils, increased blood pressure and heart rate, nausea, "goose bumps," muscular weakness, and hyperthermia.

PCP (phencyclidine) is a potent analgesic and anesthetic used in veterinary medicine. In humans it also produces stimulation of the central nervous system (CNS). Other properties include CNS depression and anesthesia. It was introduced in the 1950s as an anesthetic and was quickly discontinued because it produced delirium. This drug became popular in the mid 1970s as an illicit hallucinogenic drug used by smoking or snorting.

A. Approach these clients in a calm, nonthreatening manner and refrain form overstimulating them. The nursing assessment includes asking the client what drug(s) he or she has used, the duration, frequency, and last time used. Document this information and assess the client continuously for signs of psychosis, physical aggression, or seizures, and monitor physical symptoms such as hypertension, hyperthermia, and cardiopulmonary failure. For a more detailed discussion on the nursing assessment see pages 30 and 46.

B. Clinical symptoms of hallucinogen intoxication include drowsiness, paresthesia, inner tension, and labile emotions such as inappropriate crying or laughing. These clients may express feelings of euphoria and may experience visual illusions (e.g., colors and sounds), extreme tension, anxiety, and "panic" episodes with feelings of depersonalization. These symptoms may abate in approximately 12 hours (half-life in man is usually 3 hours). Clients may respond differently to various psychedelic agents depending on the agent, dose, and their metabolism. Some of these clients experience altered memory states with chronic use. There is no evidence of withdrawal phenomena from these agents, even though the user may experience "bad" or "good" trips or flashbacks. Fatal accidents may be related to overdose and suicides. Deaths have resulted from cardiopulmonary failure and hyperthermia in test animals. PCP produces paresthesia, drowsiness, apathy, increased heart rate, hypersalivation, increased blood pressure, and hyperthermia. Chronic use produces changes in personality: apathy, social withdrawal, violent behaviors related to delirium, and confusion. Other side-effects include muscular rigidity and diaphoresis, and altered mental states manifested by changes in body image and hostile, bizarre behavior.

C. Provide a quiet, well-lighted environment to minimize illusions, agitation, and irritability. There is a risk that the client may become psychotic and violent toward himself (e.g., self-mutilation) or others. The nurse may need to "talk" the client down in an effort to decrease anxiety and violent behavior.

D. Medications such as Ativan or Valium may be administered to deal with extreme anxiety and panic states.

E. If the patient exhibits symptoms of psychosis and extreme agitation, a neuroleptic agent such as Haldol may be prescribed.

F. An acute LSD overdose produces cardiopulmonary failure and suicidal behavior, which may be related to severe depression and psychosis. PCP may produce self-mutilation and aggressive violent behavior toward self and/or others, seizures, and increased salivation that may require immediate life-support measures, such as suctioning and treatment of central nervous system depression. Other symptoms of acute overdose include delirium.

G. These clients must be closely monitored for delirium, extreme psychosis, and violent behavior. Prepare to restrain these clients and decrease sensory stimulation.

References

Domino EF. Neurobiology of phencyclidine: an update. In: Petersen RC, Stillman RC, eds. PCP phencyclidine abuse: an appraisal. Washington, DC: National Institute of Drug Abuse, Department of Health, Education, and Welfare (Publication No ADM 78-728). US Government Printing Office, 1978:18–43.

Jaffe JH. Drug addiction and drug abuse. In: Gilman AG, Goodman LS, Rall TW, Murad F, eds. Goodman and Gilman's the pharmacological basis of therapeutics. 7th ed. New York: Macmillan, 1986:532–581.

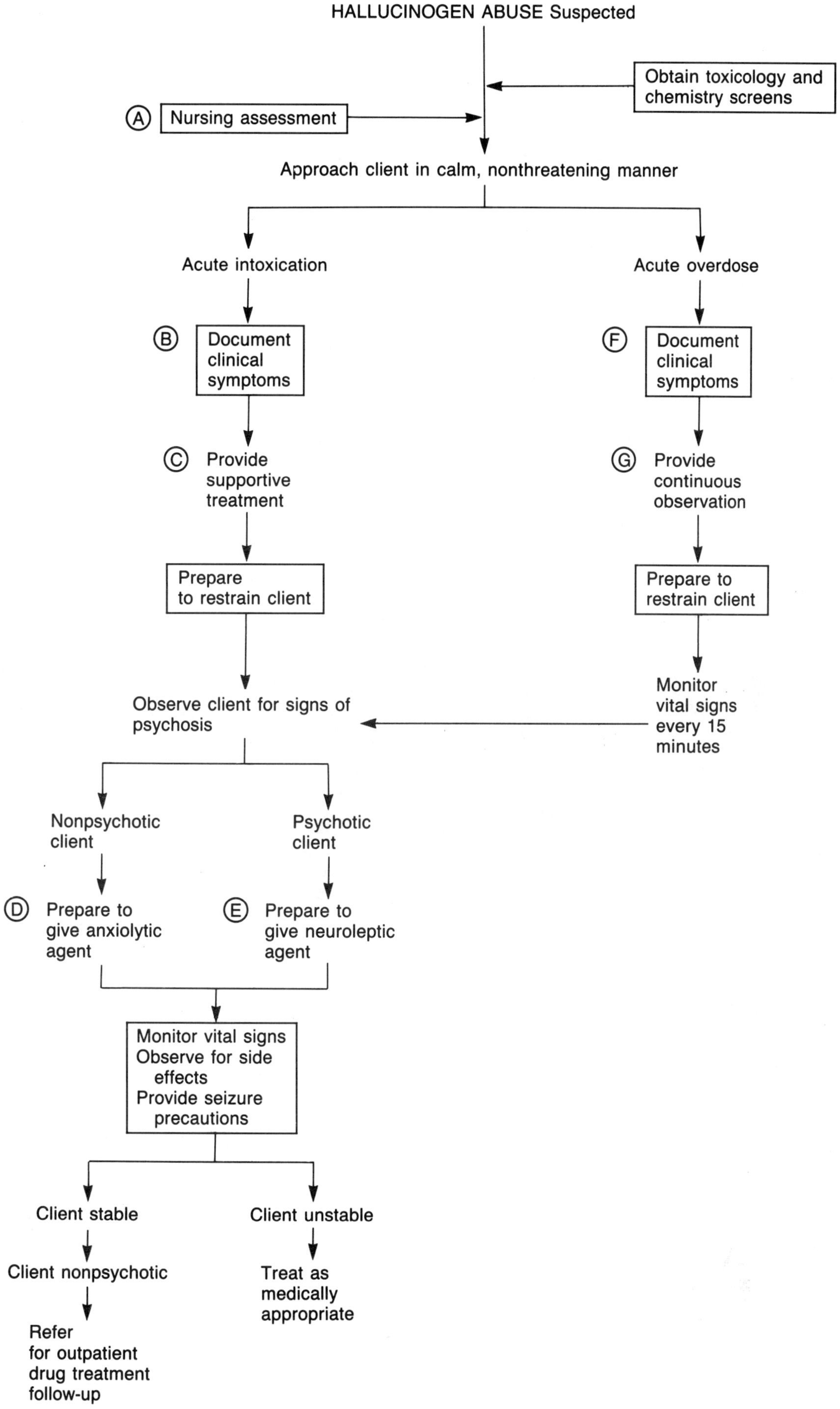
HALLUCINOGEN ABUSE Suspected
Obtain toxicology and chemistry screens
Ⓐ Nursing assessment
Approach client in calm, nonthreatening manner
Acute intoxication
Ⓑ Document clinical symptoms
Ⓒ Provide supportive treatment
Prepare to restrain client
Observe client for signs of psychosis
Nonpsychotic client
Ⓓ Prepare to give anxiolytic agent
Psychotic client
Ⓔ Prepare to give neuroleptic agent
Monitor vital signs
Observe for side effects
Provide seizure precautions
Client stable
Client nonpsychotic
Refer for outpatient drug treatment follow-up
Client unstable
Treat as medically appropriate
Acute overdose
Ⓕ Document clinical symptoms
Ⓖ Provide continuous observation
Prepare to restrain client
Monitor vital signs every 15 minutes

COCAINE ABUSE

Deborah Antai-Otong

A. The National Institute on Drug Abuse (NIDA) in 1985 estimated that approximately 6 million Americans were "current" users of cocaine (had used cocaine within the past 30 days), which was up from 1.6 million users, documented in 1977. They also reported that approximately 3 million users were dependent on cocaine. Another interesting finding documented in 1986 by Kleber and Gawin showed that cocaine emergency room visits had increased by 350 percent between 1976 and 1981 and 75 percent between 1981 and 1983. They also showed that there is an average of 2 to 4 years between first cocaine use and need for medical treatment, thus making it difficult for clients to recognize the hazards of cocaine. Cocaine is often referred to as coke, lady, and snow. It usually is sold as a white powder or in "rock" form, and its purity varies. It may be injected, "snorted," or "freebased" (smoked, usually with a pipe).

B. The nursing assessment must include a complete physical examination to determine the route, last dose, duration, and past drug or alcohol treatment. Clients who present in emergency rooms often exhibit symptoms similar to those seen in amphetamine abuse (p 34) or central nervous system (CNS) stimulation. Toxicology, blood, and urine screens are essential. Clients with histories of cocaine use report euphoria and often severe depression, especially following long-term use. For further discussion of nursing assessment see "Major Depressive Episodes" (p 46), and "Narcotic Abuse" (p 32).

C. The clinical signs and symptoms of cocaine toxicity or intoxication are the same as those seen with other CNS stimulants and include increased anxiety, paranoia, hypertension, hyperthermia, dilated pupils, tremors, diaphoresis, chest pains, and convulsions. These clients often present in emergency rooms in need of immediate medical attention and suffer severe symptoms that include unconsciousness, ventricular arrhythmias, seizures, and cardiopulmonary arrests that cause death.

D. The clinical signs and symptoms of cocaine withdrawal include craving, prolonged sleep, fatigue, and severe depression. These symptoms are often seen in clients with prolonged cocaine use. Abrupt cessation often causes increased agitation and restless. For further discussion of withdrawal symptoms, see "Amphetamine Abuse" (p 34).

E. Cocaine-induced delirium and delusional disorders can be precipitated 24 hours after initial use. For further discussion on this disorder, see "Amphetamine Abuse" (p 34).

References

Jaffe JH. Drug addiction and drug abuse. In: Gilman AG, Goodman LS, Rall TW, Murad F, eds. Goodman and Gilman's the pharmacological basis of therapeutics. 7th ed. New York: Macmillan, 1985:532–581.

Kleber HD. Introduction to cocaine abuse: historical, epidemiological and psychological perspectives. J Clin Psychiatry 1988; 49(Suppl):3–6.

Kleber HD, Gawin FH. Cocaine. In: American Psychiatric Association review. Vol 5. Washington, DC: American Psychiatric Association, 1986:160–185.

Millerman RB. Evaluation and clinical management of cocaine abusers. J Clin Psychiatry 1988; 49(Suppl):27–33.

National Household Survey. Rockville, MD: National Institute on Drug Abuse, 1985.

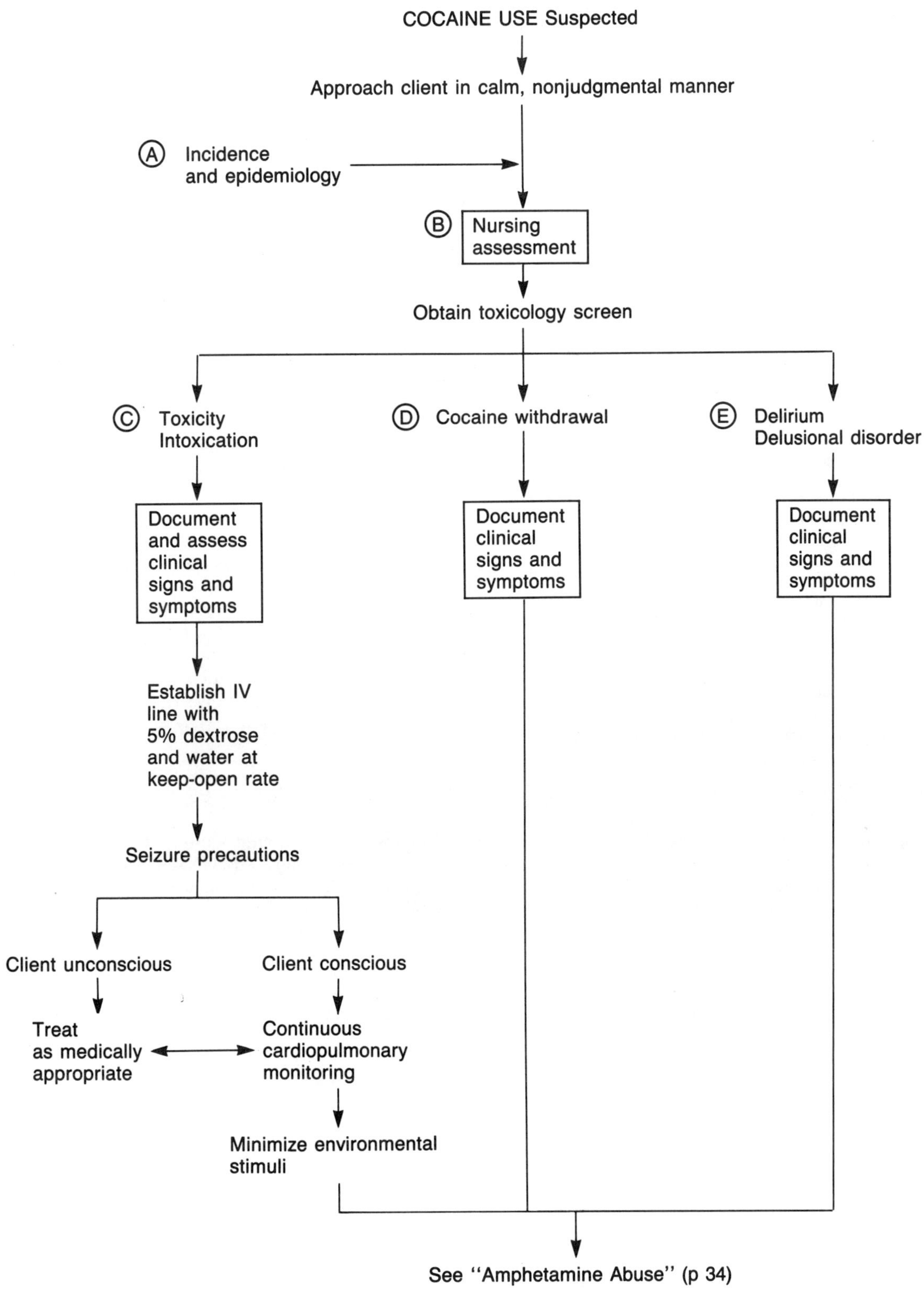
COCAINE USE Suspected
Approach client in calm, nonjudgmental manner
(A) Incidence and epidemiology
(B) Nursing assessment
Obtain toxicology screen
(C) Toxicity Intoxication
(D) Cocaine withdrawal
(E) Delirium Delusional disorder
Document and assess clinical signs and symptoms
Document clinical signs and symptoms
Document clinical signs and symptoms
Establish IV line with 5% dextrose and water at keep-open rate
Seizure precautions
Client unconscious
Client conscious
Treat as medically appropriate
Continuous cardiopulmonary monitoring
Minimize environmental stimuli
See "Amphetamine Abuse" (p 34)

SEDATIVE AND HYPNOTIC ABUSE

Deborah Antai-Otong

A. For a discussion of history taking on clients with substance abuse, see "Alchohol Abuse" (p 30). Substance abuse has produced profound effects on today's society. Studies have shown how individuals, families, and communities have been destroyed by this malignancy. Detection of substance abuse requires thorough history-taking skills and astute observations by the nurse. Family members and significant others must be included during this process to verify and clarify the client's information. Observation of family dynamics reveals pertinent information about the system's level of functioning and degree of adaptive behaviors.

B. For a discussion of nursing assessment of the client with a history of substance abuse, see "Narcotic Abuse" (p 32).

C. Central nervous system (CNS) intoxication from depressants is manifested by ataxia, slurred speech, impairment of memory and judgment, and drowsiness. Most CNS depressants are orally ingested, and intoxication results from a gradual increase in doses over a duration that produces physical dependency and tolerance. Other forms of intoxication can be produced by large doses of ingestions with or without alcohol. Moderate intoxication is similar to alcohol intoxication.

D. The client must be continuously monitored and assessed for signs and symptoms of CNS overdose (poisoning). Initially, symptoms of overdose may range from lethargy to unconsciousness; overdose symptoms constitute a medical emergency. The significance of overdose or suspected overdose represents a major problem because of the high incidence of mortality, ranging from 0.5 percent to 12 percent. Suicide attempt must always be suspected in the client with central nervous system overdoses, especially when barbiturates are used.

E. Withdrawal from CNS depressants results from cessation of long-term moderate-to-heavy use of one of these agents. Symptoms of withdrawal may begin several weeks after cessation and include tachycardia, diaphoresis, irritability, coarse tremors of the hands, and grand mal seizures. Seizures may occur 2 to 3 days after last use of short-acting barbiturates and after 7 to 8 days with long-acting benzodiazepines. Seizure precautions must be provided, and the client must be observed and monitored continuously. Another complication of withdrawal is delirium, which usually occurs 4 to 7 days after last use or reduction in dose. It is manifested by tactile hallucinations, extreme anxiety, paranoia, and agitation. This constitutes a medical emergency because of physical reactions, manifested mainly by tachycardia, hyperthermia, hypertension, and cardiopulmonary arrest, which may cause death. Some hallucinations may persist for several months and are equivalent to alcohol hallucinosis.

References

Jaffe JH. Drug addiction and drug abuse. In: Gilman AG, Goodman LS, Rall TW, Murad F, eds. Goodman and Gilman's the pharmacological basis of therapeutics. 7th ed. New York: Macmillan, 1985:532–581.

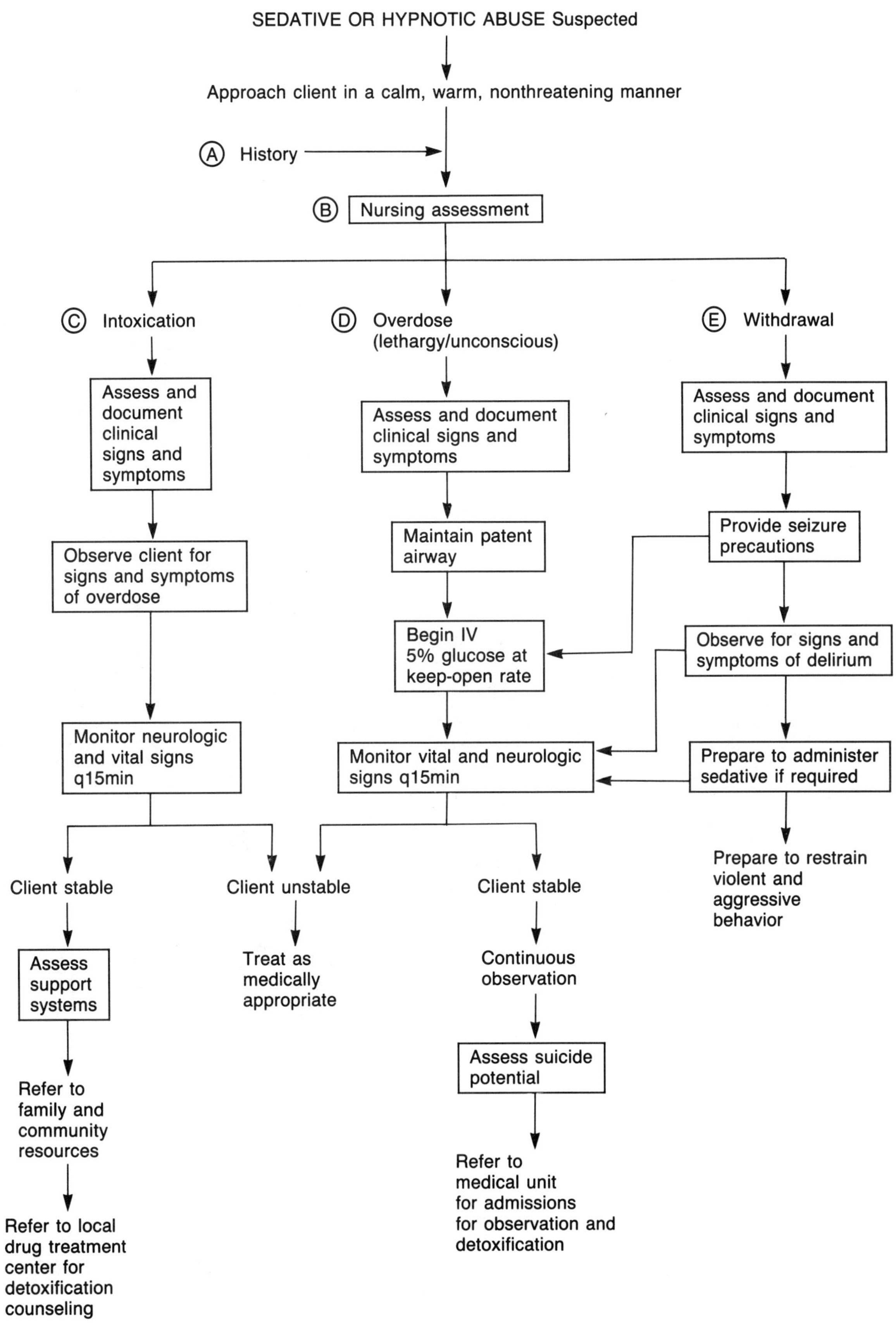
SEDATIVE OR HYPNOTIC ABUSE Suspected
Approach client in a calm, warm, nonthreatening manner
(A) History
(B) Nursing assessment
(C) Intoxication
Assess and document clinical signs and symptoms
Observe client for signs and symptoms of overdose
Monitor neurologic and vital signs q15min
Client stable
Assess support systems
Refer to family and community resources
Refer to local drug treatment center for detoxification counseling
Client unstable
Treat as medically appropriate
(D) Overdose (lethargy/unconscious)
Assess and document clinical signs and symptoms
Maintain patent airway
Begin IV 5% glucose at keep-open rate
Monitor vital and neurologic signs q15min
Client stable
Continuous observation
Assess suicide potential
Refer to medical unit for admissions for observation and detoxification
(E) Withdrawal
Assess and document clinical signs and symptoms
Provide seizure precautions
Observe for signs and symptoms of delirium
Prepare to administer sedative if required
Prepare to restrain violent and aggressive behavior

SUICIDE ATTEMPT*

Deborah Antai-Otong

A. The history must include the method by which the client tried to commit suicide, e.g., an object used to cut the wrist, chemicals, or drugs. This history must also include the reasons for the attempt, e.g., recent loss, terminal or chronic illness, auditory hallucinations, or personality disorders. Previous suicide attempts must be documented. A family history of suicide is a strong indicator of risk. An alcohol and drug history also increases the suicide risk. Past and present psychiatric treatment must be included, and the nurse should look for symptoms of depression and schizophrenia. Current medications must be documented, especially if the client has been taking antidepressants. A toxicology screen may reveal ingested substances and the results should be included in the initial history.

B. The initial nursing assessment should include the client's physical status. The vital signs, appearance, appearance of the wounds, and neurologic signs must be included. It is also essential to determine whether the overdose was a suicide attempt or an accident. Sometimes older or confused clients forget and take too many pills, and this possibility needs to be ruled out. The mental status must also be assessed and should focus on the presence of hallucinations, delusions, and appropriateness of affect. The client must be approached in a calm, concerned, and nonjudgmental manner. He must be continuously assessed for changes in both physical and mental status and must also be constantly assessed for suicidal risk.

C. Initially the clinical assessment of a conscious patient who has overdosed includes an acknowledgment of ingestion of a drug or chemical. The manifestations may vary depending upon the drug and the length of time since ingestion. The symptoms may vary from drowsiness, confusion, and blurred vision to hypotension and cardiac arrhythmias. Initial treatment should include gastric lavage and continuous monitoring for convulsions and arrhythmias.

D. The client must be continuously assessed and monitored for suicide, and this includes listening to what he is saying, particularly if he threatens to try again and has a plan; individuals who have recently made a suicide attempt are likely to try again within 24 to 48 hours. Direct questions should be asked, such as "Are you still having thoughts about killing yourself?" The suicide risk is increased in individuals who have sustained a recent loss and who have few support systems.

E. The clinical assessment in an unconscious patient who has overdosed should include any history that can be elicited and notations about unresponsiveness, possible respiratory depression, hypotension or hypertension, and dilated or constricted pupils. There may also be cardiac arrhythmias or convulsions. It is essential to maintain a patent airway and provide continuous cardiac monitoring.

F. If the client has a cut wrist, note the presence of active bleeding and whether it is a self-inflicted wound, and include a note about the weapon used.

G. The wound should be cleaned and a pressure dressing applied. Pulses distal to the wound must be checked every 15 minutes. Vital signs must be monitored closely.

H. A history of tetanus immunization must be obtained.

References

Hoff LA. People in crisis. Menlo Park, CA: Addison-Wesley, 1978.

Johnson BS. Psychiatric mental health nursing: adaptation & growth. Philadelphia: JB Lippincott, 1986:536–546.

Lanros NE. Assessment and intervention: emergency nursing. 2nd ed. Bowie, MD: Robert J. Brady, 1983:493.

Taylor CM. Mereness' essentials of psychiatric nursing. 11th ed. St. Louis: CV Mosby, 1982:278–281.

* Reprinted from Mancini ME. Decision making in emergency nursing. Toronto: BC Decker, 1987.

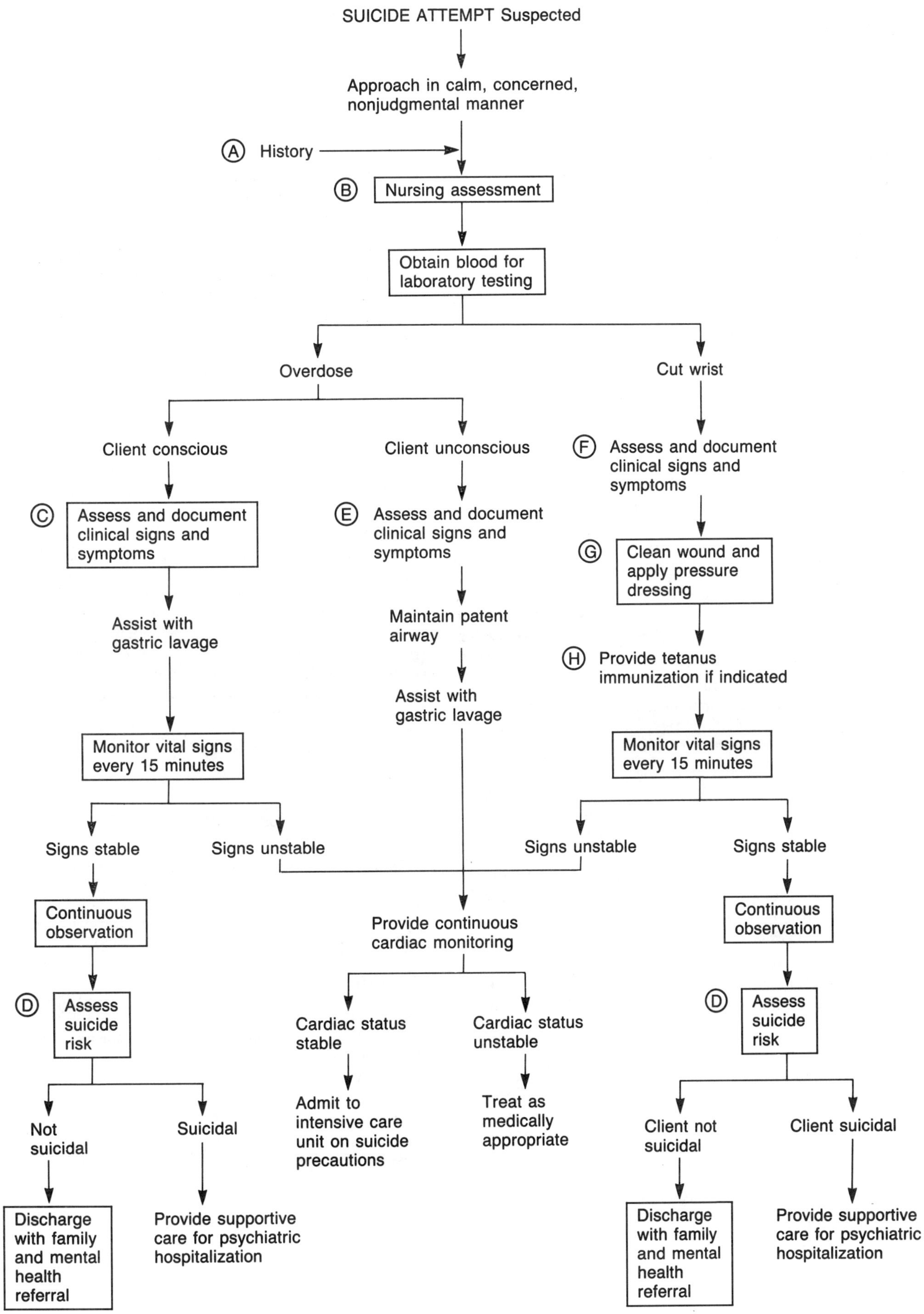
SUICIDE ATTEMPT Suspected
Approach in calm, concerned, nonjudgmental manner
Ⓐ History
Ⓑ Nursing assessment
Obtain blood for laboratory testing
Overdose
Cut wrist
Client conscious
Client unconscious
Ⓒ Assess and document clinical signs and symptoms
Assist with gastric lavage
Monitor vital signs every 15 minutes
Signs stable
Signs unstable
Continuous observation
Ⓓ Assess suicide risk
Not suicidal
Suicidal
Discharge with family and mental health referral
Provide supportive care for psychiatric hospitalization
Ⓔ Assess and document clinical signs and symptoms
Maintain patent airway
Assist with gastric lavage
Provide continuous cardiac monitoring
Cardiac status stable
Cardiac status unstable
Admit to intensive care unit on suicide precautions
Treat as medically appropriate
Ⓕ Assess and document clinical signs and symptoms
Ⓖ Clean wound and apply pressure dressing
Ⓗ Provide tetanus immunization if indicated
Monitor vital signs every 15 minutes
Signs unstable
Signs stable
Continuous observation
Ⓓ Assess suicide risk
Client not suicidal
Client suicidal
Discharge with family and mental health referral
Provide supportive care for psychiatric hospitalization

MANIA*

Deborah Antai-Otong

A. The history is essential and should include both a psychiatric and a medical history. The psychiatric history should include current and past treatment, particularly current medication. The medication history must include the length of time the medication has been taken and the dosage so that a neuroleptic syndrome can be ruled out. A drug and alcohol history is essential in making an accurate diagnosis. The psychiatric history must also include any family psychiatric history, especially regarding schizophrenia and manic-depressive illness. The medical history must include current and past treatment, including medications and familial medical illnesses. This information will be useful in ruling out medical problems as a source of psychosis, e.g., hyperthyroidism, diabetes, or respiratory problems.

B. The initial nursing assessment should include the client's mental status, including hallucinations, delusions, and congruence of mood and conversation. The vital signs should be assessed if possible. The gait, rate of speech, and appropriateness of affect are also important.

C. A schizophrenic client may exhibit explosive overactivity, auditory hallucinations, and sometimes persecutory delusions. There is usually incongruence between affect and ideas expressed, and the individual's affect is usually flat or blunted.

D. Antipsychotic medication usually produces sedation within minutes after an intramuscular injection. The drug quickly decreases agitation, rage, and overall reactivity to sensory stimuli. If symptoms persist, the dose may be repeated every 60 minutes until sedation occurs.

E. The clinical signs and symptoms of atypical psychosis can be similar to those of schizophrenia and mania, but usually the history of symptoms is different. These symptoms may be brought on by several factors, including drugs and alcohol toxicity or withdrawal. Symptoms can also be brought on by medications and medical problems, e.g., hyperthyroidism, diabetes mellitus, and electrolyte imbalance.

F. Toxicology screens provide essential data about the presence of drugs or alcohol. If the client has positive results on the toxicology screen, appropriate medical care is necessary while continuing the psychiatric evaluation. The chemistry laboratory can assist the emergency department staff in ruling out metabolic or electrolyte imbalance that may contribute to psychosis.

G. The clinical signs and symptoms of mania include physical restlessness, marked irritability, inflated self-esteem, rapid speech, and flight of ideas. The psychiatric history will reveal recurrences and a family history, and these symptoms will have existed for at least one week.

H. All antipsychotic medications have the potential to produce a wide range of side effects, including dystonia and extrapyramidal symptoms, which can occur any time after administration of the first dose. These symptoms range from uncoordinated movements of the neck, face, tongue, chest, or extremities to backward rolling of the eyes. Other symptoms include painful twisting of the back and neck. These symptoms are extremely frightening to the client and staff. They can be treated by the intravenous or intramuscular administration of diphenhydramine (Benadryl) or benztropine (Cogentin). Other side effects include orthostatic hypotension and reflex tachycardia. It is essential that the blood pressure and pulse be taken before each dose, in both lying and standing positions if feasible. Another reaction to these drugs is the malignant neuroleptic syndrome, manifested initially by a rapid deterioration in level of consciousness, hyperthermia, diaphoresis, and tachycardia.

References

Antai-Otong DJ. Psychopharmacology. In: Johnson BS, ed. Psychiatric mental health nursing: adaptation and growth. Philadelphia: JB Lippincott, 1986:245–262.

Burgess AW. Psychiatric nursing in the hospital and community. 3rd ed. Englewood Cliffs, NJ: Prentice-Hall, 1981:368–381.

Harris E. Extrapyramidal side-effects of antipsychotic medications. Am J Nurs 1981; 81:1324–1328.

Manfreda ML, Krampitz SD. Psychiatric nursing. 10th ed. Philadelphia: FA Davis, 1977.

Taylor CM. Mereness' essentials of psychiatric nursing. 11th ed. St. Louis: CV Mosby, 1982:271–273.

* Reprinted from Mancini ME. Decision making in emergency nursing. Toronto: BC Decker, 1987.

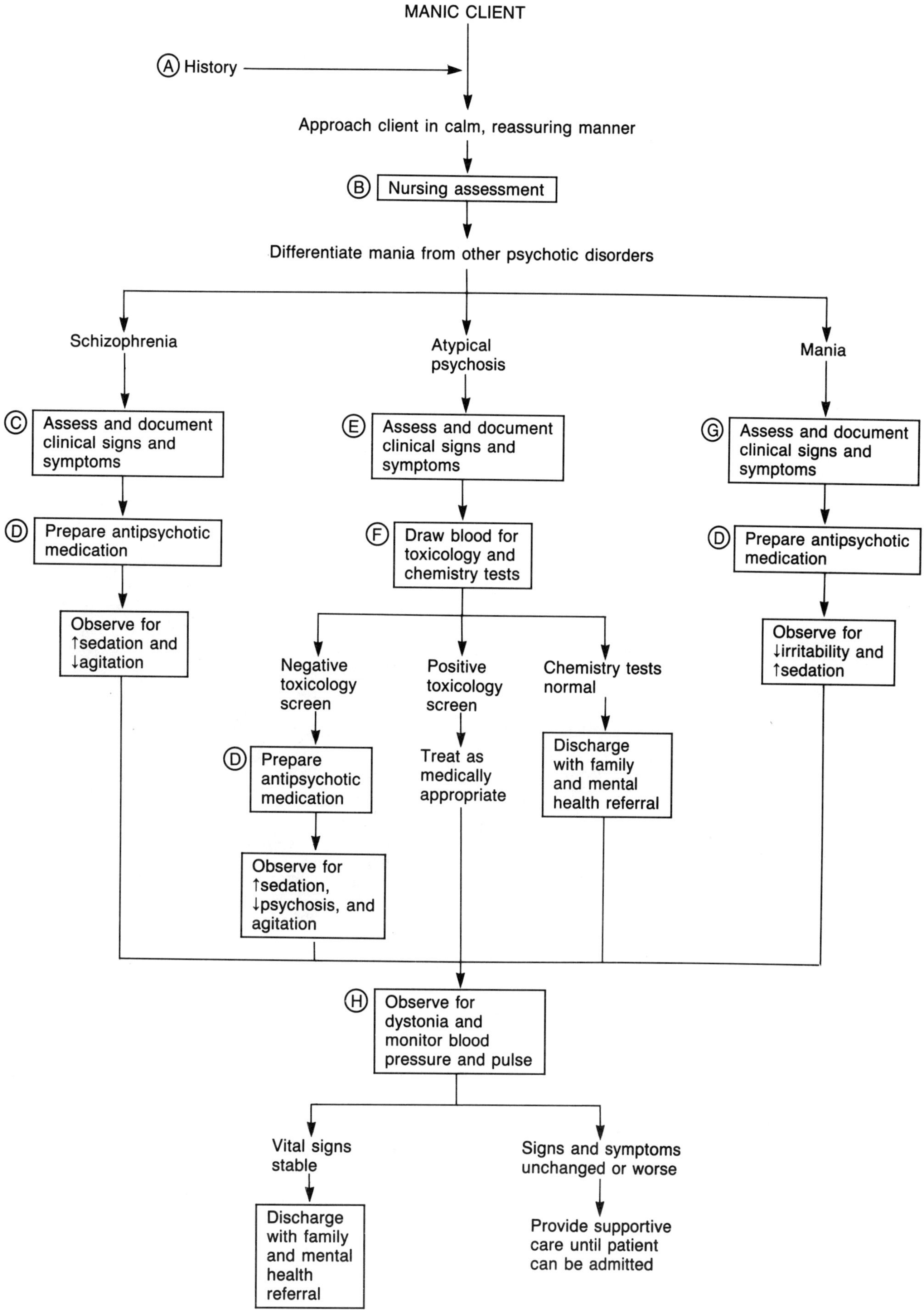
MANIC CLIENT
(A) History
Approach client in calm, reassuring manner
(B) Nursing assessment
Differentiate mania from other psychotic disorders
Schizophrenia
Atypical psychosis
Mania
(C) Assess and document clinical signs and symptoms
(D) Prepare antipsychotic medication
Observe for ↑sedation and ↓agitation
(E) Assess and document clinical signs and symptoms
(F) Draw blood for toxicology and chemistry tests
Negative toxicology screen
(D) Prepare antipsychotic medication
Observe for ↑sedation, ↓psychosis, and agitation
Positive toxicology screen
Treat as medically appropriate
Chemistry tests normal
Discharge with family and mental health referral
(G) Assess and document clinical signs and symptoms
(D) Prepare antipsychotic medication
Observe for ↓irritability and ↑sedation
(H) Observe for dystonia and monitor blood pressure and pulse
Vital signs stable
Discharge with family and mental health referral
Signs and symptoms unchanged or worse
Provide supportive care until patient can be admitted

MAJOR DEPRESSIVE EPISODES

Deborah Antai-Otong

Clients with major depression represent a large population in psychiatric nursing. Frequently, clients suffering from depression have several themes. They complain of feeling helpless and worthless and that they have no control over their lives. Depressed clients often focus on the negative rather than the positive and are pessimistic about their situation improving. These individuals also tend to overgeneralize and have distorted cognitions. Sometimes these distortions produce maladaptive coping skills and behaviors. Clients suffering from depression tend to isolate themselves from family members and feel alone. These individuals have a high risk for suicide. If depression is not treated appropriately there is also a risk of psychosis, which also increases the risk of suicide and dysfunction.

A. The history begins by asking the client and family members about recent stressors or significant life-style changes over the past 6 to 12 months. Assess the client's past and present capabilities, and document past and present psychiatric treatment. Investigate a family history of depression, and the client's and family members' substance abuse history. Include the client's current support system, level of functioning over the past year, and suicide attempts. Be aware that depressed patients in certain age groups respond to questions differently. For instance, older clients may complain of somatic problems that mimic vegetative symptoms of depression, i.e., fatigue, poor appetite, and weight loss rather than emotional pain; younger clients may be willing to talk about depression with little persuasion. Family members and significant others are important during this initial and ongoing interviews. They can verify and clarify information provided by the client. The nurse can also observe family dynamics during the data collecting phase. A recent physical examination is essential to rule out an organic etiology for all depressed clients.

B. The nursing assessment includes data from the history and documents symptoms of major depression. Manifestations of this disorder include fatigue, decrease or significant changes in appetite, weight loss or gain, poor concentration, decreased motivation, decreased libido, marked loss of interest or pleasure in everyday activities, possible agitation, and preoccupation with death or suicide. There is a high risk of suicide among depressed clients, especially those experiencing multiple and significant losses. Other circumstances that increase suicide risk include, psychosis, substance abuse, and lack of support systems. Older white males and adolescents represent the highest risk groups. Assessing clients at risk for suicide is an ongoing process, and when suicide potential is identified, steps must be taken to provide safety. Family members must be aware of the symptoms of suicide potential. For further discussion on assessing the suicidal client, see "Suicide Attempt" (p 42). Mental status is an essential part of the nursing assessment. Depressed clients must be continuously observed for changes in mental status, suicide potential, psychosis, and worsening of depression. Immediate hospitalization must be considered when they are identified.

C. Psychiatric consultation is essential when major depression is identified, because these clients are at risk for suicide. Collaboration allows the nurse to discuss findings from the assessment with the psychiatrist and develop objective treatment planning. The physician may need to further evaluate the client for antidepressant medication or immediate hospitalization.

References

American Psychiatric Association. Diagnostic and statistical manual of mental disorders. 3rd ed. Washington, DC: American Psychiatric Association, 1987:218–230.

Antai-Otong D. When your patient is depressed. Nursing '88 1988; 18:70–72.

Beck AT. Cognitive therapy and emotional disorders. New York: International Universities Press, 1976.

Beck AT, Rush JA, Shaw BF, et al. Cognitive therapy of depression. New York: The Guilford Press, 1979.

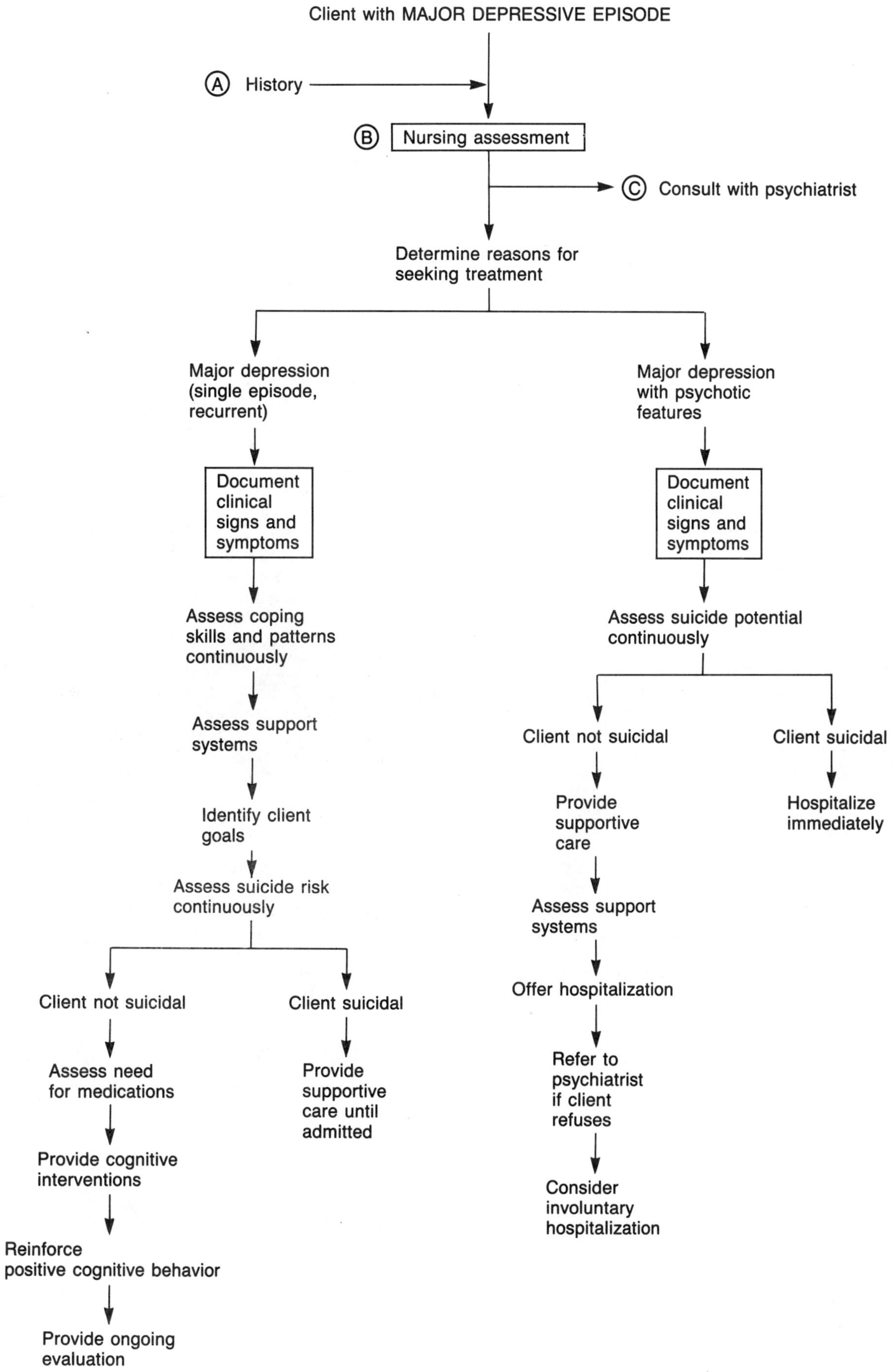
Client with MAJOR DEPRESSIVE EPISODE
(A) History
(B) Nursing assessment
(C) Consult with psychiatrist
Determine reasons for seeking treatment
Major depression (single episode, recurrent)
Major depression with psychotic features
Document clinical signs and symptoms
Document clinical signs and symptoms
Assess coping skills and patterns continuously
Assess suicide potential continuously
Assess support systems
Client not suicidal
Client suicidal
Identify client goals
Provide supportive care
Hospitalize immediately
Assess suicide risk continuously
Assess support systems
Offer hospitalization
Client not suicidal
Client suicidal
Assess need for medications
Provide supportive care until admitted
Refer to psychiatrist if client refuses
Provide cognitive interventions
Consider involuntary hospitalization
Reinforce positive cognitive behavior
Provide ongoing evaluation

DYSTHYMIC DISORDER

Deborah Antai-Otong

A. Clients with histories of dysthymia or dysthymic disorder reveal chronic depression and difficulty experiencing pleasure in life. This form of depression lacks the vegetative symptoms often seen in major depressive disorders, such as decreased libido, lack of energy, or severe weight loss resulting from poor appetite. It is essential to assess and document whether the client has had these symptoms in the past. History taking must also include whether the client has symptoms of other affective disorders, such as bipolar disorder (mania, p 44). Include in the history any family history of psychiatric problems and treatment; the client's present and past psychiatric treatment, including reasons for seeking treatment, response to treatment, and medications; and medical history, listing medications and current diagnoses and treatment. Substance abuse and treatment for both the client and family members must also be documented. Document the course and duration of the current illness, and address maladaptive behaviors and coping patterns. Investigate job history, current marital status, available support systems, and suicide history for the client and family members.

B. When clients seek treatment complaining of depression, one of the initial questions must be the client's expectations from treatment. Since the responsibility for seeking treatment lies with the client, asking these questions helps the client identify problems and goals for treatment. A complete physical examination is essential to rule out an organic basis for the presenting depressive symptoms. Assess the mental status continuously throughout treatment. Assess and document the client's response to treatment and side effects from medications.

C. Clients with dysthymia often experience crises because of maladaptive coping skills and lack of support systems. If the crisis is not resolved, symptoms of major depression may evolve. When major depression is suspected, suicide potential and risk must be assessed on an ongoing basis (see "Major Depressive Episodes" [p 46] and "Suicide Attempt" [p 42]).

D. Clients frequently seek treatment requesting medication. Antidepressant drugs may be prescribed to alleviate vegetative symptoms of depression. However, clients must understand that medications will not solve all their problems. Teaching plans must be initiated to address the expected and undesirable side effects of their medication.

E. Interventions that may be used for dysthymic disorders include focusing on distorted cognitive issues and maladaptive behaviors. Cognitive interventions are therapeutic approaches that apply specific techniques to modify thought processes. These techniques focus on distorted thought processes that are illogical and negative. Cognitive therapy allows the nurse to play an active role in modifying these cognitions and assisting the client in developing adaptive behaviors and coping skills. The client actively participates in therapy, gains improved problem-solving skills, deals with precipitating stressors more realistically, and learns to focus on strengths and positive attributes rather than weaknesses and negative ones. These interventions increase the client's self-esteem and promote confidence in dealing with everyday problems (see "Cognitive Therapy," p 108).

F. Continuous evaluation of progress must be documented and shared with the client and positive reinforcement of positive adaptive behavior must be an ongoing process. These interventions are essential to alter distorted cognitions and depression.

References

Aguilera DC, Messick JM. Crisis intervention: theory and methodology. 5th ed. St. Louis: CV Mosby, 1986.

American Psychiatric Association. Diagnostic and statistical manual of mental disorders. 3rd ed. Washington, DC: American Psychiatric Association, 1987:230–233.

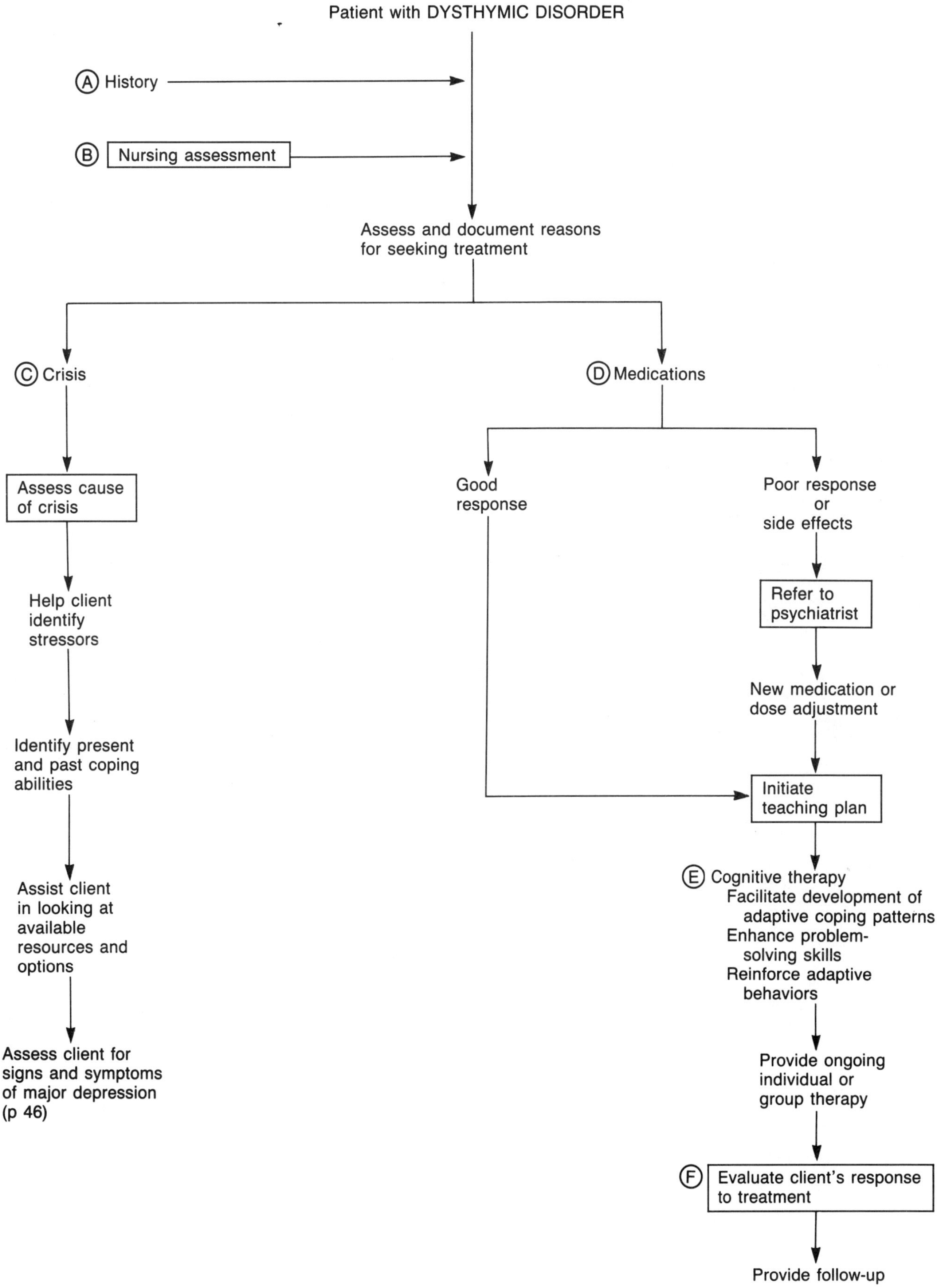
Patient with DYSTHYMIC DISORDER
(A) History
(B) Nursing assessment
Assess and document reasons for seeking treatment
(C) Crisis
Assess cause of crisis
Help client identify stressors
Identify present and past coping abilities
Assist client in looking at available resources and options
Assess client for signs and symptoms of major depression (p 46)
(D) Medications
Good response
Poor response or side effects
Refer to psychiatrist
New medication or dose adjustment
Initiate teaching plan
(E) Cognitive therapy
Facilitate development of adaptive coping patterns
Enhance problem-solving skills
Reinforce adaptive behaviors
Provide ongoing individual or group therapy
(F) Evaluate client's response to treatment
Provide follow-up

CYCLOTHYMIC DISORDER

Deborah Antai-Otong

A. Clients with cyclothymic disorder present with a history of hypomania alternating with periods of depression or loss of interest or pleasure. This disorder is not characterized by the significant social or occupational dysfunction that is frequently seen in the manic phase of bipolar disorders. Refer to "Dysthymic Disorder" (p 48) for a discussion of dysthymia and history taking, and to "Major Depressive Episodes" (p 46) and "Mania" (p 44) for assessment information. These individuals rarely experience marked impairments that require psychiatric interventions. Observations for signs of major affective disorders (i.e., mania or major depression) must be made by the nurse.

B. Since these clients rarely become dysfunctional in social areas, a thorough assessment must be made to determine reasons for seeking treatment at this time. Sometimes crises can be precipitated by ineffective coping patterns. The nurse must determine what the client expects from treatment and assist in helping the client identify realistic treatment goals. If the client exhibits symptoms of a crisis, brief, supportive crisis intervention is needed. However, if the client presents with symptoms that suggest a mood disorder (e.g., decreased sleep, appetite, libido, and energy), more aggressive intervention may be needed, including evaluation for medications, psychotherapy, and as with any crisis situation, assessment for suicide potential.

C. Symptoms that may suggest mania include rapid, tangential, and pressured speech, recent history of decreased need for sleep, decreased concentration, easy distractability, grandiose and persecutory delusions, feelings of entitlement, restlessness, and elated, elevated mood. These clients rarely seek treatment and are often brought in by family members or significant others.

References

American Psychiatric Association. Diagnostic and statistical manual of mental disorders. 3rd ed. Washington, DC: American Psychiatric Association, 1987:226–228.

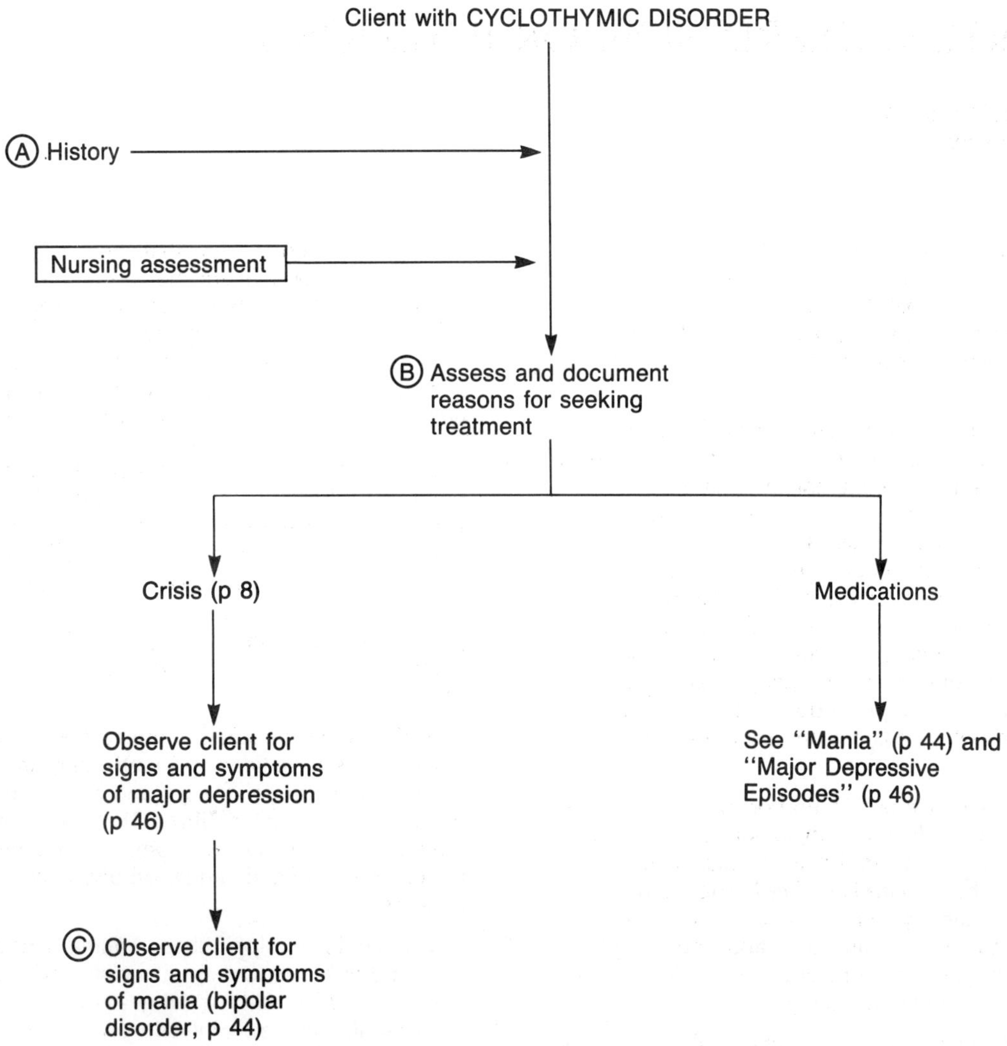
Client with CYCLOTHYMIC DISORDER
Ⓐ History
Nursing assessment
Ⓑ Assess and document reasons for seeking treatment
Crisis (p 8)
Medications
Observe client for signs and symptoms of major depression (p 46)
See "Mania" (p 44) and "Major Depressive Episodes" (p 46)
Ⓒ Observe client for signs and symptoms of mania (bipolar disorder, p 44)

POSTPARTUM DEPRESSION OR PSYCHOSIS

M.T. Mildred Carswell
Diane T. Brisson

The puerperium may be complicated by mental health problems ranging from transitory periods of depression to severe mental illness. More than half of these illnesses are affective reactions with depression predominating. Schizophrenic reactions occur primarily in younger women and adolescents.

A. Note the maternal and neonatal physical health status and the particulars of the most recent birth experience, e.g., cesarean birth or a traumatic vaginal birth. Ascertain whether the mother's perception of this birth is in accord with reality. Previous psychological dysfunction in the puerperium and/or at other times is an important predictor. Associated factors include current marital stress, single motherhood, whether this pregnancy was planned and/or wanted, and whether abortion was ever considered. Emotional and/or geographic separation from the mother's family or support systems should also be noted, as well as a family history of puerperal psychosis.

B. Observe for evidence of rejection or overprotection. A lack of affect, no evident warmth, avoidance, or oversolicitude is common, as are difficulty and discomfort when feeding and/or holding the baby. Restlessness and insomnia are also frequently found despite the client's feeling tired and fatigued. An unkempt appearance with a slumped posture is common, as are alterations in nutrition: anorexia or constant eating.

C. Coping style is ineffective because of an inability to adapt to situational crises. Fear of responsibility leads to difficulty in learning interpersonal and social skills necessary for the achievement of autonomy and maturity. The decision to have a baby may result from an effort to resolve a troubled marriage or to overcome a sense of inferiority, or it may be an act of defiance. Cognition is impaired by anxiety and ambivalence, resulting in unsound and irrational decisions.

D. Often the client has a history of a traumatic relationship with her own mother, leaving her without an acceptable model of mothering. Now that she is responsible for a passive, dependent infant she gets little satisfaction because of the lack of interpersonal feedback between herself and the baby, leading her to see herself as a bad mother. Hostility toward men and fear of being trapped in a bad marriage also may leave her highly anxious and with no clear indicators of mastery of her new role.

E. In addition to the usual adjustment following childbirth, emotional illness greatly stresses family functioning. A useful framework for family assessment is found in Wright and Leahey's work (see references). Ineffective functioning is common, with disrupted routines, closed communication, circular arguments, lack of or inappropriate problem solving, role conflict, inconsistent methods of control, false beliefs, and misdirected alliances and coalitions.

F. The client's self-concept is dominated by her lack of self-esteem and self-confidence. A particularly unrealistic self-ideal, a distorted self-image, and a general feeling of emptiness are usual findings. The reality of the baby threatens her already compromised self-concept, leading to feelings of guilt, anger, ambivalence, and powerlessness.

G. Generalized physiologic stress, trauma, sepsis, dehydration, and/or blood loss are associated with mental illness. A sudden fall of progesterone and estrogen withdrawal, elevated prolactin levels, and increasing levels of corticosteroids intrapartum and immediately postpartum which decrease markedly, have all been implicated in depression. Sleep disorders, particularly of stage IV sleep, are associated with fluctuating levels of other hormones during pregnancy, parturition, and the puerperium. The secretion, metabolism, and excretion of biogenic amines as well as a reduction in receptor sensitivity have been linked to affective disorders. Substance abuse, excess analgesia, or severe metabolic disorders are associated with toxic delirium (which is uncommon). Psychosis secondary to alcoholism or syphilis is rare.

POSTPARTAL CLIENT EXHIBITING DYSFUNCTIONAL BEHAVIOR AND/OR PSYCHOSIS

Ⓐ History

Ⓑ Nursing assessment

Assess influencing factors

Ⓒ Coping style

- Ineffective in dealing with crisis, change, or illness
- Avoids responsibility
- Disturbance in judgment
- Impaired cognition

Ⓓ Role model reflection

- Traumatic childhood relationship with mother
- Conflicting internalized images of mothering
- Hostile feelings toward men

Ⓔ Family functioning and/or supports

- Poor communication
- Poor problem solving
- Role conflict

Ⓕ Self-concept

- Motivational conflict regarding the process of motherhood
- Sense of emptiness
- Pervasive feelings of guilt, anger (p 190), powerlessness (p 184)

Ⓖ Biologic

- Generalized physiologic stress
- Sepsis
- Dehydration, blood loss
- Toxic delirium

Cont'd on p 55

H. Behaviors range from mild to severe. In role taking, an inability to care for or avoidance of the infant, or even outright neglect, verbal aggression, and physical harm may be seen. Thought processes may vary from slight impairment of memory to faulty judgment, thoughts of suicide and/or infanticide to delusions and hallucinations in which the birth is denied as well as the pregnancy. A miraculous, virginal birth with voices ordering her to kill herself and/or her baby may be reported. The baby is believed to be a monster or already dead. Confusion, disorientation, and incoherence are very ominous signs. Perceptions of self may include poor self-esteem, guilt, powerlessness, or failure. Ambivalence toward the infant and the infant's father may occur, as well as feelings of estrangement from her own body (e.g., forgetting to wash). The presence of the baby is overwhelming. Intense anxiety and agitation, angry outbursts, restlessness, and insomnia, or total lethargy and/or stupor are among the most severe findings. Notable are dependent behaviors toward her mother and the staff, relinquishing responsibility for infant care to them. Other behaviors include clinging and aimless wandering, seemingly waiting for help and direction.

I. Following improvement in the mother's psychological condition, a meeting is held with the family and the health-care team for discharge planning. This includes establishing a schedule of carefully supervised baby's visits to the unit, which gradually increase in length. Indicators of bonding are noted, such as an en-face position and calling the baby by name as well as competence in feeding and caring for the baby. The nurse remains within sight of the baby at all times, teaching, praising, and encouraging the mother in her efforts. Family members, particularly the father, are also supported and counseled.

References

Bobak IM, Jensen MD, Zalar MK. Maternity and gynecologic care: the nurse and the family. 4th ed. St. Louis: CV Mosby, 1989:863–871.

Hewat RJ. Difficult adjustment to parental role. In: Knor ER, ed. Decision making in obstetrical nursing. Toronto: BC Decker, 1987:202–203.

Hurt LD, Ray CP. Postpartum disorders: mother-infant bonding on a psychiatric unit. J Psychosoc Nurs 1985; 23(2):15–20.

Kerfoot KM, Buckwalter KC. Postpartum affective disorders: the manias and depression of childbirth. Nurs Forum 1981; 20:297–317.

Winn H. Postpartum mental disorders. In: Sciarra JJ, Zatuchni GI, eds. Gynecology and obstetrics. Vol 6. Fertility regulation, psychosomatic problems, and human sexuality. Philadelphia: JB Lippincott, 1988.

Wright LM, Leahey M. Nurses and families: a guide to family assessment and intervention. Philadelphia: FA Davis, 1984.

Zare-Parsi M, Hoffman BF. Postpartum mental disorders. Can Ment Health 1989; 37(1):13–16.

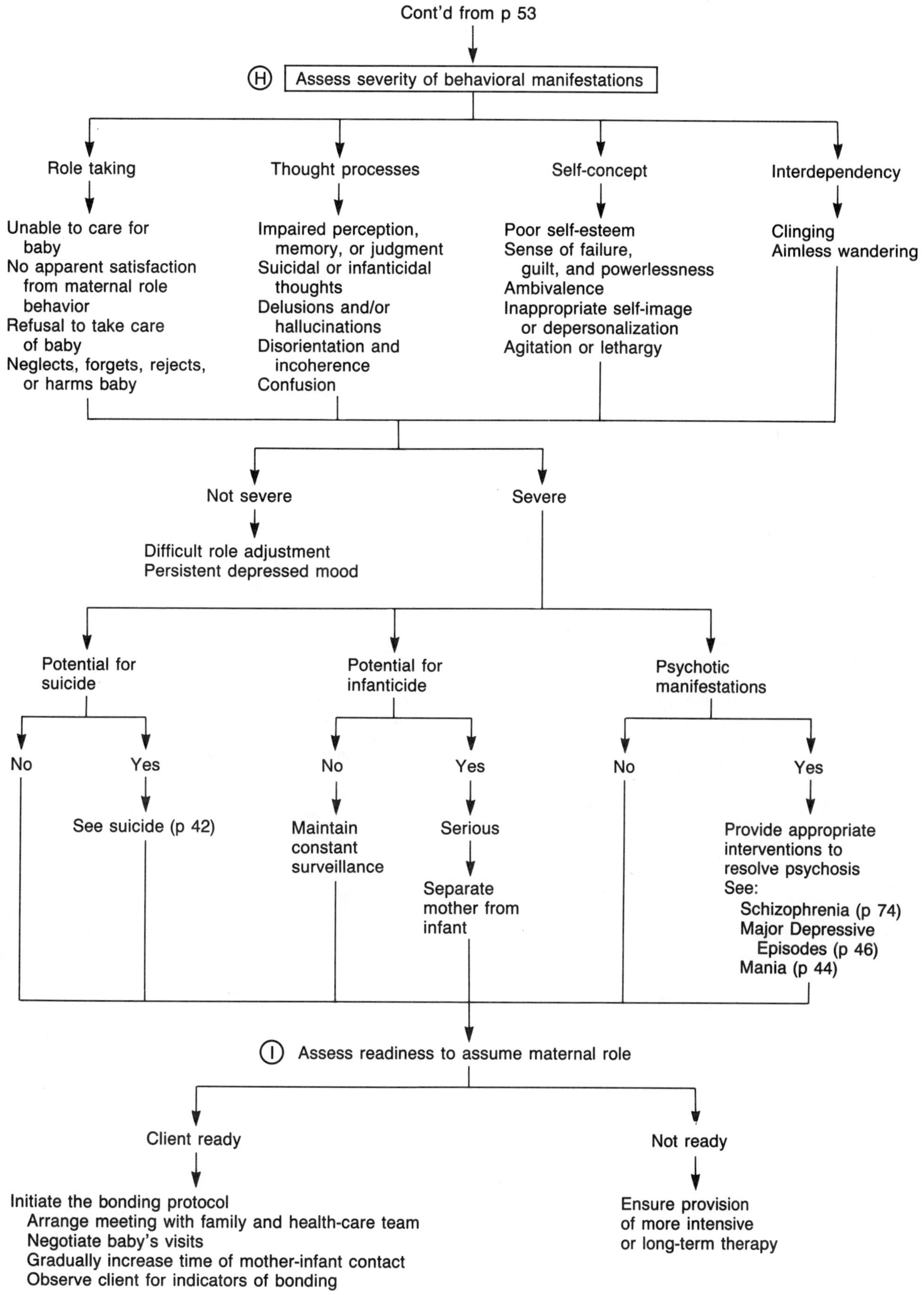
Cont'd from p 53
(H) Assess severity of behavioral manifestations
Role taking
Unable to care for baby
No apparent satisfaction from maternal role behavior
Refusal to take care of baby
Neglects, forgets, rejects, or harms baby
Thought processes
Impaired perception, memory, or judgment
Suicidal or infanticidal thoughts
Delusions and/or hallucinations
Disorientation and incoherence
Confusion
Self-concept
Poor self-esteem
Sense of failure, guilt, and powerlessness
Ambivalence
Inappropriate self-image or depersonalization
Agitation or lethargy
Interdependency
Clinging
Aimless wandering
Not severe
Difficult role adjustment
Persistent depressed mood
Severe
Potential for suicide
No
Yes
See suicide (p 42)
Potential for infanticide
No
Maintain constant surveillance
Yes
Serious
Separate mother from infant
Psychotic manifestations
No
Yes
Provide appropriate interventions to resolve psychosis
See:
Schizophrenia (p 74)
Major Depressive Episodes (p 46)
Mania (p 44)
(I) Assess readiness to assume maternal role
Client ready
Initiate the bonding protocol
Arrange meeting with family and health-care team
Negotiate baby's visits
Gradually increase time of mother-infant contact
Observe client for indicators of bonding
Not ready
Ensure provision of more intensive or long-term therapy

DYSPHORIC MOOD IN THE ELDERLY CLIENT

Ann C. Beckingham

Dysphoric mood can be described as loss of interest or pleasure in all or almost all usual activities and pastimes. The client may describe the symptoms as feeling low, blue, irritable, sad, or down in the dumps.

A. The history includes items relating to significant environment and community factors, i.e., urban versus rural areas, institutionalized versus noninstitutionalized elderly, marital status, and ethnic groups.

B. The populations that can be identified as being at high risk are the young-old, 60 to 74 years of age, and the old-old, 75 years of age and over. Questions to be asked relate to the symptoms of aging, and who are the normally functioning elderly? Sociodemographic variables such as sex, marital status, financial status, and level of education are influential factors.

C. Assessment of needs in the elderly is multifaceted and multidimensional. Self-assessments of personal health and dysphoric mood by elderly persons seem to be based largely upon how they compare themselves with peers of their age, sex, and perhaps expectations others have of their health. Some distinct characteristics differentiate the physical, social, and mental functioning of individuals in terms of specific concepts. Physical health may refer to strength and activity, and mental health (versus mental illness) to feelings and mood. Conceptual approaches and methods of needs assessment may be categorized as rational, empirical, or relativistic. Needs assessment is the initial component in the evaluation process and provides baseline data about the current status of the individual or system being evaluated. The baseline data form the basis against which comparisons of the outcomes and consequences of subsequent decisions are measured. There are also nursing models that may be used for assessment (see pp 16 and 24).

D. Needs assessment including the area of dysphoric mood is a major concern in decision making and planning for services for older people. The nurse must take into account the distinct and differing needs of the young-old and the old-old age group. Two versions of the Depression Adjective Check List (DACL) were developed, and have been used in assessing dysphoric/depressive mood. One lists adjectives that describe how the person feels "now—today" (the state version), and adjectives that describe how the person feels "in general" (the trait version). In each version there are three lists composed of 34 adjectives that the person completes. For more complete information the reader is referred to Beckingham (1988) and Lubin and Rinck (1986).

E. Assessment, reassessment, and evaluation data and feedback from the environment and client can assist nurses and other health professionals to collaboratively reach the decision that change is needed as well as what kind of change to implement. Focus on health promotion and primary prevention to help the elderly client maintain the optimal level of functioning.

F. If the client is at risk and depressed, referral to a physician for treatment is required. For a discussion of nursing interventions, identify the disorder and refer to the relevant chapter (see "Major Depressive Episodes," p 46).

References

Beckingham A. Self-perceived health status and dysphoric mood in an elderly Canadian population. Dissertation thesis. Unpublished.

Blazer DG, Williams CD. The epidemiology of dysphoria and depression in an elderly population. Am J Psychiatry 1980; 37:439–444.

Fillenbaum GG. The well-being of the elderly. Approaches to multidimensional assessment. Geneva: World Health Organization, 1984.

Lubin BL, Rinck CM. Assessment of mood and affect in the elderly. The depression adjective check list and the multiple affect check list. In: Brink TL, ed. Clinical gerontology: a guide to assessment and intervention. New York: Hayward Press, 1986.

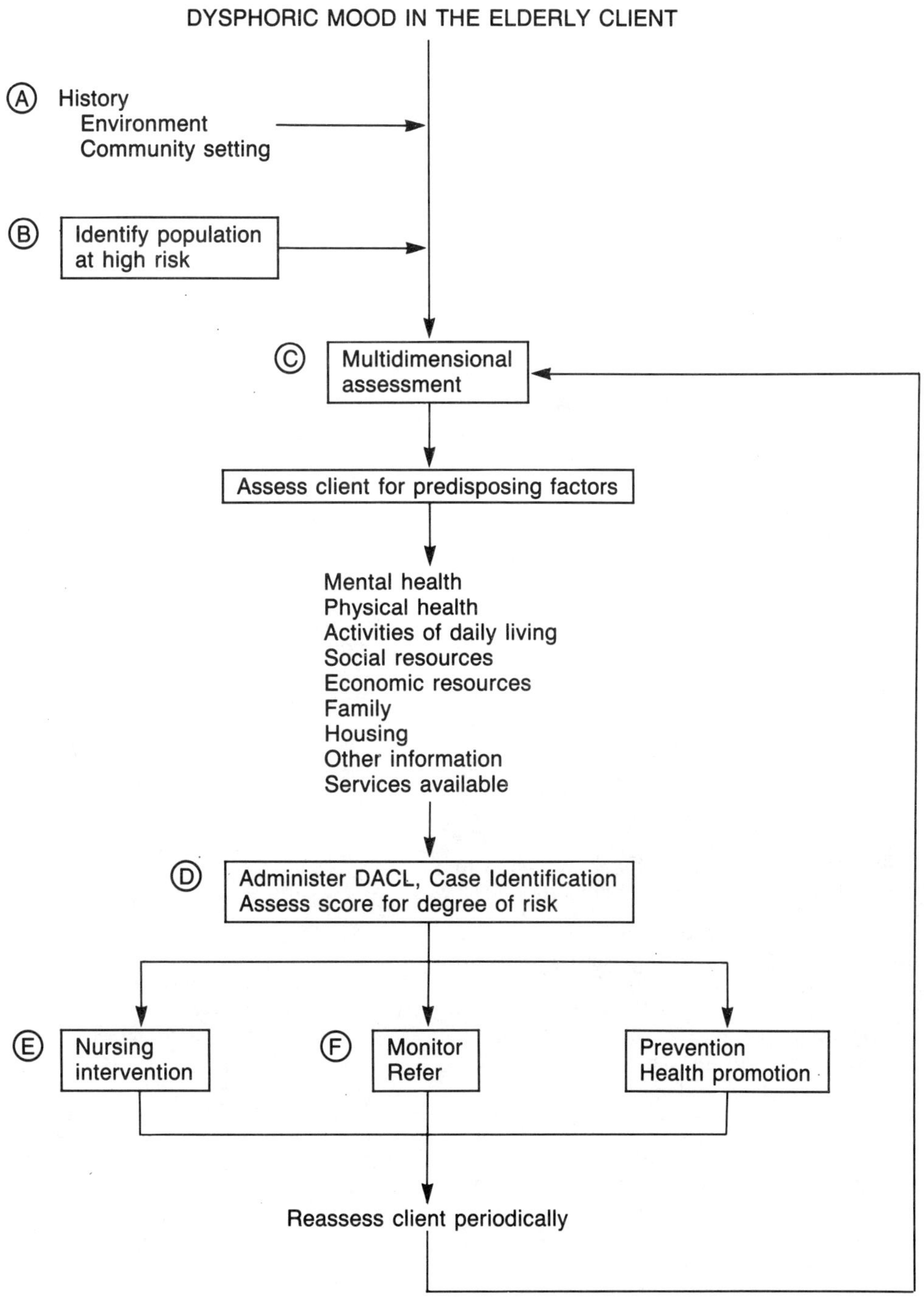
DYSPHORIC MOOD IN THE ELDERLY CLIENT
Ⓐ History
Environment
Community setting
Ⓑ Identify population at high risk
Ⓒ Multidimensional assessment
Assess client for predisposing factors
Mental health
Physical health
Activities of daily living
Social resources
Economic resources
Family
Housing
Other information
Services available
Ⓓ Administer DACL, Case Identification
Assess score for degree of risk
Ⓔ Nursing intervention
Ⓕ Monitor
Refer
Prevention
Health promotion
Reassess client periodically

CHILD WITH DEPRESSION

Erlinda T. Morales-Mann

A. Like adults, children and adolescents become depressed but exhibit varying behaviors at different ages and stages of their developmental growth. Depression in children is thought to be a reaction to loss, either loss of an object or a state of well-being. This loss leads to feelings of diminished self-esteem, helplessness, anger, hostility, grief, self-deprecation, and depression.

B. The nurse must convey an attentive, accepting, nonjudgmental attitude throughout all interviews. The assessment should focus on complaint(s) and difficulty(ies) the child or adolescent has, current medications, level of functioning in the home, school, and other relevant settings, assessment of suicidal ideation or intention, assessment of social support systems, history of previous problems (drug or alcohol ingestion, suicide attempts, stressful precipitating events), and a screening for physiologic and other psychiatric problems. A thorough family, school, peer, and medical history must be obtained from appropriate sources or from other social agencies.

C. Whenever a child presents with behavior patterns consistent with childhood depression, it is important to involve the psychiatrist very early in the evaluation. The depressed child who has somatic complaints (i.e., headache, stomach ache, diarrhea, vomiting, dizziness) must be referred for a thorough medical evaluation to rule out an organic basis for these complaints.

D. The most frequent depressive feature is a negative self-image. The child looks depressed and feels unloved and rejected. Depressed adolescents are sensitive and tend to overreact to any criticism with heightened self-condemnation. Other depressive features are found in cases of school phobia (p 150), school failure, and somatic complaints. Somatic complaints are seen to be surface manifestations that obscure depressive feelings.

E. Many children who are depressed demonstrate behavior patterns with aggressive features such as fighting, biting, bullying, and teasing. At times aggression is displayed by lighting matches, defecating or urinating in inappropriate places, or extreme negativism. Adolescents use acting out and denial as a way of handling problems. Acts such as promiscuity, cheating, theft, physical assault, violence, masochism, drug or alcohol abuse, and running away from home represent ways of relieving painful, depressive feelings. Delinquents usually suffer from a severely impoverished self-image and profound feelings of emptiness. Because of painful feelings of inadequacy, the adolescent attempts to prove that he or she is tough and fearless by being the most aggressive one in the group and engaging in dangerous activity.

F. Behavior patterns in the family of the child with depression greatly influence the child's difficulties. There is a high incidence of parental depression, with the child identifying with the depressed parent. Like the children, the parents have difficulty handling aggression and hostility. Often the parents fuse aggression and hostility and direct it toward the child as a helpless object. Various forms of parental rejection are observed in the depressed child's family. Emotional as well as physical neglect is evident in many cases. Other forms of parental rejection of the child are scapegoating, favoring other children, and getting the least attention and the most punishment among the children.

G. Suicide in childhood and adolescence is associated more frequently with a diagnosis of depression than with any other psychiatric diagnosis. Suicide is often precipitated by seemingly trivial events. It is important to assess the nature and intensity of depressive feelings as well as the danger of behaviors acted out to ward off painful feelings. Certain areas, such as the methods selected to harm self, seriousness of intent, previous and present level of stress, history of previous attempts, family history of suicide or dangerous violent behaviors, and the child's present mental status must be explored. If the child's safety is in doubt, hospital admission is recommended (see "Suicide Attempt," p 42).

H. Assessment and treatment of the child and family can be accomplished in an outpatient setting, but severely acting-out and suicidal children are often helped by a period of hospitalization, which enables the multidisciplinary team to evaluate the child in an objective setting away from home and family, often the focus of his problems. A flexible therapeutic approach is recommended, using different types of therapy (family, individual, or group) separately, sequentially, or in conjunction, according to the situation and individual needs of the child. The nurse assists in the treatment plan as a therapist or cotherapist if he or she has had extensive training in child development and therapy. The therapist must develop an honest, frank, and nonjudgmental relationship with the child in which the expression and exploration of his painful feelings through play or words lead to discovering alternate ways of relieving unwanted feelings. It is imperative to have the family actively involved in the therapeutic process, especially if the child is living at home. Family therapy reflects the premise that the child's pathology often arises from the family system's inability to communicate and relate to each other. The therapist assists the family to focus on the problem areas that involve them all. This is done by identifying those aspects of family life that are marked by a high degree of anxiety, hostility, and confusion. By demonstration and explanation the therapist creates the possibility of alternative behavior and encourages the family members to increase the number of ways in which they interact. In a hospital setting, the multidisciplinary team provides the child with a structured therapeutic milieu to influence behavior and encourage wholesome relationships and re-educational experiences. The team works in unison to individualize the treatment approach to raise the child's self-esteem through teaching of skills and provision of success experiences. Treatment may include antidepressant, antianxiety, and antipsychotic medications, depending on exhibited behaviors.

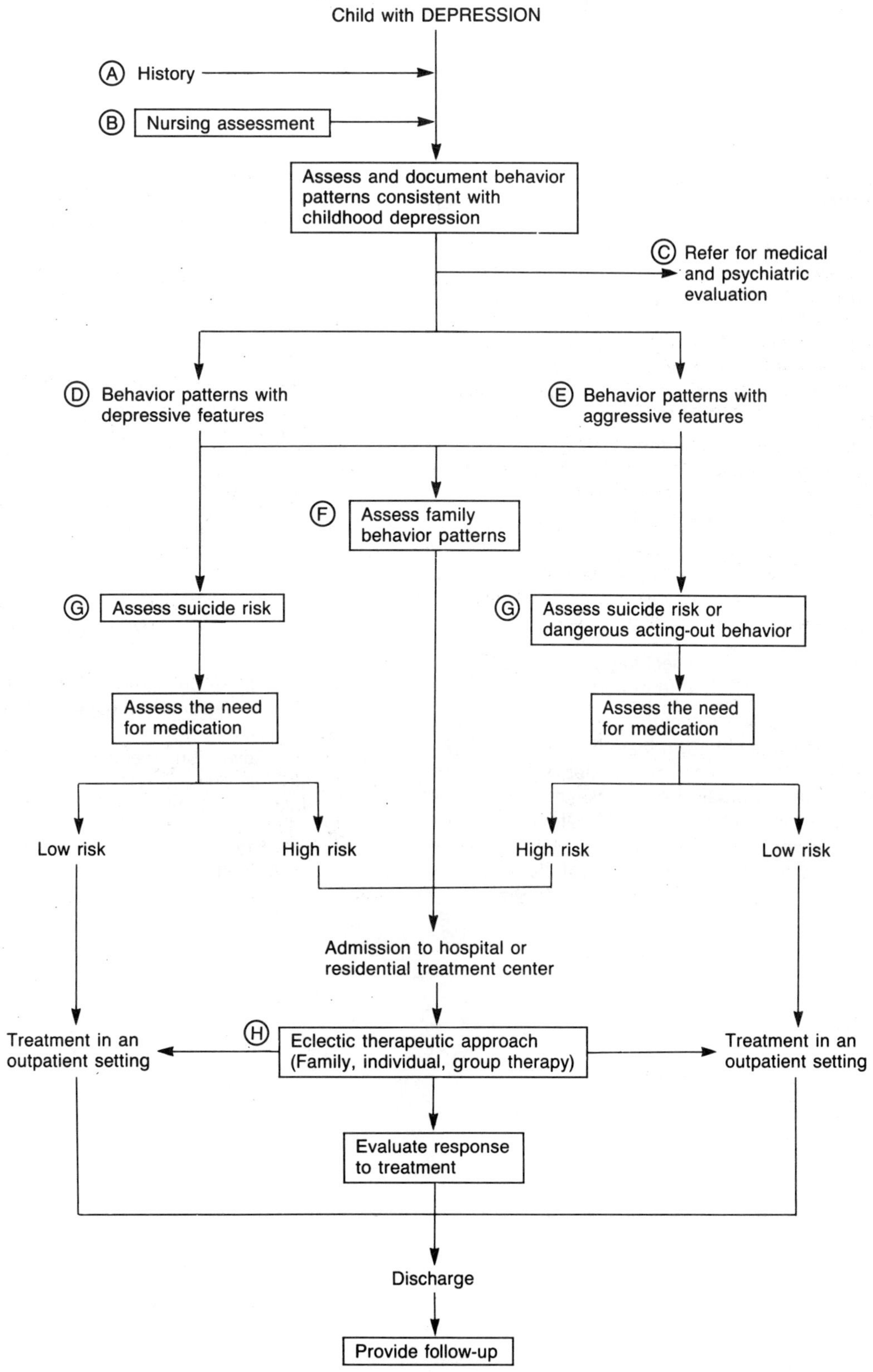

References

Brady MA. Childhood depression: development of a screening tool. Pediatr Nurs 1984; 10:225–235.

Cantwell DP, Carlson GA, eds. Affective disorders in childhood and adolescence. New York: Spectrum Publications, 1983.

Cantwell DP. Depressive disorders in children. Psychiatr Clin North Am 1985; 8:779–789.

Nelms BC. Assessing childhood depression: do parents and children agree. Pediatr Nurs 1986; 12:23–26.

Rhine MC. Children at risk for depression. Am J Nurs 1986; 12:1378–1382.

GENERALIZED ANXIETY DISORDER

Deborah Antai-Otong

A. Generalized anxiety disorder (GAD) produces symptoms that mimic major medical problems. Clients often present in the emergency room complaining of having a heart attack or "feeling like they are going to die." Symptoms of this disorder include palpitations, shortness of breath, dizziness, restlessness, and paresthesia. Clients diagnosed with GAD must have a complete medical examination to rule out an organic basis for their complaints, and the history must include current medications, duration of course, and compliance. Often these clients are referred to psychiatry for evaluation. Nursing responsibilities include gathering information about present and past psychiatric treatment, history of substance abuse for client and family members, and current stressors.

B. The nursing assessment focuses on assimilating medical and psychiatric histories to identify the client's current needs and expectations. A mental status examination and the client's current and past coping and adaptive patterns must be assessed.

C. Determine the reasons for seeking treatment and assist the client to identify short-term and realistic goals.

D. Cognitive therapy is useful in treating anxiety disorders. It involves assisting clients to learn how to identify distorted self-statements, the related anxiety reactions, and the accompanying physical reactions (i.e., diaphoresis, racing heart, and shortness of breath). Often progressive muscle relaxation (p 118) is used in conjunction with cognitive therapy to enhance the client's skills. This technique allows nurses to use imagery (p 120) as a means to help clients progressively relax their muscles and reduce tension and stress. It also allows the nurse to facilitate a "body-mind connection" and helps the client learn ways to deal more effectively with anxiety-evoking situations. For further discussion of cognitive therapy, see p 108.

E. Medications often used to treat anxiety disorders include the benzodiazepines and tricyclic antidepressants. Benzodiazepines can produce side effects that include psychological and physical dependence, and tricyclic antidepressants may have anticholinergic effects and affect the cardiovascular system. The desired and untoward effects of these agents must be discussed with clients and their families.

References

Antai-Otong DJ. Psychopharmacology. In: Johnson BS, ed. Psychiatric nursing: adaptation and growth. 2nd ed. Philadelphia: JB Lippincott, 1989:268–294.

Kolkmeir LG. Relaxation: opening the door to change. In: Dossey BM, Keegan L, Guzzetta CE, Kolkmeir LG, eds. Holistic nursing: a handbook for practice. Rockville, MD: Aspen, 1988:195–222.

Lachman VD. Stress management: a manual for nurses. New York: Grune & Stratton, 1983.

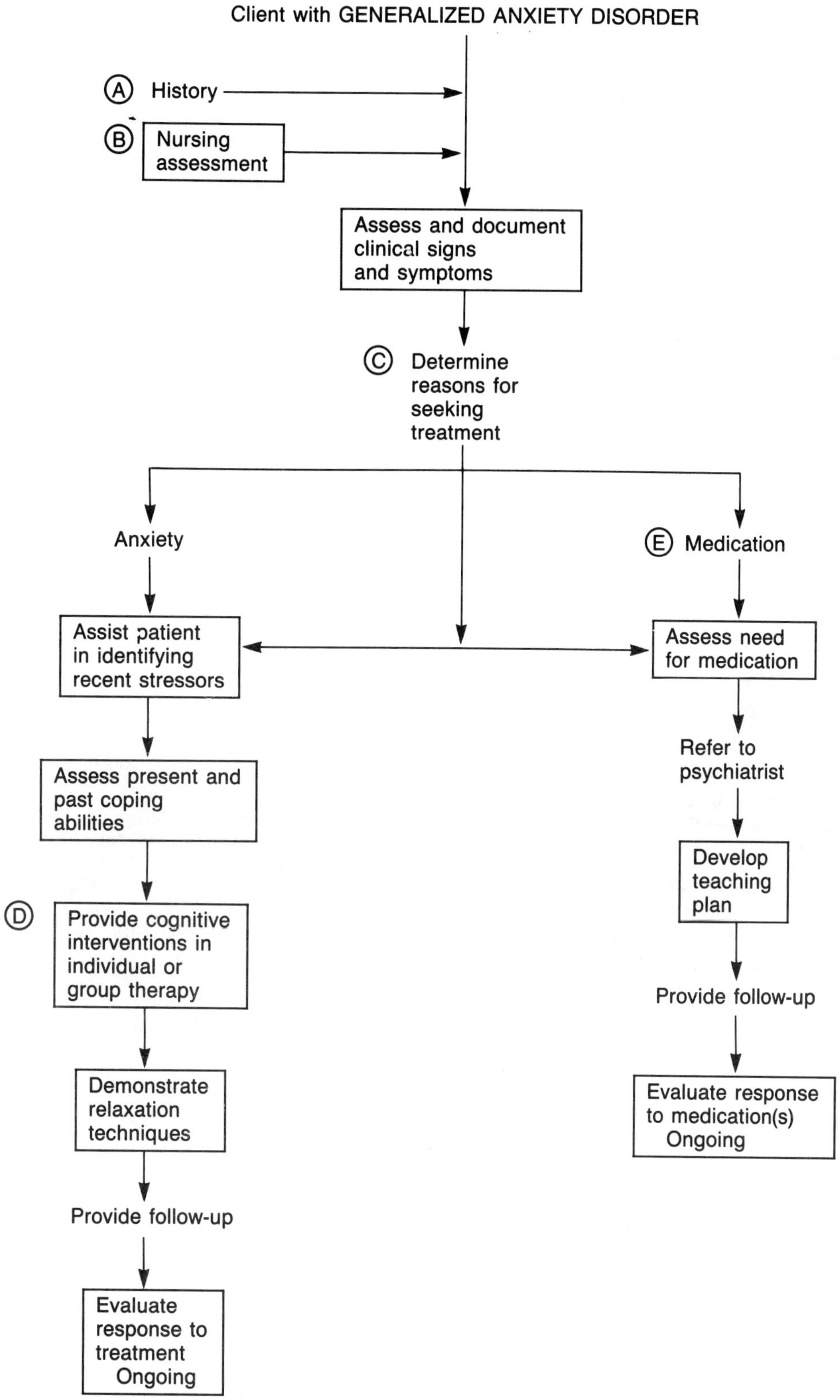
Client with GENERALIZED ANXIETY DISORDER
A History
B Nursing assessment
Assess and document clinical signs and symptoms
C Determine reasons for seeking treatment
Anxiety
E Medication
Assist patient in identifying recent stressors
Assess need for medication
Assess present and past coping abilities
Refer to psychiatrist
Develop teaching plan
D Provide cognitive interventions in individual or group therapy
Provide follow-up
Demonstrate relaxation techniques
Evaluate response to medication(s) Ongoing
Provide follow-up
Evaluate response to treatment Ongoing

AGORAPHOBIA

Deborah Antai-Otong

A. Clients with agoraphobia often complain of fears of being in open spaces, from which their altered perception causes them to believe that escape is difficult. Many of these individuals have developed coping mechanisms that produce avoidance behavior. Depending on the severity of the agoraphobia, the client's dysfunction ranges from being able to pursue a relatively normal lifestyle to being a recluse (housebound). Sometimes this disorder is accompanied by panic attacks, which are manifested by shortness of breath, chest pain, paresthesias, dizziness, and palpitations. During the history, questions about these symptoms need to be addressed. If panic attacks occur, ask the client about the frequency, duration, and precipitating stressors. A recent complete physical examination is imperative to rule out an organic basis for the symptoms. The history must also include the client's current medications, previous psychiatric treatment, substance abuse history, and family history of psychiatric treatment and substance abuse.

B. For a discussion of nursing assessment for generalized anxiety disorders, see page 60. Clients with agoraphobia frequently experience feelings of alienation, helplessness, and hopelessness, which may precipitate major depression. The client should be assessed and treated appropriately. When major depression is identified (p 46), a suicidal assessment (p 42) must be initiated and followed up continuously.

C. Relaxation therapy is frequently used to treat anxiety disorders (see p 118). This intervention utilizes progressive muscle relaxation by focusing on a comforting imagery, which reduces internal tension. The client can be taught to relax under stressful conditions, allowing facilitation of a tranquil and calm state. Music may also be used during this intervention. Relaxation tapes are useful for client use at home.

D. Systematic desensitization (p 124) is another technique that is useful in reducing anxiety-provoking events. This method utilizes both physical and mental relaxation and imagery. During this process, clients are encouraged to rehearse visualization of a comforting place or event when the phobia is encountered. Frequent visualization of the phobia and comforting event assists the client to reduce the reactions evoked by the phobia. Provide frequent positive reinforcement of adaptive behavior and improved coping skills. Breathing exercises assist the client to reduce the physical reactions to the phobia. Family members can help by recognizing the client's phobias and reinforcing positive adaptive behaviors and providing comfort and support when the client relapses.

E. For discussion of medications used for anxiety disorders, see page 60.

References

Byrne PP, Unde TW. Exogenous factors in panic disorders: clinical and research implications. J Clin Psychiatry 1988; 49:56–61.

Dossey BM. Imagery: awakening the inner healer. In: Dossey BM, Keegan L, Guzzetta CE, Kolkmeir LG, eds. Holistic nursing: a handbook for practice. Rockville, MD: Aspen, 1988:223–261.

Meichenbaum D. Cognitive-behavior modification. New York: Plenum, 1979.

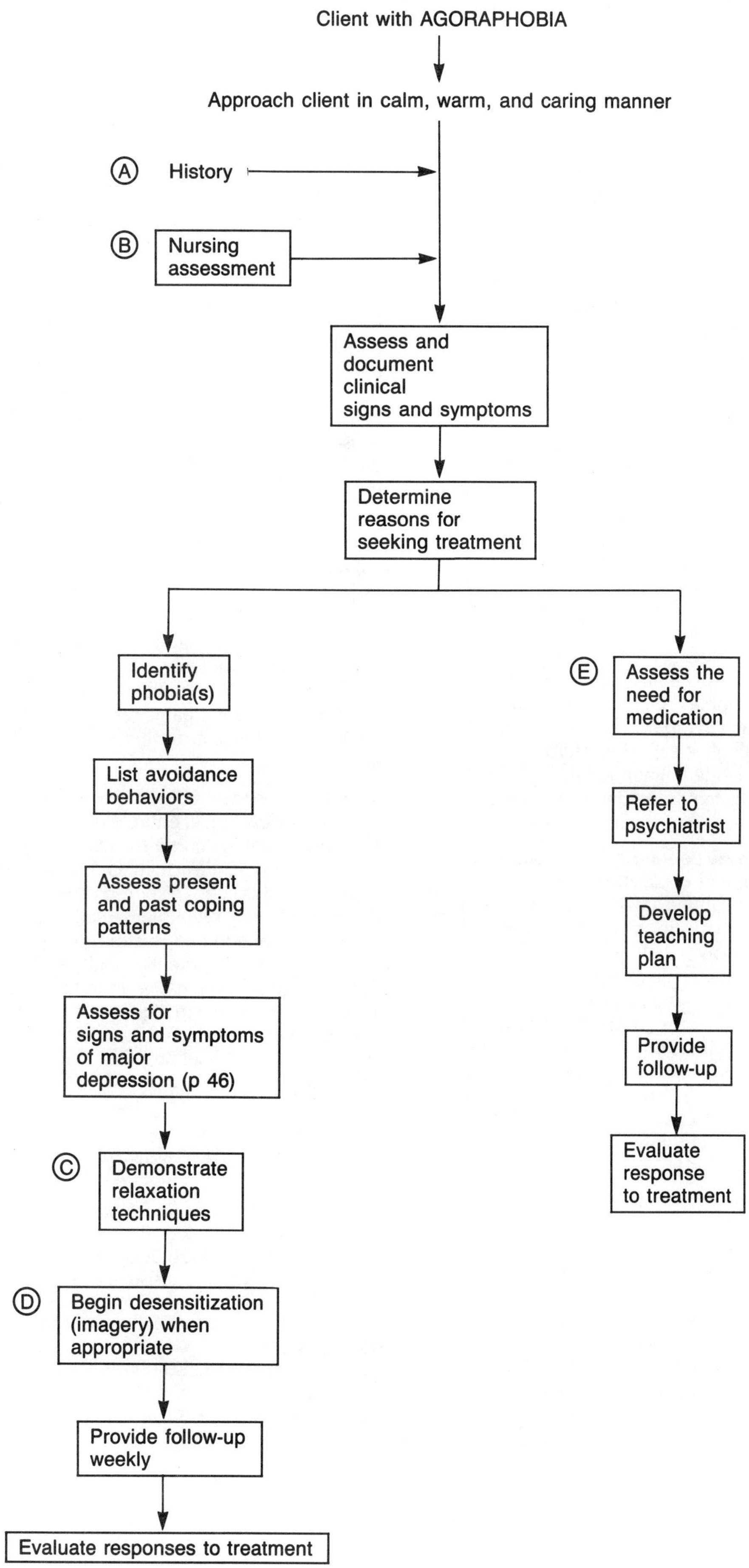
Client with AGORAPHOBIA
Approach client in calm, warm, and caring manner
Ⓐ History
Ⓑ Nursing assessment
Assess and document clinical signs and symptoms
Determine reasons for seeking treatment
Identify phobia(s)
List avoidance behaviors
Assess present and past coping patterns
Assess for signs and symptoms of major depression (p 46)
Ⓒ Demonstrate relaxation techniques
Ⓓ Begin desensitization (imagery) when appropriate
Provide follow-up weekly
Evaluate responses to treatment
Ⓔ Assess the need for medication
Refer to psychiatrist
Develop teaching plan
Provide follow-up
Evaluate response to treatment

OBSESSIVE-COMPULSIVE DISORDERS

Diane T. Brisson

An obsession is a powerful, incessant, ego-alien, unwanted, uncontrollable, and internally induced thought. Simultaneously, the client feels an irrational urge to act out or avoid certain situations and desperately tries to resist or fight these impulses. Urges and attempts to control them result in compulsive behavior consisting of repetitive, stereotyped acts or rituals that tend to neutralize the unwanted thought, thus providing temporary and partial relief from anxiety. Obsessive-compulsive traits are built-in patterns of preoccupation with perfection, fear of failure, and loss of control.

A. Obsessive-compulsive episodes account for about 5 percent of all diagnosed psychiatric conditions. Obsessions are often about dirt and contamination, sex, religion, aggression, orderliness, and death. Cleaning and checking are the most common compulsions, although such behaviors as dressing-undressing, praying, and touching objects also occur. Onset is predominantly in adolescence or early adulthood and can often be linked to a precise stressful event. The client seeks consultation when exhausted physically and mentally by the burden of the rituals. Suicidal thoughts are common. Furthermore, the family and the social atmosphere are greatly affected, with some members reluctantly participating in the compulsive routine in order to be supportive and helpful. The client with obsessive character traits typically complains about being unhappy, chronically anxious, and having serious family problems and unsatisfying relationships at work and in society in general.

B. The client with an obsessive personality is cautious, rigid, pedictable, controlling, and conforming. Having internalized a strict judgmental and intellectualized vision of life, the client sets unrealistic standards for self and others, leading in turn to emotional inhibition and social isolation. A preoccupation with detail impairs the client's decision-making processes. Tension frequently affects the client's sleep and eating patterns. Incessant ruminations and urges to act out, which are emotionally distressing and exhausting, are experienced. Skin integrity may be affected by too frequent washings or repetitive kneelings. Although intelligent and aware of the senselessness of the rituals, the client cannot oppose them and becomes upset and angry if prevented.

C. From a psychoanalytic point of view, obsessive-compulsive neurosis is a regression and fixation to the pre-oedipal anal-sadistic phase. The superego inhibits the sadistic tendencies and attempts to repress anxiety, guilt, and hostility. Isolation, denial, undoing, and reaction formation are additional ego defenses forming protection against insight. From the behavioral perspective, obsessions are conditioned stimuli to anxiety. Here, anxiety-provoking stimuli are paired with neutral ones, so obsessional thoughts gain the capacity to arouse anxiety. The person discovers that certain behaviors reduce or neutralize the anxiety attached to an obsession, even if they are unpleasant and senseless.

D. The planning of a particular therapeutic program will depend on many factors such as the nature of the psychiatric conceptual framework shared by the team, whether it be biologic, psychoanalytic, interpersonal, behavioral, or a combination of these; the areas of competence and specialization of professionals; the resources and time available; and finally, the client's particular needs. Neurotic obsessive-compulsive clients are treated on either an inpatient or an outpatient basis; therapy is usually short-term and intensive in nature. The client with an obsessional personality can benefit from a long-term therapeutic program, either as an outpatient or in a community-based facility.

E. The obsessive-compulsive client might not be an ideal candidate for insight therapy, because of the inner resistance to focusing on feelings and deep motivations. At first, chemotherapy and the maintenance of a therapeutic environment may be a better approach. When insight therapy is implemented, the nurse must maintain a specially nonthreatening and therapeutic atmosphere in order to prevent a panic reaction in the client. Long-term approaches can further deal with the client psychodynamics.

F. Systematic behavioral and cognitive behavioral approaches focus almost entirely on modifying the manifestations as they currently exist. Direct behavioral modifying procedures, such as desensitization (p 124), aversive conditioning, response prevention, and implosion therapy, may be implemented by specially trained nurses. In a one-to-one relationship or in a group setting, the nurse implements cognitive behavioral procedures including progressive muscle relaxation (p 118), assertiveness therapy (p 126), modeling (p 122), rehearsal, role playing, teaching positive self-talk (p 108), assignments and self-instructional guidelines, and coaching.

References

Bowman C, Spadoni A. Assertion therapy: the nurse and the psychiatric patient in an acute, short-term hospital setting. J Psychiatr Nurs Ment Health Serv 1981; 19(6):7–20.

Nemiak JC. Obsessive-compulsive neurosis. In: Freedman AM, Kaplan HI, Benjamin J, eds. Comprehensive textbook of psychiatry. Vol 2. 2nd ed. Baltimore: Williams & Wilkins, 1975:1241–1255.

Rachman SJ, Hodgson RJ. Obsession and compulsion. Englewood Cliffs, NJ: Prentice-Hall, 1980.

Ruch J. Psychology: the personal science. Belmont, CA: Wadsworth, 1984.

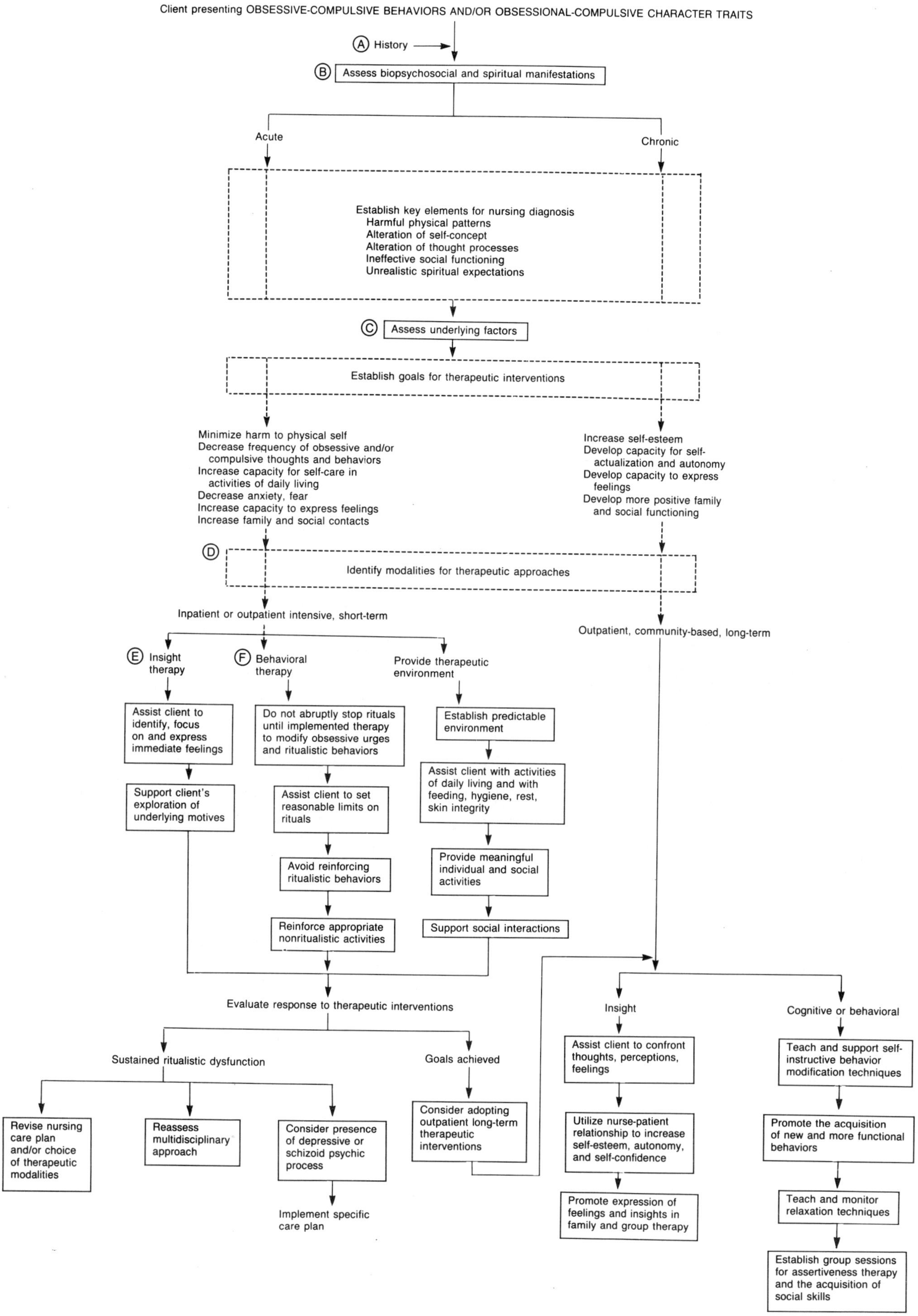
Client presenting OBSESSIVE-COMPULSIVE BEHAVIORS AND/OR OBSESSIONAL-COMPULSIVE CHARACTER TRAITS
A History
B Assess biopsychosocial and spiritual manifestations
Acute
Chronic
Establish key elements for nursing diagnosis
Harmful physical patterns
Alteration of self-concept
Alteration of thought processes
Ineffective social functioning
Unrealistic spiritual expectations
C Assess underlying factors
Establish goals for therapeutic interventions
Minimize harm to physical self
Decrease frequency of obsessive and/or compulsive thoughts and behaviors
Increase capacity for self-care in activities of daily living
Decrease anxiety, fear
Increase capacity to express feelings
Increase family and social contacts
Increase self-esteem
Develop capacity for self-actualization and autonomy
Develop capacity to express feelings
Develop more positive family and social functioning
D Identify modalities for therapeutic approaches
Inpatient or outpatient intensive, short-term
Outpatient, community-based, long-term
E Insight therapy
F Behavioral therapy
Provide therapeutic environment
Assist client to identify, focus on and express immediate feelings
Support client's exploration of underlying motives
Do not abruptly stop rituals until implemented therapy to modify obsessive urges and ritualistic behaviors
Assist client to set reasonable limits on rituals
Avoid reinforcing ritualistic behaviors
Reinforce appropriate nonritualistic activities
Establish predictable environment
Assist client with activities of daily living and with feeding, hygiene, rest, skin integrity
Provide meaningful individual and social activities
Support social interactions
Evaluate response to therapeutic interventions
Sustained ritualistic dysfunction
Goals achieved
Revise nursing care plan and/or choice of therapeutic modalities
Reassess multidisciplinary approach
Consider presence of depressive or schizoid psychic process
Implement specific care plan
Consider adopting outpatient long-term therapeutic interventions
Insight
Cognitive or behavioral
Assist client to confront thoughts, perceptions, feelings
Utilize nurse-patient relationship to increase self-esteem, autonomy, and self-confidence
Promote expression of feelings and insights in family and group therapy
Teach and support self-instructive behavior modification techniques
Promote the acquisition of new and more functional behaviors
Teach and monitor relaxation techniques
Establish group sessions for assertiveness therapy and the acquisition of social skills

POST-TRAUMATIC STRESS DISORDERS

Nancy E. Johnston

The essential feature of post-traumatic stress disorders (PTSD) is the development of characteristic symptoms after experiencing a psychologically traumatic event outside the range of usual human experience. The characteristic symptoms involve reexperiencing the traumatic event; numbing of responsiveness to, or involvement with, the external world; and other autonomic, dysphoric, or cognitive symptoms such as exaggerated startle response, difficulty concentrating, memory impairment, guilt feelings, depression, irritability, and sleep difficulties. This syndrome has been repeatedly described after stressors such as war, natural catastrophes (e.g., earthquakes and floods), large-scale accidents such as airplane crashes, and individual traumas such as rape, auto accidents, and accidents in the home. Rape trauma syndrome is one form of PTSD.

A. It is important to assess the nature of the stressor. Intensity, severity, duration of the event, whether the event involved physical injury, and the extent to which the event was extreme or catastrophic are essential aspects. Especially important in war veterans is the exposure to, or participation in, guilt-producing activities.

B. Since not all clients who suffer identical stressors experience PTSD, it is necessary to assess personal factors. These may include age, genetic predisposition, personality traits, availability of social support, and the presence of other sources of stress.

C. Duration of the clinical manifestations provides some guidance in selecting appropriate treatment modalities.

D. Acute PTSD may be diagnosed in clients who have experienced symptoms for less than 6 months or in whom symptoms have developed within 6 months after the traumatic event. Generally, acute PTSD has a favorable prognosis and a brief, less intensive treatment approach. Symptoms often remit spontaneously and without psychiatric intervention.

E. The treatment of choice for acute PTSD is supportive psychotherapy. Encourage the client to ventilate about the event without attempting further penetration of the repressive barrier. Reinforce adaptive coping mechanisms and encourage resumption of normal activities.

F. Chronic PTSD may be diagnosed in clients whose symptoms occur over a period lasting more than 6 months, or have a latency period greater than 6 months. The more chronic the symptoms, the poorer the prognosis.

G. The initial stages of the treatment for chronic PTSD are based on an insight-oriented approach, either in individual sessions or in group therapy, to permit intrapsychic mastery of the highly charged events by enabling the client to relive the event. With the aid of the therapist, the client is able to examine the traumatic event and its specific meaning for him or her.

H. Behavioral techniques may be useful adjuncts to the psychotherapy described above. Facilitating the reexperiencing of the traumatic event may be accomplished through visualization and guided imagery techniques (p 120). Progressive relaxation and visualization techniques may also be used to systematically desensitize the client and neutralize the emotionally charged recollections of specific aspects of the traumatic events.

I. It is often helpful to offer marital (pp 164, 196) and family therapy (p 170) in order to avert the development of "vicious circles" created and fed by rage, despair, and mutual alienation. It is important to reduce the potential of the client to obtain secondary gain (reinforcement) for maladaptive behavior. The resumption of appropriate family, occupational, and social roles is actively encouraged and supported.

J. Referral for antianxiety or antidepressant medication should be made only when other approaches have failed, because of the risk of psychological or physical dependence on drugs in these clients.

References

Andreasen NC. Posttraumatic stress disorder. In: Kaplan HI, Sadock BJ, eds. Comprehensive textbook of psychiatry. 4th ed. Baltimore: Williams & Wilkins, 1985:918–924.

Bleich A, Garb R, Kottler MN. Treatment of prolonged combat reaction. Br J Psychiatry 1986; 148:493–496.

Brodsky L, et al. Post traumatic stress disorders: a tri-modal approach. Psychiatr J Univ Ottawa 1987; 12(1):41–46.

American Psychiatric Association. Diagnostic and statistical manual of mental disorders. 3rd ed. Washington, DC: American Psychiatric Association, 1987:247–253.

Grigsby JP. Single case study: the use of imagery in the treatment of posttraumatic stress disorder. J Nerv Ment Dis 1987; 175:55–59.

Sirois MB, Swift BG. Behavioral issues: understanding posttraumatic stress disorder in Vietnam veterans. J Emerg Nurs 1987; 13:290–295.

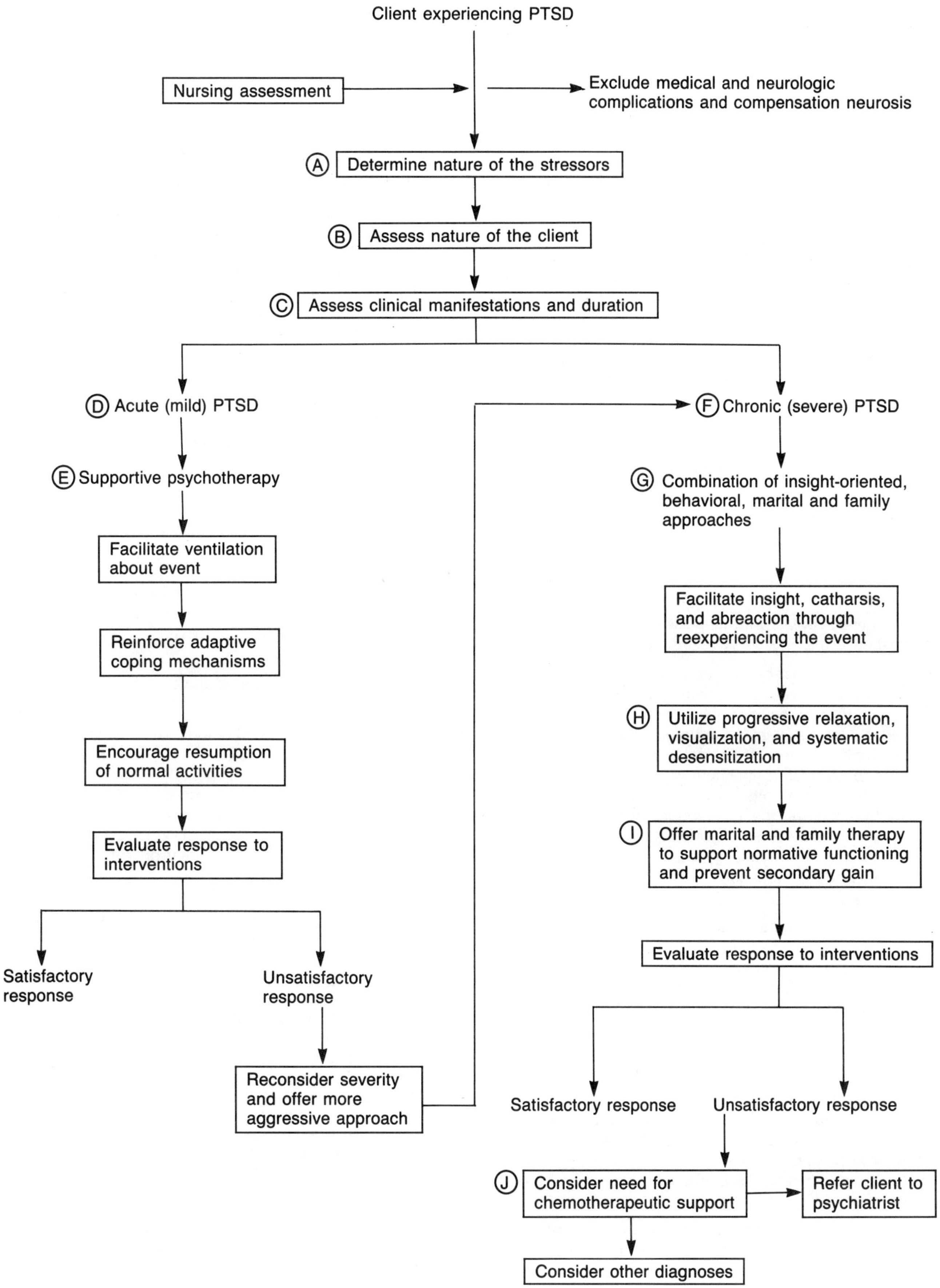
Client experiencing PTSD
Nursing assessment
Exclude medical and neurologic complications and compensation neurosis
(A) Determine nature of the stressors
(B) Assess nature of the client
(C) Assess clinical manifestations and duration
(D) Acute (mild) PTSD
(E) Supportive psychotherapy
Facilitate ventilation about event
Reinforce adaptive coping mechanisms
Encourage resumption of normal activities
Evaluate response to interventions
Satisfactory response
Unsatisfactory response
Reconsider severity and offer more aggressive approach
(F) Chronic (severe) PTSD
(G) Combination of insight-oriented, behavioral, marital and family approaches
Facilitate insight, catharsis, and abreaction through reexperiencing the event
(H) Utilize progressive relaxation, visualization, and systematic desensitization
(I) Offer marital and family therapy to support normative functioning and prevent secondary gain
Evaluate response to interventions
Satisfactory response
Unsatisfactory response
(J) Consider need for chemotherapeutic support
Refer client to psychiatrist
Consider other diagnoses

MULTIPLE PERSONALITY DISORDER

Nancy E. Johnston

A. Multiple personality disorder (MPD) is defined as the existence within the person of two or more distinct personalities or personality states. At least two of these personality states recurrently take full control of the person's behavior. Informal diagnostic signs seen in these clients include: periods of amnesia, hypnotizability, suggestibility, and varying EEG readings, which correspond to the alternative personalities. Two predisposing factors are necessary for the development of MPD: an inborn biologic and psychological capacity to dissociate and a history of repeated exposure to an inconsistently stressful environment, usually sexual and/or physical abuse.

B. Treatment is carried out most effectively using a multidisciplinary team approach. Frequently nurses work closely with an attending psychiatrist, psychologist, social worker, and occupational therapist to develop the plan of care.

C. Essential to the treatment process is the development of a therapeutic relationship in which the need for feelings of safety and security are addressed. Trust must be established so that the client including the subpersonalities will be able to disclose memories and express needs. Frequently contact with subpersonalities may be accomplished using relaxation techniques or hypnosis.

D. Once contact has been established with the subpersonalities it is important to articulate the goals for therapy. Depending on the level of trust and motivation and the capacity of the client to undergo an intensive, inpatient psychotherapy, a decision may be made to admit the patient to hospital. If the client is not prepared to undertake this intensive process, a supportive approach aimed at strengthening the therapeutic relationship may be used. As greater trust and feelings of safety are established, the nurse-therapist reassesses the client's capacity for intensive inpatient psychotherapy.

E. During the period of hospitalization, nurses may assume primary roles that include playing an active role in the actual psychotherapeutic process or they may assume associate roles to provide supports to the therapists and offer backup care to the client during the therapist's absence. The nurse functioning in an associate role maintains regular communication with those in primary roles in order to ensure that the total approach to the client remains consistent and unambiguous.

F. Of central importance to the psychotherapeutic process is the dismantling of amnesic barriers and establishing co-consciousness with the subpersonalities. This may be done by mapping and transmitting neutral material across the amnesic barriers by conversing, writing, and audio- or videotaping.

G. Following the establishment of co-consciousness, interpersonality communication is facilitated. Effective communication among the subpersonalities is promoted in order to pave the way for sound negotiation and decision making about integrating all the personalities.

H. Frequently the roles of the subpersonalities are distinct and characteristic. They may involve roles such as the child, the helper, the angry one, and the resistive one. The nurse must avoid the temptation to reinforce compliancy and dependency and to reject anger and resistance. All personalities play an important role and must be respectfully engaged if they are to be encouraged to make the necessary compromises in order to bring about integration.

I. An essential part of therapy is assisting the client to reexperience abusive events. Through remembering, the release of dissociated material occurs. The client is then encouraged to experience anger, helplessness, and fear without dissociating.

J. Once transmission of painful memories to the original personality has occurred, negotiation among the subpersonalities to give up their identity in favor of the development of the integrated personality occurs. Facilitating the grieving process for the relinquishing subpersonalities becomes an important feature of this stage of the psychotherapeutic process.

K. Fusion occurs only when all personalities agree to be integrated. In 1984, Kluft found that the average treatment time to complete fusion was 21.6 months.

L. Following successful fusion, the goals of therapy shift to helping the client determine a new set of goals. These goals are often related to achieving greater perspective and acceptance of thoughts and feelings that are now fully experienced rather than being dissociated, and helping the client to develop new priorities for meaningful relationships and satisfying career options.

References

American Psychiatric Association. Diagnostic and statistical manual of mental disorders. 3rd ed. Washington, DC: American Psychiatric Association, 1987.

Anderson G, Ross CA. A model for psychiatric nurses working with clients who have multiple personality disorder. Can J Psychiatr Nurs 1988; 29(4):13–18.

Anderson G, Ross CA. Strategies for working with a patient who has a multiple personality disorder. Arch Psychiatr Nurs 1988; 11:236–243.

Bornn E. Multiple personality disorder. Can Nurse 1988; 84(9):16–19.

Drew BL. Multiple personality disorder: an historical approach. Arch Psychiatr Nurs 1988; 11:227–230.

Lego S. Multiple personality disorder: an interpersonal approach to etiology, treatment and nursing care. Arch Psychiatr Nurs 1988; 11:231–235.

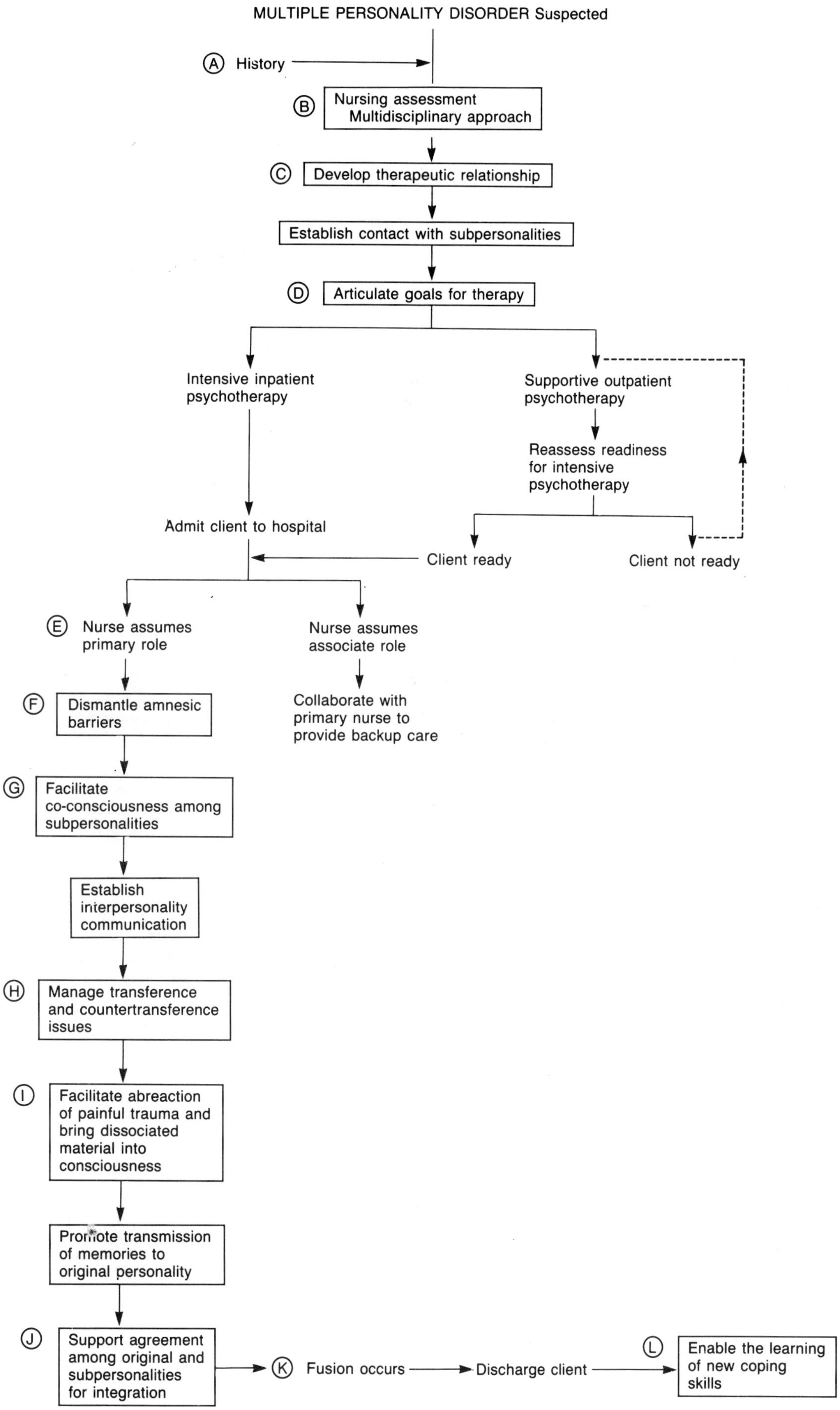
MULTIPLE PERSONALITY DISORDER Suspected
(A) History
(B) Nursing assessment
Multidisciplinary approach
(C) Develop therapeutic relationship
Establish contact with subpersonalities
(D) Articulate goals for therapy
Intensive inpatient psychotherapy
Supportive outpatient psychotherapy
Reassess readiness for intensive psychotherapy
Admit client to hospital
Client ready
Client not ready
(E) Nurse assumes primary role
Nurse assumes associate role
(F) Dismantle amnesic barriers
Collaborate with primary nurse to provide backup care
(G) Facilitate co-consciousness among subpersonalities
Establish interpersonality communication
(H) Manage transference and countertransference issues
(I) Facilitate abreaction of painful trauma and bring dissociated material into consciousness
Promote transmission of memories to original personality
(J) Support agreement among original and subpersonalities for integration
(K) Fusion occurs
Discharge client
(L) Enable the learning of new coping skills

PSYCHOSOMATIC DISORDERS

Deborah Antai-Otong

A. Psychosomatic disorders are defined as physiologic responses triggered by psychological factors. Prolonged stress reactions and maladaptive coping skills play a major role in these disorders. Stress may be generated from cultural, environmental, and socioeconomic sources. Some individuals are predisposed to psychosomatic illness by biological and psychosocial factors. Clients must be approached in a calm, organized manner, and the nurse should focus on identifying present and past stressors, their meaning to the client, and current coping patterns. Assess the client's immediate support systems, available resources, and reasons for seeking treatment.

B. Stress plays a major part in these disorders, which have been labeled by Seyle as general adaptation syndrome (GAS). He identified three stages of this syndrome: stage 1 begins when the stressor is encountered, stage 2 is characterized by the individual trying to use available resources to promote homeostasis, and stage 3 results from the client exhausting both physiologic and psychological resources. If stage 3 is not resolved, death will ensue.

C. The client develops psychophysiologic reactions when stage 3 is not resolved, such as angina, asthma, or gastrointestinal disturbances. Maladaptive coping patterns prolong these physical reactions and cause biological, psychological, and sociological dysfunction.

D. Biological responses often result from prolonged stimulation of the autonomic nervous system and include coronary artery disease, peptic ulcer disease, and skin ailments. Other research suggests that the immune system responses may be decreased, predisposing the client to numerous illnesses. Nursing goals include maintaining physical integrity and minimizing exacerbations.

E. Sociological responses involve the client's inability to recognize the long-term effects of prolonged stress and the associated psychological and biological reactions. Maladaptive coping patterns often lead to regression and adopting the "sick role," and the client often complains of feeling helpless and powerless. These clients tend to focus on their physical condition and alienate family members and significant others, thereby becoming more susceptible to depression. Major nursing goals include strengthening support systems, teaching the client more adaptive coping patterns, and helping the client to understand conditions that affect health.

F. Psychological responses often result from learned adaptive behavioral patterns, and certain personality types may be predisposed to some of these responses. Researchers have identified individuals with type A personality as those who demonstrate a high incidence of coronary artery disease. They tend to be rigid, controlling, ambitious, and achievement oriented. These clients are often described as cold and aloof, and they have difficulty recognizing the relationship between increased stress and somatic problems. Nursing goals include cognitive interventions to deal with distorted thinking and teaching these clients stress-reducing techniques.

G. Biofeedback is a muscle relaxation technique taught by using a machine that assists clients to identify physical reactions that suggest stress and relaxation. Imagery is often used as part of this technique. Electrical impulses induced by the client's physiologic responses are detected by the machine and displayed on a monitor. Because the reactions can be observed visually, this technique can be used to teach clients how to control their blood pressure, heart rate, skin temperature, and muscle tension.

References

Knapp DH. Current theoretical concepts in psychosomatic medicine. In: Kaplan HI, Sadock BJ, eds. Comprehensive textbook of psychiatry. 4th ed. Baltimore: Williams & Wilkins, 1985:1113–1121.

Selye H. The stress of life. New York: McGraw-Hill, 1956.

Seyle H. Stress without distress. New York: New American Library, 1974.

Stuart GW, Sundeen SJ. Principles and practice of psychiatric nursing. St. Louis: CV Mosby, 1987:376–393.

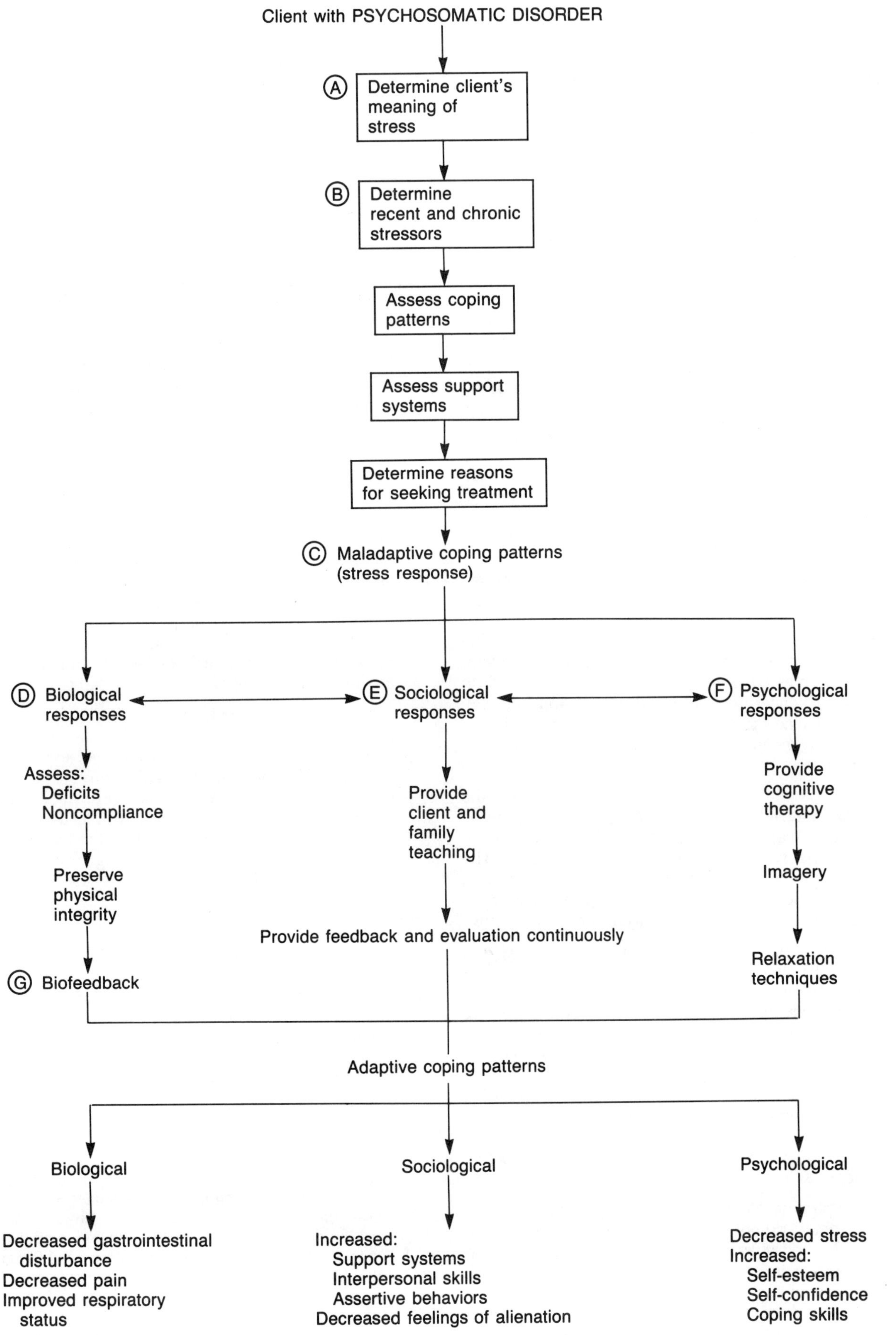
Client with PSYCHOSOMATIC DISORDER
(A) Determine client's meaning of stress
(B) Determine recent and chronic stressors
Assess coping patterns
Assess support systems
Determine reasons for seeking treatment
(C) Maladaptive coping patterns (stress response)
(D) Biological responses
(E) Sociological responses
(F) Psychological responses
Assess:
Deficits
Noncompliance
Preserve physical integrity
(G) Biofeedback
Provide client and family teaching
Provide feedback and evaluation continuously
Provide cognitive therapy
Imagery
Relaxation techniques
Adaptive coping patterns
Biological
Sociological
Psychological
Decreased gastrointestinal disturbance
Decreased pain
Improved respiratory status
Increased:
Support systems
Interpersonal skills
Assertive behaviors
Decreased feelings of alienation
Decreased stress
Increased:
Self-esteem
Self-confidence
Coping skills

EXPRESSED EMOTION: ASSESSING AND PROMOTING FAMILY SUPPORT FOR THE SCHIZOPHRENIC CLIENT

Nancy E. Johnston

The need for involvement of families with their schizophrenic members has become an increasing concern, particularly in an era of reduced hospital stays and the paucity of acceptable living alternatives in the community. Ways of helping the family cope with a chronically mentally ill member at home without seriously jeopardizing the mental and social adaptation of other family members are critically needed.

A. In order to predict the risk of the index client for relapse, it is important to assess ambient or persisting stress in the client's everyday living situation, especially the attitudes and personalities of key caregiver(s). Relatives who express critical comments, are hostile, or who are markedly overinvolved provide a less-than-optimal climate for client recovery. Assess the level of deficit and social inadequacy exhibited by the client. Clients exhibiting florid and "negative" or deficit symptoms are obvious sources of family stress. Families confronting other concomitant sources of stress such as marital dysfunction, physical or mental illness, and/or financial and social difficulties experience high levels of burden that may reduce their ability to cope effectively with the problems posed by the schizophrenic member. The term "high expressed emotion" has been developed to describe high levels of distress, dissatisfaction, and concern about the client by family members. Frequently one key family member expresses the greatest degree of distress.

B. Attempt to reduce the symptoms of the client that the family caregivers find so distressing. Florid, psychotic symptoms may often be brought under better control by readjusting types and dosages of medications. The nurse's role involves communicating and collaborating with members of the health-care team responsible for determining maintenance medication administration.

C. If the family expressed emotion, criticism, hostility, and overinvolvement remain high despite effective psychopharmacologic approaches, advise less face-to-face contact between the client and the key caregiver expressing the highest level of discontent. This may involve negotiating with the family to bring more tolerant, less involved members to the fore and supporting the distressed member to divert his or her attention elsewhere. Supporting the family, and especially the most distressed member, to expand the range of social contacts and personal interests may be a particularly effective therapeutic strategy.

D. When pharmacologic approaches and reduced face-to-face contact do not reduce family distress, consider an intensive behavioral family approach. A number of psychosocial strategies may be deployed to reduce the risk of exacerbation of florid symptoms, promote social functioning, and reduce the handicaps associated with the negative features of schizophrenia. These include: (1) educating the client and the family about the stress-related biologic nature of schizophrenia and the importance of prophylactic treatment, so that they can actively support the treatment plan; (2) enhancing the efficiency of client problem-solving functions to deal with environmental stress and social rehabilitation; (3) enhancing the efficiency of family problem-solving so that maximal functional improvements for each member of the family can be obtained; and (4) training to develop coping strategies that are effective in contending with the residual symptoms of schizophrenia and other persisting stresses in the social environment.

E. Should deleterious levels of discontent continue to be directed toward the client, consider whether the client's and family's needs might be better served by temporarily removing the index client from the home. The degree of respite provided should correspond to the degree of relief required for the family to achieve or maintain satisfactory levels of tolerance and patience when dealing with its schizophrenic member. In families with a high level of discontent, residential living on a short-term basis may be necessary. For other families a day treatment modality or an occasional weekend respite may afford adequate interim relief.

F. When it becomes obvious that living with his or her family can only be accomplished at great cost (i.e., risk of relapse) for the client and when it involves severe and debilitating hardship for the family, prolonged separation may be the only effective option. Every attempt must be made to view the separation as an effective and consensual decision. Refrain from ascribing blame to any family member and facilitate planning for ongoing but limited family contact.

References

Brown GW, Birley JLT, Wing JK. Influence of family life on the course of schizophrenic disorders: a replication. Br J Psychiatry 1972; 121:241–258.

Falloon IRH, Boyd JL, McGill CW. Family care of schizophrenia. New York: Guilford Press, 1984.

Hatfield AB, Spaniol L, Zipple AM. Expressed emotion: a family perspective. Schizophrenia Bull 1987; 13:221–226.

Lachance R. Schizophrenic family process. Can J Psychiatr Nursing 1987; 28(4):9–14.

Mintz LI, Liberman RP, Miklowitz DJ, Mintz J. Expressed emotion: a call for partnership among relatives, patients and professionals. Schizophrenia Bull 1987; 13:227–235.

Runions J, Prudo R. Problem behaviours encountered by families living with a schizophrenic member. Can J Psychiatry 1983; 28:382–386.

Strachan AM, Leff JP, Goldstein J, Doane JA, Burtt C. Emotional attitudes and direct communication in the families of schizophrenics: a cross-national replication. Br J Psychiatry 1986; 149:279–287.

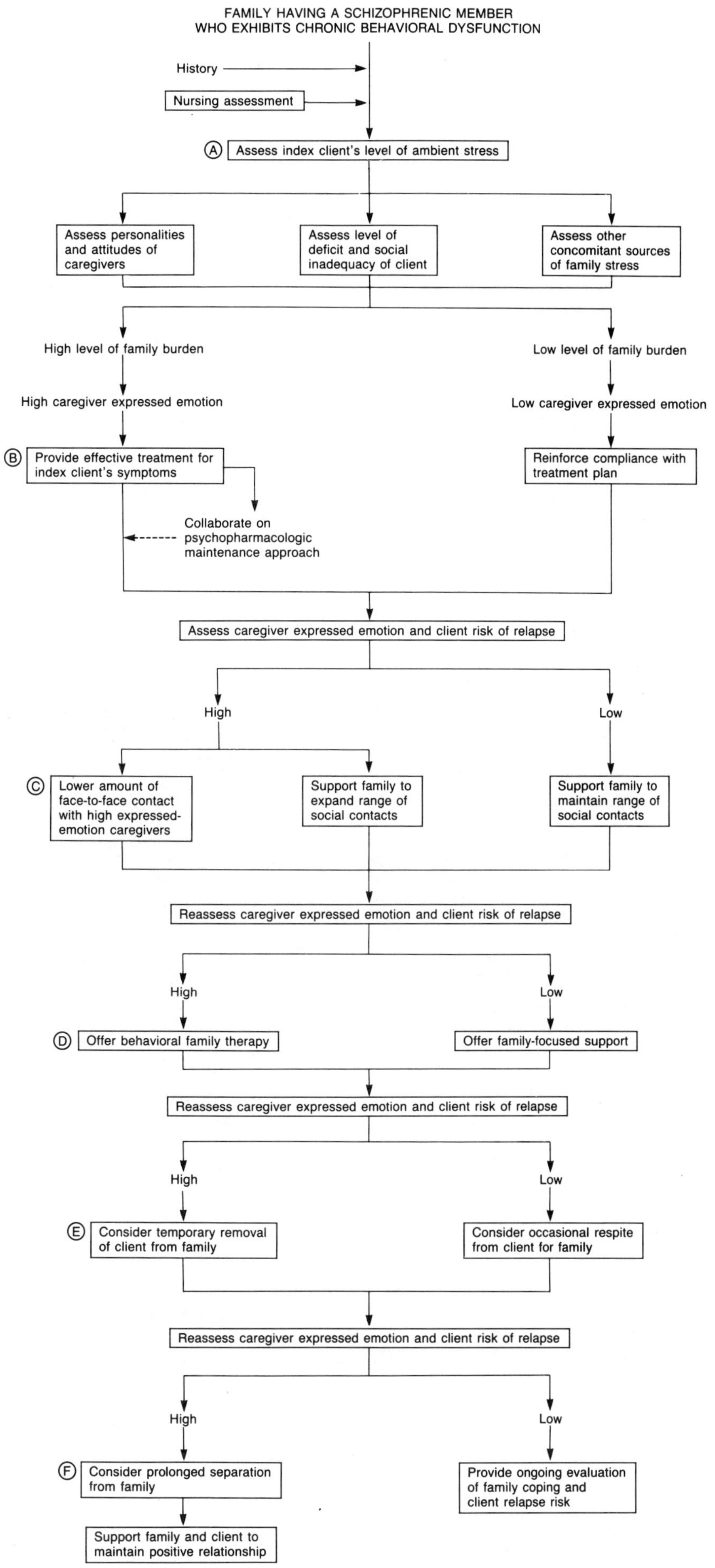

FAMILY HAVING A SCHIZOPHRENIC MEMBER WHO EXHIBITS CHRONIC BEHAVIORAL DYSFUNCTION
History
Nursing assessment
Ⓐ Assess index client's level of ambient stress
Assess personalities and attitudes of caregivers
Assess level of deficit and social inadequacy of client
Assess other concomitant sources of family stress
High level of family burden
High caregiver expressed emotion
Ⓑ Provide effective treatment for index client's symptoms
Collaborate on psychopharmacologic maintenance approach
Low level of family burden
Low caregiver expressed emotion
Reinforce compliance with treatment plan
Assess caregiver expressed emotion and client risk of relapse
High
Low
Ⓒ Lower amount of face-to-face contact with high expressed-emotion caregivers
Support family to expand range of social contacts
Support family to maintain range of social contacts
Reassess caregiver expressed emotion and client risk of relapse
High
Low
Ⓓ Offer behavioral family therapy
Offer family-focused support
Reassess caregiver expressed emotion and client risk of relapse
High
Low
Ⓔ Consider temporary removal of client from family
Consider occasional respite from client for family
Reassess caregiver expressed emotion and client risk of relapse
High
Low
Ⓕ Consider prolonged separation from family
Support family and client to maintain positive relationship
Provide ongoing evaluation of family coping and client relapse risk

INTERVENING WITH THE ACUTELY ILL SCHIZOPHRENIC CLIENT AND FAMILY

Nancy E. Johnston

A. At the time a schizophrenic client enters the hospital, he or she may be enduring a terrifying and bewildering subjective experience characterized by fragmented and bizarre thinking, delusions, and hallucinations. These cognitive distortions may be accompanied by extreme emotional states including anxiety, fear, and panic and may find expression in withdrawal or destructive acts directed toward the self, others, or the environment.

B. When the client has demonstrated thinking or behavior that indicates a high risk for aggressive acts, when no insight into the problem exists, or when a strong resistance to remaining in the hospital is expressed, it may be necessary to commit the client involuntarily for assessment. The nurse is responsible for verifying the client's status, whether voluntary or involuntary, with the medical team in attendance. If necessary, interventions can then be deployed to protect the client from self-destructive acts and to ensure that the potential for aggression toward others is minimized. Appropriate protective measures may include removal of all objects that could be used to inflict harm, reduction of environmental stimuli, constant care, surveillance protocols, and administration of neuroleptic drugs. Measures to ensure the safety of other clients are then implemented. These may include restricted or heavily supervised contact with the distressed client.

C. The most effective intervention to reduce anxiety and secure confidence and cooperation is the establishment of a reassuring nurse-client relationship. Approach the client in a calm and nonthreatening manner that conveys caring, protection, and understanding.

D. Trust is deepened by explaining in advance how and for what reason events related to treatment and unit routines will occur, in order to reduce the element of surprise and minimize the client's fear and suspicion.

E. Of particular importance in promoting trust, reducing confusion, and securing cooperation is the development of an approach that maintains continuity and consistency. Since the implementation of the treatment plan typically involves many disciplines, it often becomes the nurse's responsibility to coordinate the care. Accordingly, the nurse must have a clear grasp of those duties that fall within nursing's domain as well as those that may be addressed in a collaborative, multidisciplinary context.

F. Consistency is best achieved by one nurse being primarily responsible for the day-to-day implementation of the care plan. In this intensive one-to-one context, the nurse consolidates her relationship with the client and is in the best position to report on the effectiveness of the treatment plan. The effectiveness of psychopharmacologic approaches and changes in the client's mental status are communicated to the team so that effective medical care can be instituted and maintained.

G. Because of the intimate and trusting nature of the nurse-client relationship, the nurse understands the nature of the client's subjective experience and how and why the client may be perplexed and frightened by certain phenomena. Acting as a mediator between the client's inner experience and objective reality, the nurse interprets and clarifies events in a way that can be most easily assimilated. In this way, the client's beliefs are acknowledged without colluding in the delusions, thereby gradually enabling the client to bring a level of questioning to beliefs that had been firmly held. The nurse also contributes to the multidisciplinary team approach by conveying information gained by frequent contact with concerned family members. Thus, family support is offered by drawing on family strengths, minimizing guilt, and enabling the piecing together of a developmental and family history.

H. Once the sensorium is clear, anxiety is contained within manageable limits, and the medical diagnosis is established, consider the readiness of the client and family for information. In consultation with other members of the team, impart information on the nature of the illness and its treatment.

I. When floridly psychotic symptoms are in abeyance, concentrate subsequent effort on shaping the client's behavior toward adaptive functioning. To eliminate bizarre and strange mannerisms, selectively reinforce communications and behavior that are reality oriented. Encourage the client to participate in group, recreational, and occupational activities that emphasize positive coping skills. Offer opportunities to learn how to develop a home climate that will offer the client and family the best chance of successful recovery and adaptation.

J. Because a reappearance of some symptoms is expected as the client anticipates separation and discharge, prepare the client for the termination of the relationship. Review positive accomplishments and encourage integration of the meaning of the illness. Attempt to maintain continuity and consistency in care by involving the client and family in discharge planning and by introducing them to professionals who will be involved in the provision of continuing care.

References

Corden A. Schizophrenia: the search for therapeutic responses. Nurs Times 1988; 84(3):50–52.

Dawson D, Blum HM, Bartolucci G. Schizophrenia in focus: guidelines for treatment and rehabilitation. New York: Human Sciences Press, 1983.

Greenberg L, Fine SB, Cohen C, et al. An interdisciplinary psychoeducation program for schizophrenic patients and their families in an acute care setting. Hosp Commun Psychiatry 1988; 39:277–282.

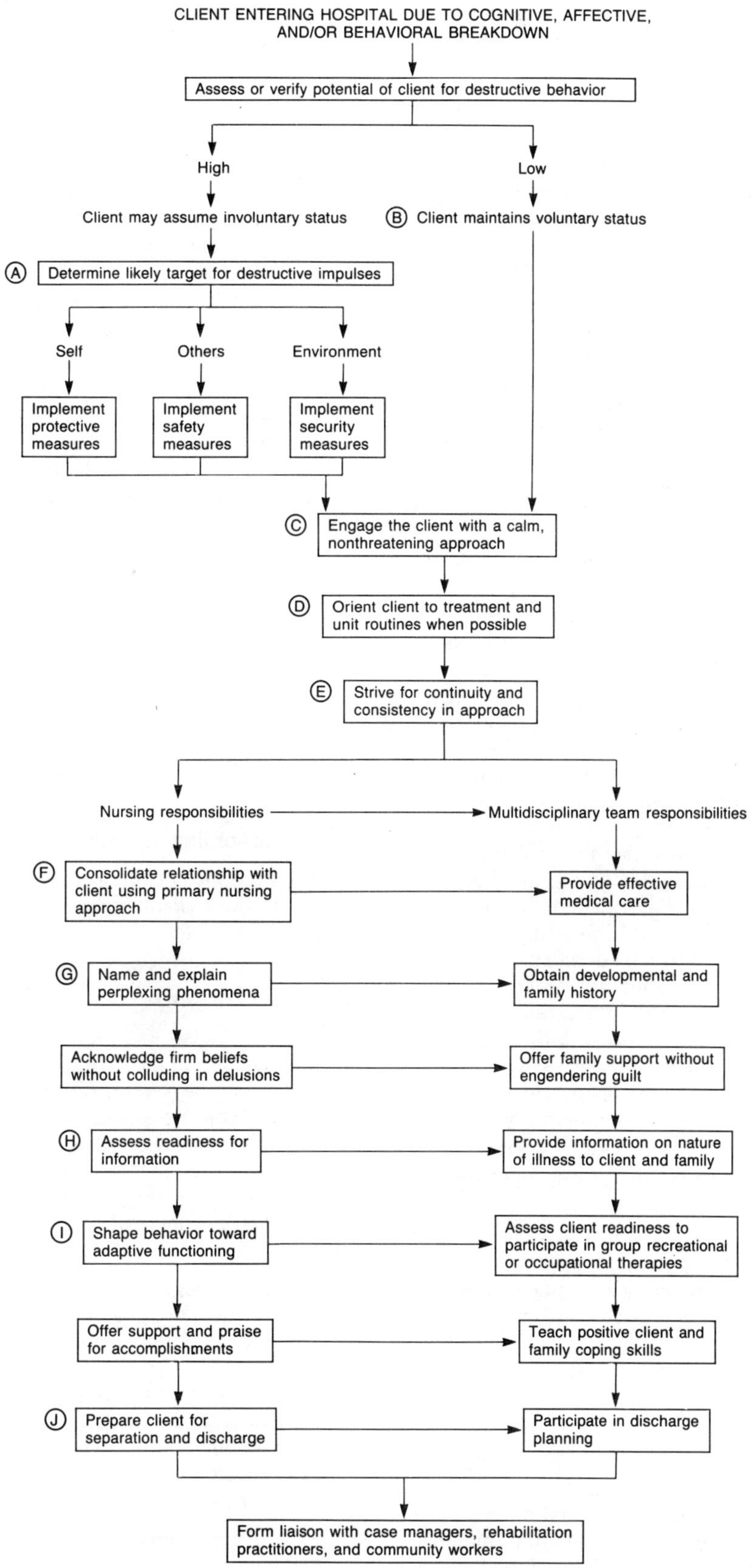

Khan A, Cohen S, Chiles J, et al. Therapeutic role of a psychiatric intensive care unit in acute psychosis. Comprehens Psychiatry 1987; 28:264–269.

Murray RB, Huelskoetter MMW. Psychiatric/mental health nursing: giving emotional care. 2nd ed. Norwalk, CT: Appleton and Lange, 1987:489–529.

Torrey EF. Excerpts from surviving schizophrenia. Princeton, NJ: ER Squibb & Sons, 1984.

CATATONIA AND NEUROLEPTIC MALIGNANT SYNDROME*

Karen Perkins

A. Rapid and accurate identification of the underlying cause and appropriate medical and nursing management of the catatonic client are particularly challenging. Catatonia is a syndrome whose symptoms include mutism, catatonic negativism, stupor or excitement, posturing, rigidity, and occasionally catalepsy. Catatonia may be due to either an organic or a functional disorder. Many medical illnesses present as catatonic stupor, whereas acute delirium may present as catatonic excitement. Toxic states and acute neurologic disorders presenting with catatonic symptoms render the patient at risk for medical complications, including death. Another and frequently lethal (20 to 30 percent) syndrome, the neuroleptic malignant syndrome, may initially present with catatonia-like symptoms. This syndrome is caused by neuroleptic drugs, especially such high-potency drugs as Haldol and Prolixin. The neuroleptic malignant syndrome may develop following one dose of neuroleptic medication, or 2 weeks or even years of neuroleptic treatment may be required for it to develop. The primary symptoms of the neuroleptic malignant syndrome include muscular rigidity, a rising temperature culminating in a high fever, and autonomic symptoms. Secondary symptoms include impaired breathing, muteness, autonomic hyperactivity, diaphoresis, tachypnea, agitation, and electrolyte and metabolic abnormalities. Tremor may also be present (not usually seen in catatonia). Rigidity and restlessness develop prior to increased fever. The patient becomes increasingly stuporous and may exhibit wide swings in blood pressure. Mortality is usually due to dehydration, aspiration, hypotension, or respiratory failure. The history should include recent medical symptoms and treatments, a thorough medication history, a drug use and abuse history, exposure to toxic substances, exposure to prolonged high temperature, and any psychiatric history, including medication regimens. Obviously this history must be obtained from family, friends, and co-workers, if the patient's condition precludes verbal communication.

B. Clinical assessment includes frequent assessment of vital signs with careful attention to temperature increases and increasing hypotension. Laboratory tests include electrolyte levels, a complete blood count, calcium, glucose, BUN, and creatinine levels, liver function tests, and a toxicology screen sensitive for phencyclidine (PCP).

C. Because catatonia can result from so many different causes, the diagnostic process must be systematic. Known psychiatric clients require differential diagnosis just as any nonpsychiatric client does. Withhold neuroleptic drugs until a definitive diagnosis has been made. Be prepared to assist with lumbar puncture, electroencephalography, or transfer for a CT scan if the history and physical examination indicate a need. In the neuroleptic malignant syndrome, the levels of muscle enzymes such as creatine phosphokinase and aldolase are elevated secondary to myonecrosis. An electroencephalogram may be ordered to help rule out or confirm organic delirium or excited catatonia. A lumbar puncture is performed if there is a fever and concomitant leukocytosis.

D. Psychiatric causes include affective disorder (both manic and depressive), conversion reaction, and schizophrenia. Affective disorders account for most psychiatric cases of catatonia. Electroconvulsive therapy is the treatment of choice, but usually emergency department treatment consists of neuroleptic medications. Schizophrenia is also treated with neuroleptic drugs. The conversion disordered client may respond to smelling salts and the suggestion that he is all right.

E. Metabolic causes include hypercalcemia, hepatic encephalopathy, acute intermittent porphyria, pellagra, and diabetic ketoacidosis. Manage the client according to the physician's directions. The client may require hospitalization.

F. Neurologic causes include parkinsonism, lesions of the basal ganglia, acute encephalitis, and postictal states. Treat according to institutional policy.

G. If neuroleptic catatonia is suspected, benztropine, 2 mg intravenously or intramuscularly, can be given and repeated in 30 minutes. Two doses should provide symptomatic relief.

H. For a discussion of chemical dependence see pages 30 to 41.

I. The first step in the treatment of the neuroleptic malignant syndrome is to stop administration of all neuroleptic drugs. A complete assessment of vital signs is indicated every 15 minutes or more frequently. The cardinal sign of the syndrome, besides muscle rigidity, is an ever increasing temperature. Follow institutional policy or the physician's orders concerning rapid cooling of the patient with a very high temperature.

J. Dantrolene is given orally or intravenously in doses of 0.8 to 1.0 mg per kilogram of body weight every 6 hours. (Therapy is continued for 2 weeks because of the risk of relapse.) Therapy with bromocriptine, 2.5 mg, is started twice a day, and the dosage is gradually increased to 5 mg three times a day. The patient should show improvement within 2 hours after initial treatment. These two drugs are still considered experimental and may be used singly or in combination.

K. Because the neuroleptic malignant syndrome is not readily diagnosed in its earliest stages, by the time the diagnosis is made and treatment has begun the syndrome may have progressed to the point at which the patient must be hospitalized for 5 to 20 days for supportive nursing care and medical management.

* Reprinted from: Mancini ME. Decision making in emergency nursing. Toronto: BC Decker, 1987.

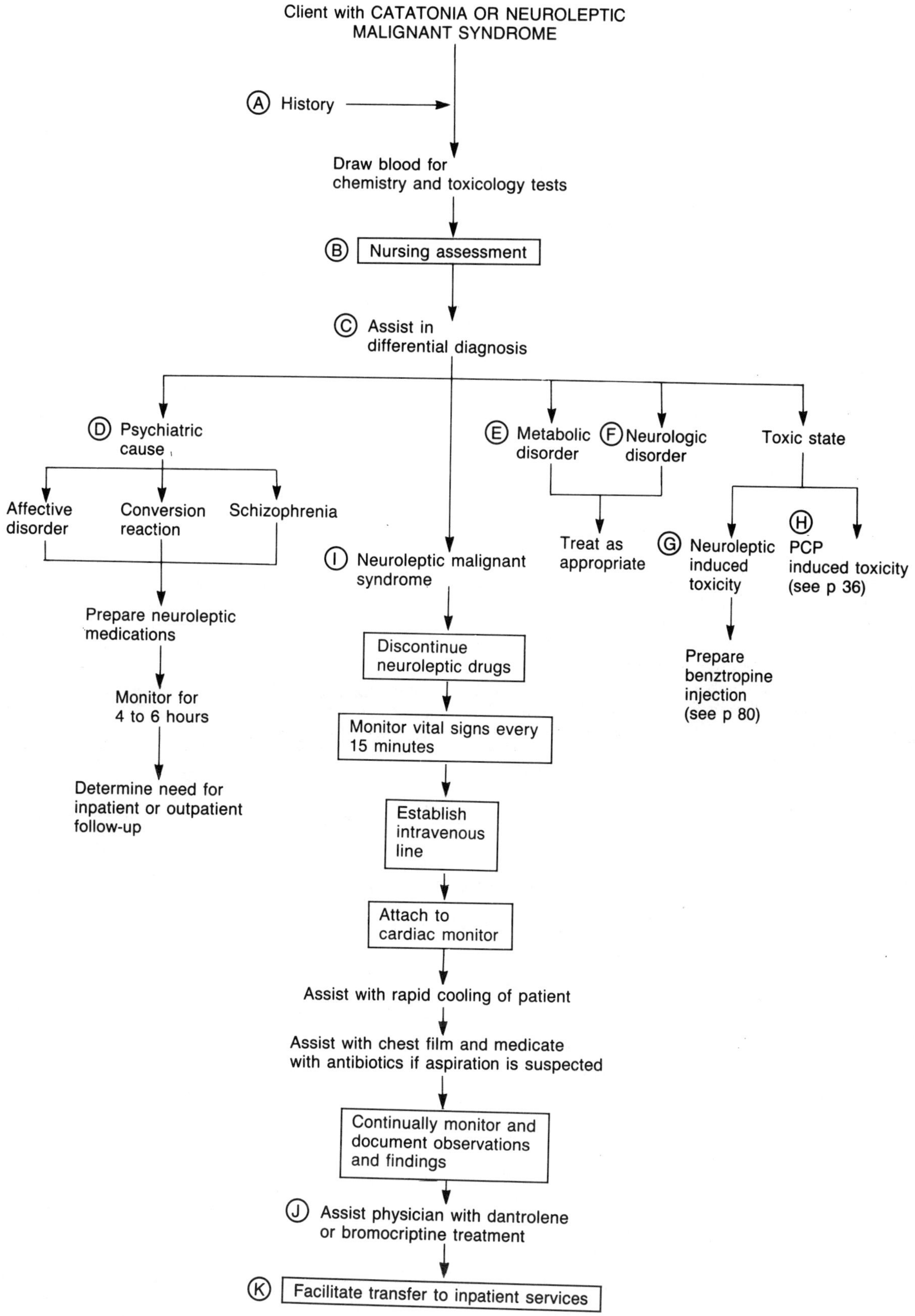

References

Cahill MC, Arana GW. Navigating neuroleptic malignant syndrome. Am J Nurs 1986, 86:671–673.

Hyman SE. Manual of psychiatric emergencies. Boston: Little, Brown, 1984:99–105.

Keltner NL, McIntyer CW. Neuroleptic malignant syndrome. J Neurosurg Nurs 1985; 17:362–366.

EXTRAPYRAMIDAL SIDE-EFFECTS

Deborah Antai-Otong

Extrapyramidal side-effects (EPS) represent the neurologic side-effects of neuroleptic agents used to treat psychotic disorders. Agents that produce the highest incidence of side-effects include the high-potency piperazine group (Prolixin Decanoate) and the group of phenothiazines and butyrophenones (haloperidol). The major symptoms include pseudoparkinsonism (40 percent of all EPS) and dystonias, dyskinesias, and akathisias (50 percent).

A. The nursing assessment includes documenting the type of neuroleptic (antipsychotic) agent, dose, duration of treatment, and reasons for taking the medication. Assess as well the subjective symptoms experienced by patients.

B. Clinical signs and symptoms of EPS include pseudoparkinsonism, akathisia, and dystonia. These symptoms are extremely embarrassing and frightening to patients and must be assessed and treated as soon as possible to prevent poor medication compliance and recurrent psychosis. Pseudoparkinsonian symptoms may occur 5 to 30 days after the initial dose of the neuroleptic agent and include resting tremors, drooling, shuffling gait, mask-like facial expression, psychomotor retardation, rigidity, and "pill rolling" movements. Symptoms of akathisia may occur within 5 to 60 days after initial treatment and include subjective feelings of restlessness, inability to sit still, and pacing. Symptoms of dystonias and dyskinesias may occur hours to 5 days after the initial dose and are manifested by facial grimacing, tightening of neck and back muscles, and oculogyric crisis.

C. The nurse may be ordered to administer a parenteral anticholinergic agent such as diphenhydramine (Benadryl) 25 to 50 mg intramuscularly or benztropine mesylate (Cogentin) 1 to 2 mg intramuscularly or intravenously slowly, to treat EPS (see "Dystonic Reaction," p 80). The client's vital signs must be monitored as well as his response to treatment. The nurse must also monitor clients for side-effects from these anticholinergic agents, such as sedation, dizziness, delirium, and confusion. If the client's symptoms respond to parenteral anticholinergic agents, the physician usually discharges the client after prescribing an oral preparation for several days or an indefinite period of time.

References

Antai-Otong DJ. Psychopharmacology. In: Johnson BS, ed. Psychiatric mental health nursing: adaptation and growth. 2nd ed. Philadelphia: JB Lippincott, 1989:268–294.

Appleton WS. Fourth psychoactive drug usage guide. J Clin Psychiatry 1982; 43:12–27.

Baldessarini RJ. Drugs and treatment of psychiatric disorders. In: Gilman AG, Goodman LS, Rall TW, Murad F, eds. Goodman and Gilman's the pharmacological basis of therapeutics. 7th ed. New York: Macmillan, 1985:387–445.

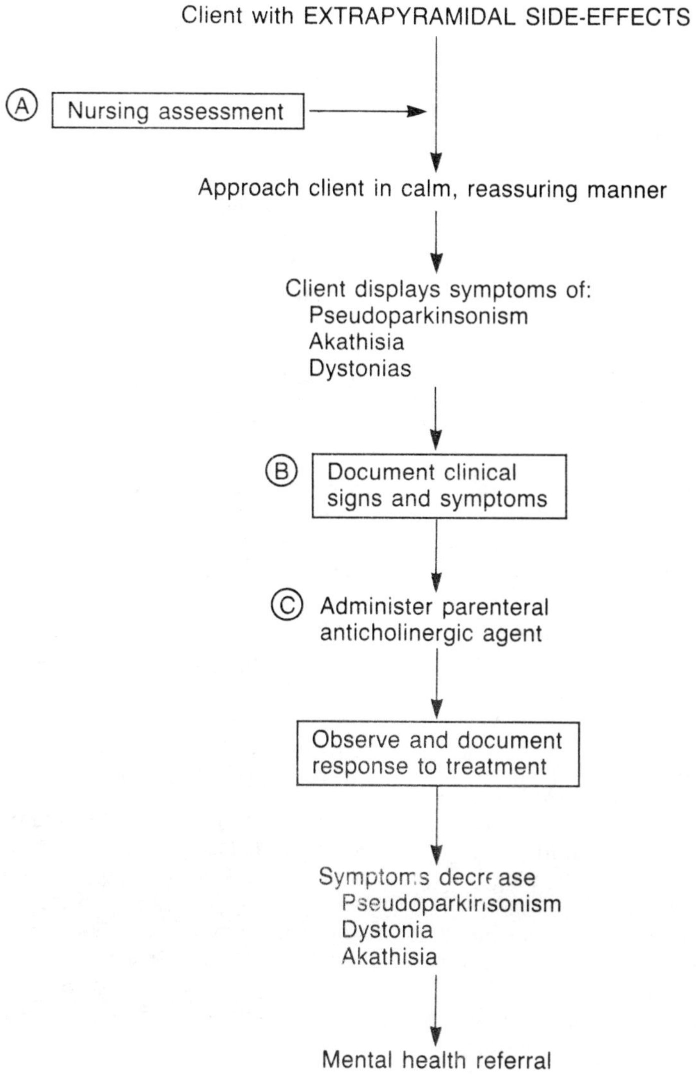
Client with EXTRAPYRAMIDAL SIDE-EFFECTS
(A) Nursing assessment
Approach client in calm, reassuring manner
Client displays symptoms of:
Pseudoparkinsonism
Akathisia
Dystonias
(B) Document clinical signs and symptoms
(C) Administer parenteral anticholinergic agent
Observe and document response to treatment
Symptoms decrease
Pseudoparkinsonism
Dystonia
Akathisia
Mental health referral

DYSTONIC REACTION*

Karen Perkins

A. There are four groups of extrapyramidal symptoms associated with antipsychotic drugs: akathisia, tardive dyskinesia, parkinson-like responses, and dystonia. The symptoms may range in intensity from mild to severe and often lead to misdiagnosis. All nurses should be familiar with the signs and symptoms, as well as the nursing and medical management of, each group. The three most common dystonic presentations include torticollis (the head and neck are twisted into an extreme position), opisthotonos (the head and neck are hyperextended), and the oculogyric crisis (the patient cannot move his eyes from a fixed upward gaze). Laryngeal dystonia is rare but may be life threatening. All these frightening and painful conditions demand prompt assessment and treatment. There is a high incidence in young muscular males. High-potency neuroleptic drugs such as haloperidol (Haldol), thiothixene (Navane), and fluphenazine (Prolixin) are associated with higher incidences than other neuroleptic drugs. Acute dystonic reactions usually occur 1 hour to 5 days after the initiation of antipsychotic treatment or usage, but may occur at any time during treatment. The history should include the onset of symptoms, psychiatric treatment (including the type of medication taken and the dosage), and past problems with psychotropic regimens. If a client denies known antipsychotic drug ingestion, inquire about street drugs. Many clients, for a variety of reasons, are reluctant to disclose illicit drug use and must be repeatedly encouraged before they will acknowledge taking nonprescribed drugs. Children frequently develop dystonias following a single dose of prochlorperazine (Compazine) for the treatment of nausea.

B. Acute dystonic reactions have been misdiagnosed as epilepsy, meningitis, encephalitis, poliomyelitis, and tetanus. Misdiagnosis may lead to hospitalization and a host of invasive procedures. Dystonic reactions have also been misdiagnosed as the "psychotic posturing" of a schizophrenic, thereby resulting in the patient's being given antipsychotic medications, which only worsen the dystonia.

C. Many physicians feel that when a patient presents with sudden onset of an undiagnosable bizarre neurologic disorder, a trial of diphenhydramine (Benadryl), 25 to 50 mg intravenously or intramuscularly, or benztropine (Cogentin), 1 to 2 mg intravenously or intramuscularly, may prove beneficial. These drugs will not interfere with further diagnostic procedures or cause severe side effects.

D. The management of the acute dystonic reaction is the same as in C.

E. Observe, monitor, and record the client's response to treatment; a dramatic reduction in muscular spasms and almost instantaneous return of normal tone and posture are expected with intravenous treatment. Intramuscular medication usually brings marked relief within 20 to 30 minutes.

F. In the rare likelihood that the client does not respond as expected, continue to provide support and monitor and document the clinical status. Assist the physician with further diagnostic procedures, and facilitate the client's transfer to inpatient service if he is to be admitted.

G. Once a client has experienced a dystonic reaction, he may be reluctant to continue with antipsychotic treatment. A great deal of support and encouragement is needed. Help the client to understand the rationale behind the physician's orders to change or decrease medication or add an antiparkinson drug to the medication regimen. Obtain a scheduled outpatient follow-up appointment for the client as soon as possible.

References

Hyman SE. Manual of psychiatric emergencies. Boston: Little, Brown, 1984:215–217.

Rund DA, Hutzler JC. Emergency psychiatry. St. Louis: CV Mosby, 1983:288–289.

Stuart GW, Sundeen SJ. Principles and practice of psychiatric nursing. St. Louis: CV Mosby, 1983:500–503.

* Reprinted from: Mancini ME. Decision making in emergency nursing. Toronto: BC Decker, 1987.

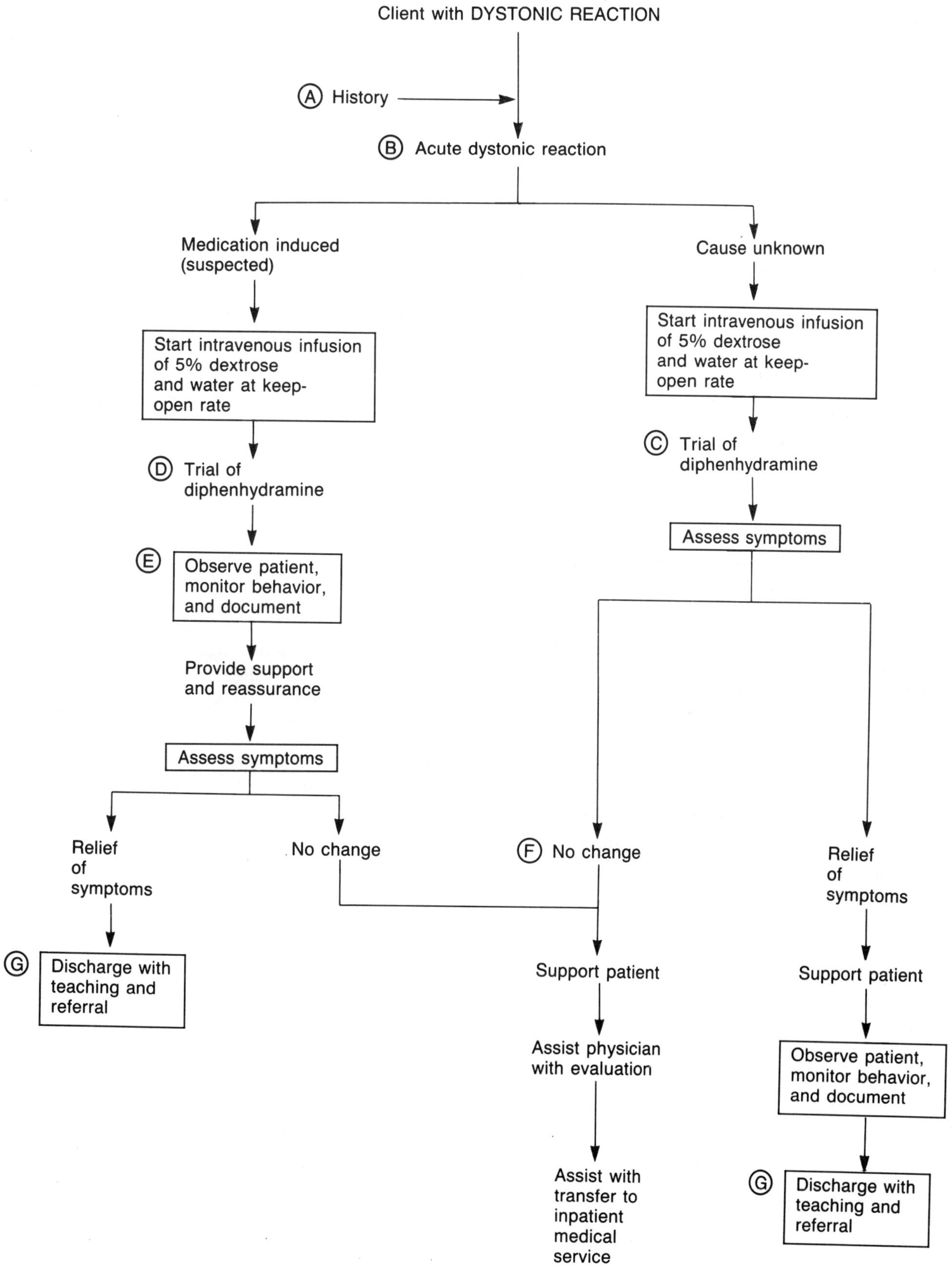
Client with DYSTONIC REACTION
(A) History
(B) Acute dystonic reaction
Medication induced (suspected)
Cause unknown
Start intravenous infusion of 5% dextrose and water at keep-open rate
Start intravenous infusion of 5% dextrose and water at keep-open rate
(D) Trial of diphenhydramine
(C) Trial of diphenhydramine
(E) Observe patient, monitor behavior, and document
Assess symptoms
Provide support and reassurance
Assess symptoms
Relief of symptoms
No change
(F) No change
Relief of symptoms
(G) Discharge with teaching and referral
Support patient
Support patient
Assist physician with evaluation
Observe patient, monitor behavior, and document
Assist with transfer to inpatient medical service
(G) Discharge with teaching and referral

EATING DISORDERS

Donna Ciliska

A. In addition to a general history, the patient should be questioned specifically about the development of symptoms, history of weight fluctuations, dieting and other past practices of weight control, sexual abuse, patient and family history of psychiatric problems such as eating disorders, depression, drug and alcohol abuse, and dependency. The nurse should probe concerns of body weight and shape, body dissatisfaction, daily pattern and amount of food intake (proportion of intake in carbohydrate, fat, and protein), and presence, frequency, and amount of binges, vomiting, laxative and diuretic use, and exercise.

B. The physical assessment should particularly include weight (do not rely on self-report), height, and assessing for presence of dehydration, calluses on the back of the hand, swollen salivary glands, muscle weakness, emaciation, bradycardia, and hypotension.

C. Multidisciplinary assessment is made by psychiatrist, psychologist, nutritionist, occupational therapist, and social worker. Laboratory investigation includes electrocardiography (ECG), complete blood count, urea nitrogen, electrolytes, urinalysis, and serum creatinine. Creatinine phosphokinase is required in patients who abuse ipecac. Decisions are made in the team as to diagnosis and appropriate treatment. About 1 percent of the female population suffers from anorexia nervosa (AN), and the same percent have bulimia nervosa (BN). However, about 50 percent of AN patients also have BN.

D. Emotional support is required particularly around meal times for AN patients. Usually, therapies cannot be effective until symptoms of starvation have been treated and some weight gain has been achieved. Treatment is directed to support of refeeding and weight restoration.

E. Inpatient care is indicated where weight loss has been greater than 25 percent of original body weight, potassium level is under 2.5 mM/L accompanied by ECG changes, or there are cardiac enzyme changes, severe dehydration, acute abdominal symptoms, presence of convulsions, or suicidal behavior. In addition, BN patients may be initially admitted to stabilize chaotic eating patterns. Therapy (group, individual, and family) is begun by the multidisciplinary team, and often includes pharmacotherapy (antidepressants, anxiolytics, antipsychotics, and appetite stimulants for AN patients). Nursing care includes monitoring of weight changes, drug effectiveness, and side effects.

F. In some communities, resources exist for day-hospital treatment. Usually, the patient is admitted from the community, but may be part of a step-down approach after emergency admission. A multidisciplinary group is involved in therapy (cognitive-behavioral and psychodynamic approaches have all been effectively used) to deal with depression, need for control, and sense of personal ineffectiveness; and in education regarding assertiveness, resistance to social expectations for thinness in women, meal planning, and clothes shopping. Most programs involve patients from breakfast time until after the evening meal, 5 days per week, for 3 weeks to 4 months. If day-hospital treatment is unavailable, the same treatment is often delivered by outpatient or community agencies.

G. Some communities offer short-term, group programs that consist of education and group therapy. Usually these groups meet 1 to 2 hours a week for 6 to 12 weeks. The education covers normal eating (quantity, quality, and pattern of intake), cultural messages for women to be thin and how to resist, effects of starvation, ineffectiveness of the binge-purge cycle in maintaining low weight, and consequences of dieting. Therapy is directed at dealing with symptoms, sense of ineffectiveness, and depression.

H. If binge-purge cycles are still occurring twice per week or more in BN patients, or if weight is chronically low in AN patients, and psychological symptoms persist, group therapy is recommended.

I. Patients may go on to individual therapy if symptom levels are still high (see E). AN is considered a chronic disease with estimates as high as 50 percent nonrecovered at 5 years after diagnosis. Less evidence is available for BN patients, but the trend is similar to AN in chronicity. Both conditions are associated with other psychiatric disorders such as affective and anxiety disorders, psychosis, interpersonal dysfunction, and substance abuse. Individual therapy may, therefore, be long and intensive. If pharmacotherapy (as in E) is instituted, the nurse must monitor compliance and be aware of the potential for abuse.

J. Self-help or professionally led support groups are valuable for the ongoing management of symptoms, maintenance of weight gains, and resistance to psychiatric comorbidity. Educational issues such as those described in G are often reinforced.

References

Eating Disorders Group, Department of Psychiatry, Toronto General Hospital. Current update: anorexia nervosa and bulimia nervosa. Toronto: Upjohn, 1988.

Fairburn CG. A cognitive-behavioral approach to the treatment of bulimia. Psychol Med 1981; 11:707–711.

Garner DM, Rockert W, Olmsted M, Johnson CL, Coscina DV. Psychoeducational principles in the treatment of bulimia and anorexia nervosa. In: Garner DM, Garfinkel PE, eds. Handbook of psychotherapy for anorexia nervosa and bulimia. New York: Guilford Press, 1985.

Hudson JI, Pope HG, Yurgelun-Todd D, Jonas JM, Frankenburg FR. A controlled study of lifetime prevalence of affective and other psychiatric disorders in bulimic outpatients. Am J Psychiatry 1987; 144:1283–1287.

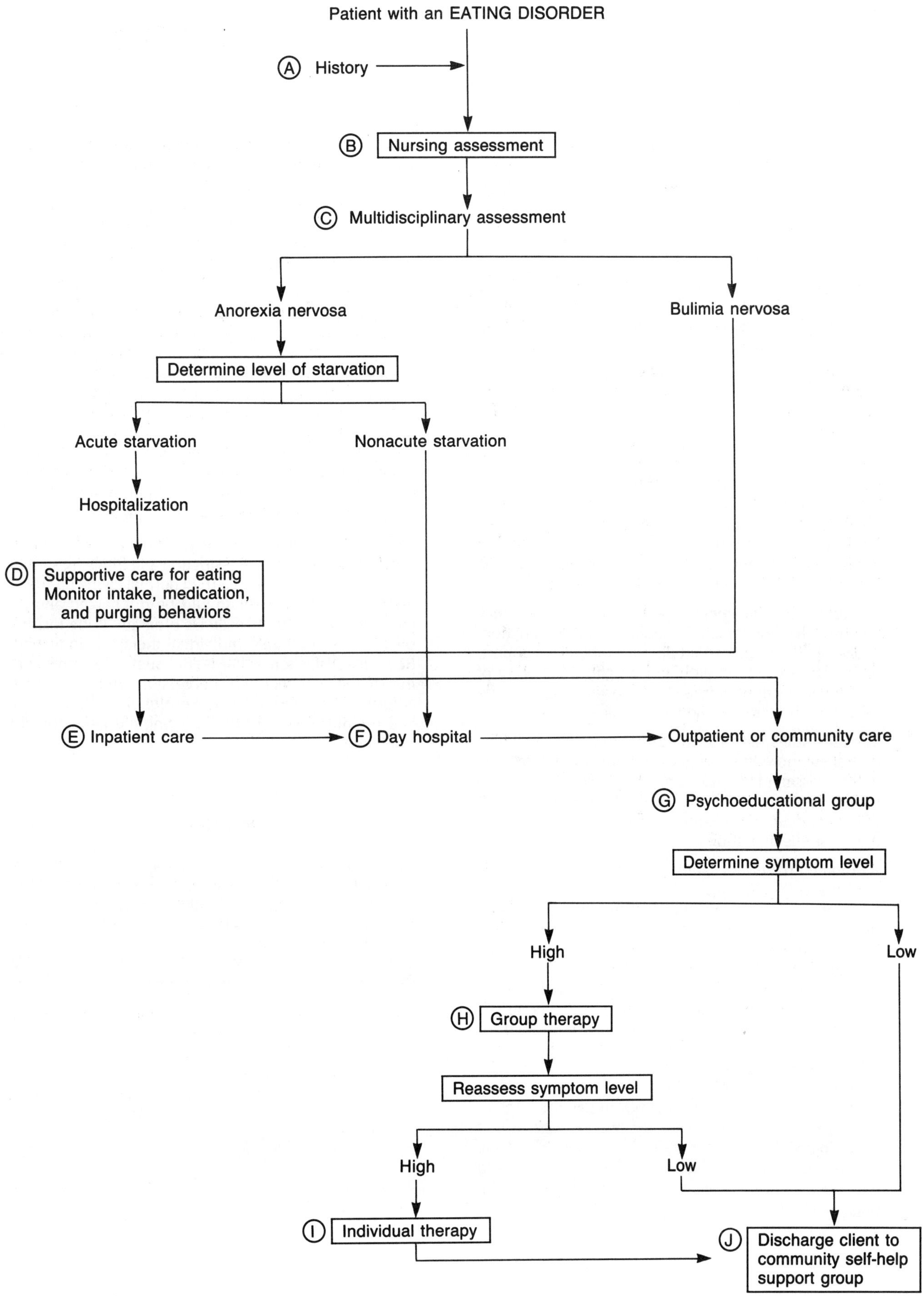

Patient with an EATING DISORDER
A History
B Nursing assessment
C Multidisciplinary assessment
Anorexia nervosa
Bulimia nervosa
Determine level of starvation
Acute starvation
Nonacute starvation
Hospitalization
D Supportive care for eating Monitor intake, medication, and purging behaviors
E Inpatient care
F Day hospital
Outpatient or community care
G Psychoeducational group
Determine symptom level
High
Low
H Group therapy
Reassess symptom level
High
Low
I Individual therapy
J Discharge client to community self-help support group

OBESITY

Donna Ciliska

A. In addition to a general history, the client should be questioned specifically about history of weight fluctuations, dieting, and other past practices of weight control, presence of binge-purge symptoms or periods of restrained eating, depression, drug and alcohol abuse and dependency, family history of weight problems, hypertension, heart disease, and diabetes mellitus. The nurse should probe concerns of body weight and shape, body dissatisfaction, daily pattern and amount of food intake (proportion of intake in carbohydrate, fat, and protein), and exercise pattern.

B. The physical assessment should particularly include height, weight (measured—do not rely on self-report), blood pressure, and measurement of waist and hips for calculation of ratio.

C. Multidisciplinary assessment is made by a psychiatrist, psychologist, nutritionist, occupational therapist, and social worker. Laboratory investigation includes particularly thyroid functioning, glucose tolerance, triglyceride levels, total cholesterol, and HDL and LDL cholesterol levels. Diagnosis and treatment of any medical disorders is primary before actual treatment of obesity.

D. If obesity is life-threatening, the treatment of choice may be hospitalization for gastric stapling, calorie restriction, and/or appetite suppressant pharmacotherapy. Support, daily measurement of girth and weight, monitoring of emotional reactions, intake, drug effectiveness, and side effects are required in the nursing care.

E. Several studies have indicated that most obese clients do not eat more than the general population. However, if the assessment of intake indicates that a client is overeating, behavior modification and education about nutrition and how to modify intake has been shown to have the most effective long-term outcome.

F. A common pattern of eating in the obese population is to restrict intake for days, or for the early part of the day, followed by a breakdown of the restriction when large quantities of food are ingested. The guilt that follows leads to more severe restriction, followed again by bingeing, and the cycle intensifies, sometimes to the point of actual bulimia nervosa. A useful treatment for this group is a psychoeducational group that meets 1 to 2 hours per week for 6 to 12 weeks. The purpose of this group is for participants to normalize eating and to reduce the importance of body weight in determining self-esteem. Education is given regarding the biological controls over weight (set-point theory), the cultural imperative for thinness in women and how to resist this message, differences in health risks associated with obesity depending on distribution of fat (abdominal obesity is associated with diabetes mellitus and heart disease; gluteal-femoral obesity is not associated with greater health risks), ineffectiveness and dangers of severe food restriction, benefits of mild exercise, self-enhancement through wardrobe and makeup choices, normal eating and how to retrain oneself to respond to hunger and satiety. Therapeutic interventions include assertiveness training, role playing, body image exercises, cognitive therapy to counteract "I'm fat, therefore, I'm a failure" thinking, and dealing with grieving over the loss of the dream to be thin.

G. As stated previously, many obese clients do not eat more than the nonobese population. They may have done so at one time in order for weight to be gained, but do not need to continue a high level of intake to maintain a high weight. These obese individuals are thought to be at "set-point" or metabolically "efficient." This group needs to be supported in a nondieting stance. Most are very nutrition conscious, but some may need education about quality and quantity of food. They should then be discharged with a referral to a community agency that would support a moderate exercise program.

H. Following participation in a psychoeducational group or hospitalization, levels of restriction and bingeing should again be assessed. If a pattern of normal eating has been established, the patient should be discharged and referred to a community exercise program. If the restrict-binge cycle continues, individual therapy is indicated. Body dissatisfaction, self-esteem issues, alternative coping strategies, concurrent depression, and social maladjustment are all addressed. Resolution of these issues, and establishment of normal eating are indicators for discharge.

References

Brownell KD, Wadden TA. Behavior therapy for obesity: modern approaches and better results. In: Brownell KD, Foreyt JP, eds. Handbook of eating disorders: physiology, psychology, and treatment of obesity, anorexia, and bulimia. New York: Basic Books, 1986.

Garner DM, Rockert W, Olmsted M, Johnson CL, Coscina DV. Psychoeducational principles in the treatment of bulimia and anorexia nervosa. In: Garner DM, Garfinkel PE, eds. Handbook of psychotherapy for anorexia nervosa and bulimia. New York: Guilford Press, 1985.

Polivy J, Herman CP. Dieting and bingeing: a causal analysis. Am Psychol 1985; 40:193–201.

Stunkard AJ, Coll M, Lindquist S, Meyers A. Obesity and eating style. Arch Gen Psychiatr 1980; 37:1127–1129.

Wing RR, Jeffrey RW. Outpatient treatment of obesity: a comparison of methodology and clinical results. Int J Obes 1979; 3:261–279.

Wooley SC, Wooley OW. Should obesity be treated at all? In: Stunkard AJ, Stellar E, eds. Eating and its disorders. New York: Raven Press, 1984.

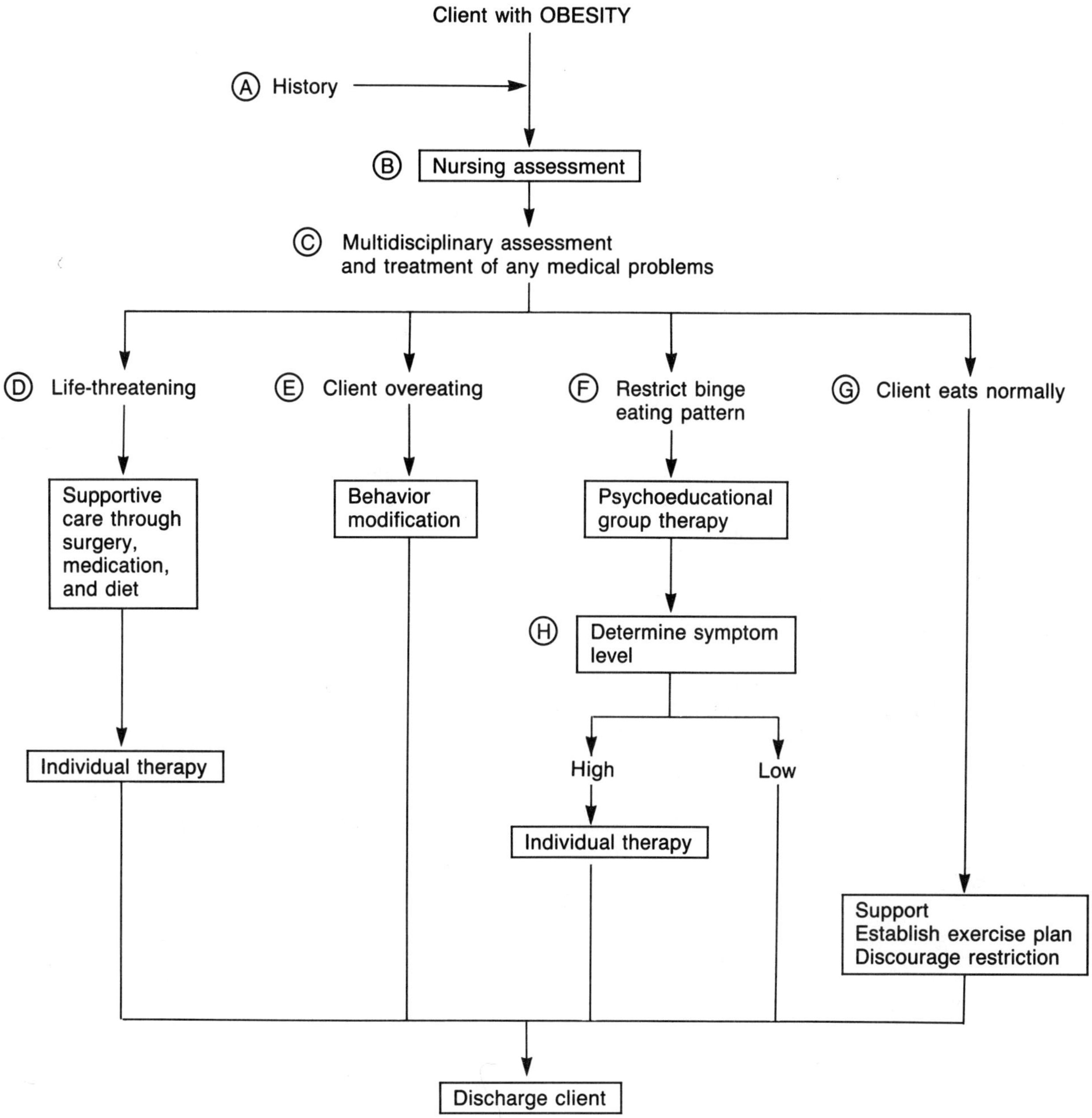
Client with OBESITY
(A) History
(B) Nursing assessment
(C) Multidisciplinary assessment and treatment of any medical problems
(D) Life-threatening
(E) Client overeating
(F) Restrict binge eating pattern
(G) Client eats normally
Supportive care through surgery, medication, and diet
Behavior modification
Psychoeducational group therapy
(H) Determine symptom level
High
Low
Individual therapy
Individual therapy
Support
Establish exercise plan
Discourage restriction
Discharge client

ANTISOCIAL PERSONALITY

Nona Flye

A. It is essential to document psychiatric and medical histories, which encompass childhood and adolescent behaviors that address issues such as truancy, incorrigibility, theft, and frequent running away. Other areas to assess include unlawful behaviors, interpersonal relationships, and authority problems. These clients often have histories of poor impulse control, low frustration tolerance, inability to profit from past experiences, and frequent deviant sexual behavior.

B. The initial nursing assessment should include the client's mental status, including the presence or absence of hallucinations or delusions, hostility, and anger. If violent behavior is anticipated, consider security back-up if the client is not psychotic and is acting out. Personality disorder should be suspected if the individual has a lifelong history of dysfunction in interpersonal, social, and occupational areas. These individuals are usually adept at explaining their histories by blaming others or unfortunate circumstances.

C. Although clients have long histories of "acting out" or "withdrawn" behaviors, most often they appear normal. They exhibit symptoms of poor judgment and poor insight and have difficulty feeling remorseful or guilty over inappropriate behaviors.

D. Clients who exhibit violent or aggressive behavior must be secluded to prevent them from hurting themselves and others. This provides physical control and prevents escalating violence in the therapeutic milieu.

E. Although Ativan has been used successfully to control violent and aggressive behavior, medications are not used on a regular basis to deal with these individuals.

F. The nurse must approach these clients in a firm, reasonable manner and set consistent and immediate limits. They must be informed that this type of behavior will not be tolerated and of the consequences should it be displayed.

References

Faucett J. Dynamics of violence. Chicago: American Medical Association, 1971.

Lion JR. Personality disorders: diagnosis and management. 2nd ed. Baltimore: Williams & Wilkins, 1981.

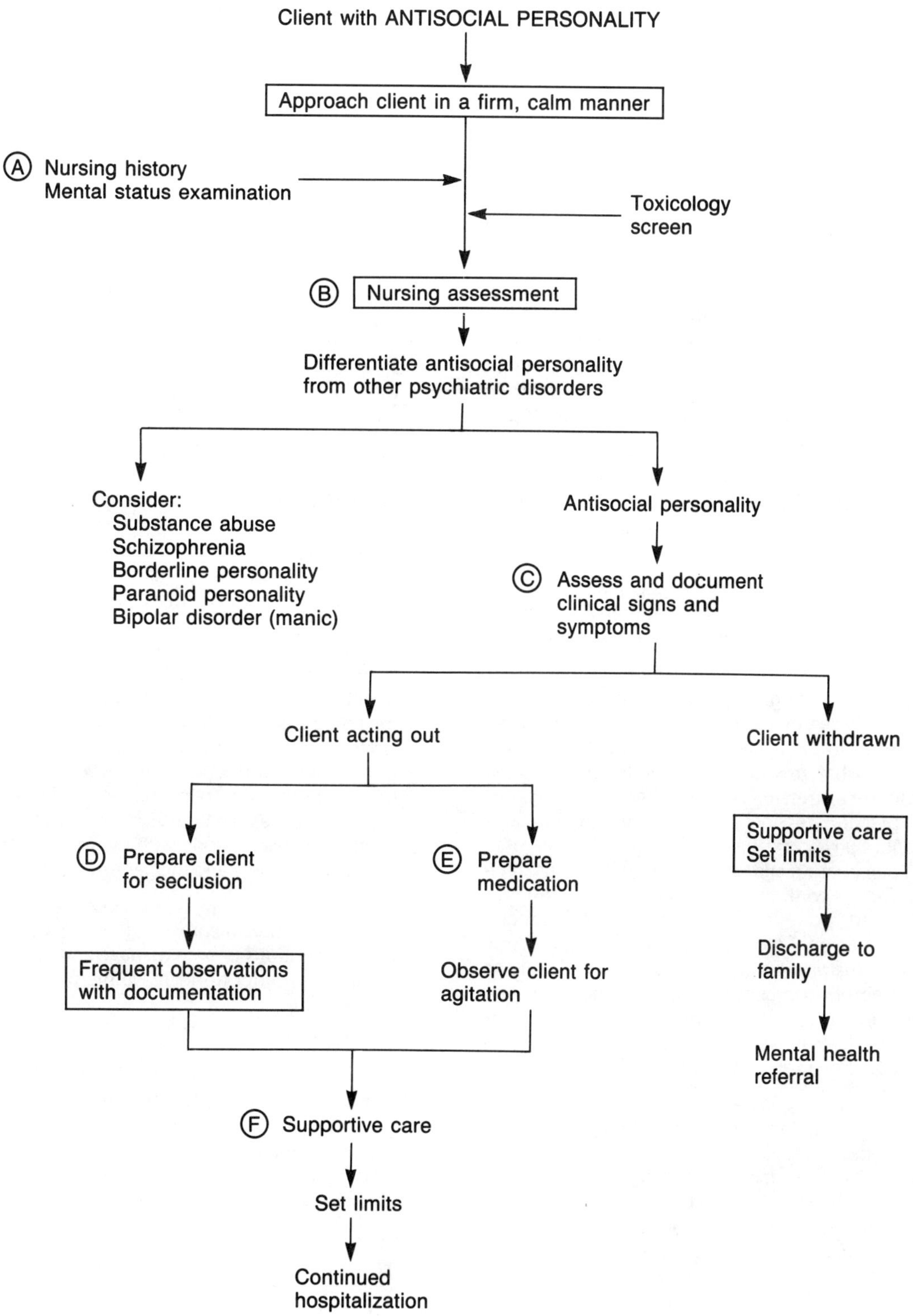
Client with ANTISOCIAL PERSONALITY
Approach client in a firm, calm manner
A Nursing history
Mental status examination
Toxicology screen
B Nursing assessment
Differentiate antisocial personality from other psychiatric disorders
Consider:
Substance abuse
Schizophrenia
Borderline personality
Paranoid personality
Bipolar disorder (manic)
Antisocial personality
C Assess and document clinical signs and symptoms
Client acting out
Client withdrawn
D Prepare client for seclusion
E Prepare medication
Supportive care
Set limits
Frequent observations with documentation
Observe client for agitation
Discharge to family
Mental health referral
F Supportive care
Set limits
Continued hospitalization

AGGRESSIVE BEHAVIOR

Mary-Lou Martin
Helen Kirkpatrick

A. Self-awareness is important for nurses who work with aggressive patients. Nurses hold expectations of themselves and of their patients; for example, the nurse may expect aggressive behavior and not assist the patient to change, or the nurse may unrealistically expect that the patient can correct or control the behavior. To develop self-awareness, the nurse must identify and work through any personal issues. Assessment of aggression is enhanced by the development of a therapeutic nurse-patient relationship (see p 98).

B. Aggressive patients create anxiety for themselves, the staff, other patients, family, and community. Aggression is a verbal or nonverbal behavior that is forceful, inappropriate, and nonadaptive.

C. The potential for aggression may be assessed by considering such risk factors as historical pattern of aggressive behavior, drug toxicity, delusional state, and physiologic disease process.

D. The nature of the patient's aggression must be assessed. What was the aggressive behavior? What cues were observed prior to the aggressive behavior? Was there a target? If yes, what or who? What were the precipitants? Where did the aggression occur? When did the aggression take place? Assessment is continuous and includes assessment of physical status, medication regimen, mental status, perceptions, and effectiveness of previous interventions. Factors contributing to patient aggression may be helplessness, powerlessness, unfamiliar environment, violation of personal space, drugs, alcohol, hallucinations, and delusions. Some patients may be unable to evaluate their environment realistically. They may perceive individuals or objects in the environment as threatening when sensory-perceptual alterations (e.g., hallucinations) or altered thought processes (e.g., delusions) are present.

E. Aggression has meaning and may be the outcome of feelings or emotions such as anxiety, fear, frustration, and anger. The challenge for nurses is to understand the meaning of the behavior for this particular patient. Aggression is frequently a behavioral response to an interpersonal situation that is anxiety producing. Aggression may be an attempt to increase self-stimulation in response to the lack of environmental stimulation, or it may represent a need to exert control when overwhelmed with feelings of powerlessness. Aggression may also be a means to get staff attention.

F. Assess the patient's repertoire of coping strategies. How does the patient cope with feelings and emotions? What effective and ineffective coping strategies has the patient used in the past? Is the patient able to identify the stressors? Does the patient have any plans to manage this stressful experience? The patient's ability to communicate may be altered by the nature of an illness or trauma. Patients may behave in the only way they can (e.g., the patient with aphasia who cannot verbalize feelings may strike out with a cane when angry). The nurse assesses the situation and assists the patient to identify needs and alternatives to the aggressive behavior.

G. Interventions are aimed where possible at assisting the patient to recognize the potential for aggression. Different etiologies direct the nurse to employ different interventions. A comprehensive assessment aids the nurse in selecting appropriate interventions that not only respond to patterns of aggressive behavior but also work to prevent it. Physical or pharmacologic intervention may be necessary; however, it may provide only temporary relief and may not prevent future episodes. Communication between nurse and patient should continue even when the patient is physically restrained or in seclusion. During interaction with the patient, the nurse should demonstrate nonthreatening behavior. The environment may also be altered to change the level of stimuli. Psychotherapy and/or counseling may assist the patient to understand the aggressive behavior. The nurse should explore each aggressive episode with the patient in order to help the patient understand the pattern and learn new coping skills.

H. Through the nursing process the nurse chooses appropriate interventions to both manage and prevent aggressive behavior in order to decrease the patient's episodes of aggression.

References

Boettcher EG. Preventing violent behavior: an integrated theoretical model for nursing. Perspect Psychiatr Care 1983; 20(2):54–58.

Lanza ML. How nurses react to patient assault. J Psychosoc Nurs 1985; 23(6):6–11.

Lion JR, Reid WH, eds. Assaults within psychiatric facilities. New York: Grune & Stratton, 1983.

Martin M-L, Kirkpatrick H. Nursing assessment of the aggressive elderly, Perspectives 1987; 11(3):8–10.

Morton PG. Staff roles and responsibilities in incidents of patient violence. Arch Psychiatr Nurs 1987; 1:280–284.

Rix G. Care plan for an aggressive person, based on Peplau's model of nursing. In: Collister B, ed. Psychiatric nursing, person to person. London: Edward Arnold, 1988.

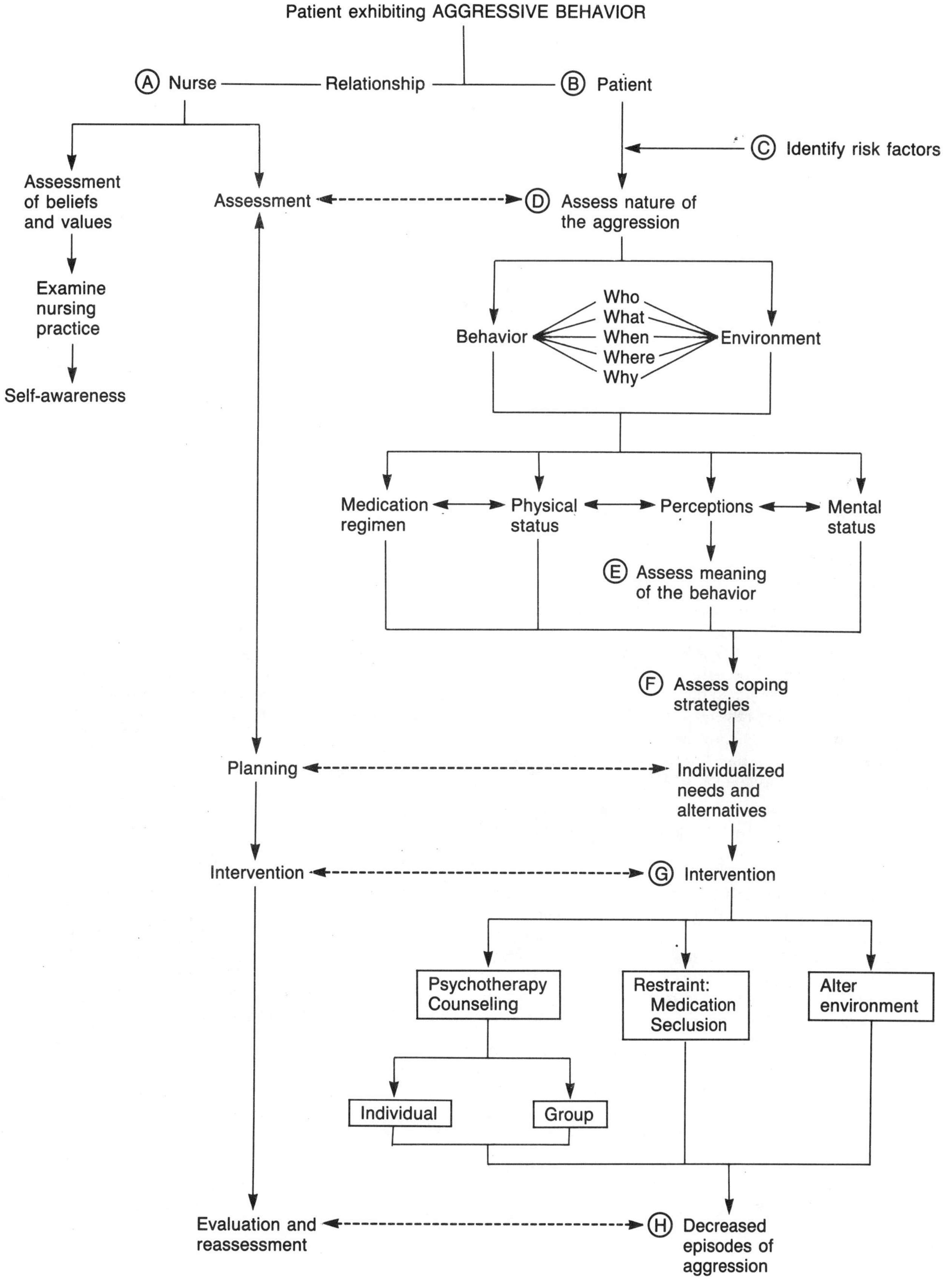
Patient exhibiting AGGRESSIVE BEHAVIOR
(A) Nurse
Relationship
(B) Patient
(C) Identify risk factors
Assessment of beliefs and values
Examine nursing practice
Self-awareness
Assessment
(D) Assess nature of the aggression
Behavior
Who
What
When
Where
Why
Environment
Medication regimen
Physical status
Perceptions
Mental status
(E) Assess meaning of the behavior
(F) Assess coping strategies
Planning
Individualized needs and alternatives
Intervention
(G) Intervention
Psychotherapy Counseling
Restraint: Medication Seclusion
Alter environment
Individual
Group
Evaluation and reassessment
(H) Decreased episodes of aggression

BORDERLINE PERSONALITY DISORDER

Jan Westwell
Elizabeth McCay

A. All interactions occurring between the nurse and client represent a combination of both the client's and nurse's personalities and experiences. The nurse-client relationship is a vehicle for both the nurse and client to understand the client's struggles. The client has a unique personality and brings an accumulation of past experiences to the nurse-client relationship. In particular, a person with a borderline personality is thought to continue the struggle of separation-individuation in this relationship. As a result, the borderline client may exhibit self-destructive behavior, a pattern of unstable and/or intense relationships, intense anger, impulsiveness, an underdeveloped sense of self, affective instability, transient psychotic episodes, chronic feelings of emptiness and boredom, and an intolerance of being alone. The nurse also has a unique personality and brings an accumulation of past experiences to the nurse-client relationship. The nurse's sense of self and clinical expertise directly influence the quality of the relationship.

B. Acting-out behavior is related to the client's inability to tolerate and/or verbalize affect. Acting-out behavior may include eloping, slashing, drinking, sexual promiscuity, and aggressive behavior. Nursing interventions are directed toward limiting the acting-out behavior in a non-punitive manner. Attention must also be given to helping the client understand the meaning of the acting-out behavior. Contracting can provide the external structure to augment ego functioning and provide an environment in which to do therapeutic work (see p 130).

C. Idealization and devaluation are components of splitting. Splitting is a primitive defense that protects the client from being overwhelmed by both the good and bad internal representations of his or her relationships with others. Consequently, the client's relationships with staff are usually characterized by rejection or idealization. Recognition of this mechanism as defensive rather than personally directed will prevent the nurse from acting on feelings of flattery or hostility. Staff will experience different parts of the client as a result of splitting and lack of object constancy.

D. Abandonment depression is experienced by the client in relation to a perceived or actual withdrawal of emotional support. This withdrawal is devastating for the client because it is reminiscent of earlier maternal abandonment. During this affective state, the client feels empty, hopeless, and is vulnerable to suicidal impulsivity. Therefore, the nurse needs to ensure the client's safety. The nurse may help the client to understand the precipitant(s) that led to this crisis. Throughout this process, the nurse provides a sense of realistic hopefulness for the client.

E. The nurse has several responsibilities that will affect the quality of his or her therapeutic work with the client. Clinical supervision is essential. Frequent multidisciplinary team meetings that promote open discussion are also necessary to prevent the chaos, confusion, and disagreement that may result from unrecognized transference and countertransference responses. Owing to the complex nature of these clients, additional reading is recommended.

F. Criteria that may affect the client's response to treatment include the fit between the nurse and the client; the degree of the client's pathology; and the expectations held. Client improvement may be manifested by a decrease in acting out, more stable relationships, and increased sense of self.

G. The client who is able to tolerate and remain engaged in a therapeutic nurse-client relationship may be a candidate for long-term insight-oriented therapy with an experienced therapist.

H. When no improvement is noted it is necessary to reassess the therapeutic relationship and the multidisciplinary team approach.

References

Adler G. Hospital treatment of borderline patient. Am J Psychiatry 1973; 130(1):32–36.

American Psychiatric Association. Diagnostic and statistical manual of mental disorders (DSM III R). Washington, DC: American Psychiatric Association, 1987.

Carser D. The defense mechanism of splitting: developmental origins, effects on staff, recommendations for nursing. J Psychiatr Nurs Mental Health Serv 1979; 17(3):21–28.

Gallop R. Escaping borderline stereotypes. J Psychosoc Nurs 1988; 26(2):16–20.

Silver D. Psychodynamics and psychotherapeutic management of the self-destructive character disordered patient. Psychiatr Clin North Am 1985; 8:357–375.

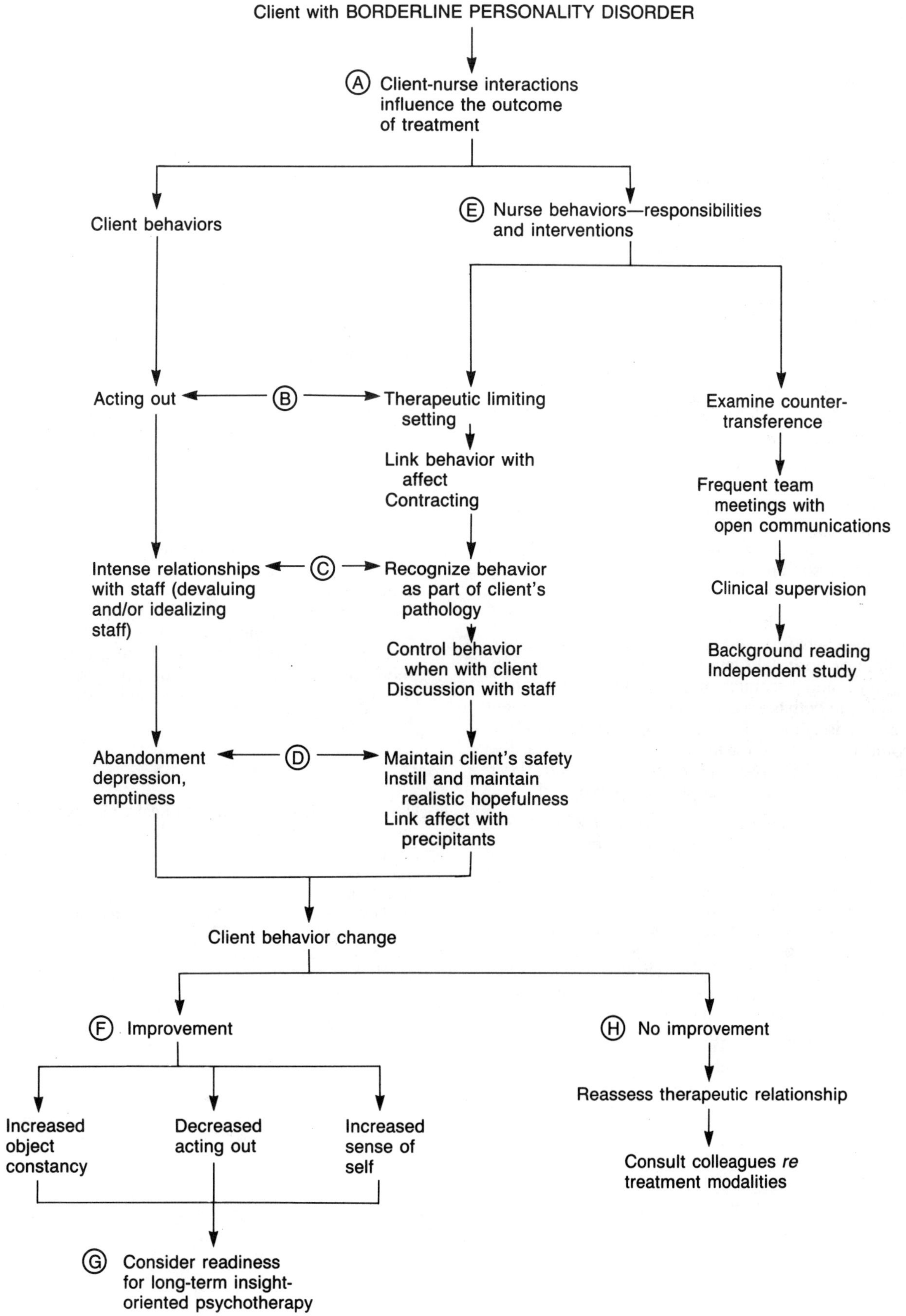
Client with BORDERLINE PERSONALITY DISORDER
(A) Client-nurse interactions influence the outcome of treatment
Client behaviors
(E) Nurse behaviors—responsibilities and interventions
Acting out
(B)
Therapeutic limiting setting
Link behavior with affect
Contracting
Examine counter-transference
Frequent team meetings with open communications
Clinical supervision
Background reading
Independent study
Intense relationships with staff (devaluing and/or idealizing staff)
(C)
Recognize behavior as part of client's pathology
Control behavior when with client
Discussion with staff
Abandonment depression, emptiness
(D)
Maintain client's safety
Instill and maintain realistic hopefulness
Link affect with precipitants
Client behavior change
(F) Improvement
(H) No improvement
Increased object constancy
Decreased acting out
Increased sense of self
Reassess therapeutic relationship
Consult colleagues *re* treatment modalities
(G) Consider readiness for long-term insight-oriented psychotherapy

PASSIVE-AGGRESSIVE PERSONALITY

Andrea Baumann

Passive-aggressive behavior is a personality disorder characterized by ineffective coping strategies such as forgetfulness, procrastination, negativism, eating disorders, or a series of unsuccessful drug overdoses. Milder, irritating habits such as habitual lateness and disruptive behavior (i.e., belching, gum cracking) may also be a sign of this maladaptive behavior. The behavior is a defensive mode of living rather than an overt psychiatric illness. The disorder is thought to result from feelings of anger that are turned inward. The manifestation of the behavior over time may be quite subtle. The client may seek help because he or she may feel ineffective and unappreciated both in the workplace and socially. It is important to develop insight into defensive behavior and develop more adaptive positive responses.

A. The disorder is thought to originate in early childhood when there was not a climate to express angry or hostile feelings in an overt and healthy fashion. The person becomes outwardly submissive and tries to control the environment by manipulative behaviors. People withdraw from the person and the behavior eventually becomes self-defeating.

B. Assessment is an important phase of the relationship when the client first presents to the therapist. There may be little or no insight into the behavior. However, unhappiness and discomfort may be expressed about relationships in both the social and work realm. Assessment of any underlying depression is important because this should be treated through counseling and supportive pharmacologic interventions. Family and individual patterns of dealing with anger should be explored.

C. Immediate treatment focuses on crisis resolution (see "Crisis State," p 8), and long-term interventions are targeted at a more adaptive approach to both social and work life. Ineffective coping behaviors must be identified and more positive behaviors reinforced. Some clients may be receptive to pointing out when passive behavior (not directly confronting the issue) is being used. However, some clients may passively resist behaviors that lead to adequate adjustment. Appropriate expression of anger and accurate identification of the maladaptive behaviors are important aspects on which to focus. Anger must be channeled away from resistance to more productive modes of behavior.

D. These clients are difficult to treat because they may provoke the therapist and prevent attempts to help them. The client-therapist interaction is frustrating because the client may resist attempts to help, and there may be a treatment impasse due to the pattern of resistance the client has set up. The nurse therapist needs to recognize and deal with his or her personal reactions in order to avoid abandoning the client.

E. Assertiveness training is helpful to reinforce autonomy, self-reliance, and general feelings of competence (see "Assertiveness Training," p 126). The use of counter-projection, time out, confrontation, role playing, and limit-setting techniques are some examples of important therapeutic approaches. Also, there may be a need for family and group therapy or long-term psychotherapy.

F. It is important to reinforce behaviors that increase the client's sense of social competence and encourage relationships that increase confidence and self-esteem and lead to more adaptive social behaviors. Termination is appropriate when the patient becomes less defensive, feels more comfortable about expressing anger, and feels more autonomous. A positive outcome is the foundation for adaptable social behaviors and insight into the maladaptive behaviors.

References

Birckhead L. Psychiatric and mental health nursing: the therapeutic use of self. Philadelphia: JB Lippincott, 1989:401–426.

Greene JA. Maladaptation: the personality disorders. In: Johnson B, ed. Adaptation and growth: psychiatric and mental health nursing. Philadelphia: JB Lippincott, 1989:374–375.

Perry C, Flannery L. Passive aggressive personality disorder. J Nerv Disord Ment Dis 1982; 170:164–173.

Rawlins R, Thomas S. Anger. In: Beck C, Rawlins R, Williams S, eds. Mental health and psychiatric nursing. St. Louis: CV Mosby, 1988:228–230.

Wilson H, Kneisl C. Psychiatric nursing. Menlo Park, CA: Addison-Wesley, 1988:573–579.

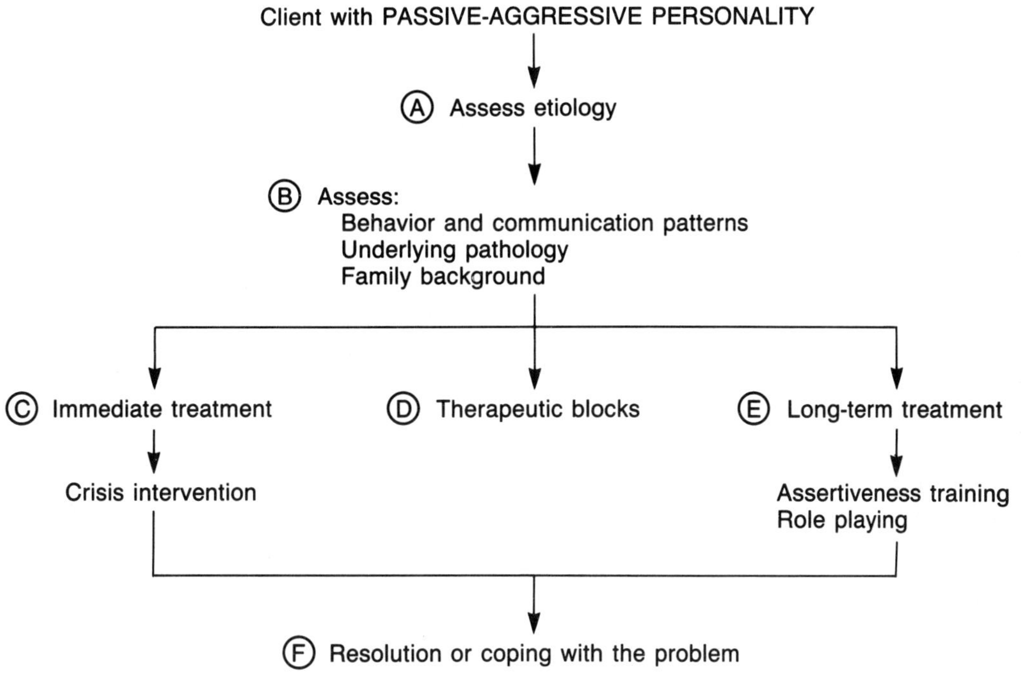
Client with PASSIVE-AGGRESSIVE PERSONALITY
Ⓐ Assess etiology
Ⓑ Assess:
Behavior and communication patterns
Underlying pathology
Family background
Ⓒ Immediate treatment
Crisis intervention
Ⓓ Therapeutic blocks
Ⓔ Long-term treatment
Assertiveness training
Role playing
Ⓕ Resolution or coping with the problem

ALZHEIMER'S DISEASE

Andrea Baumann
Marilyn E. Dewis

A. Alzheimer's disease is the most prevalent example of a chronic organic mental disorder. It is characterized by impaired intellectual function, judgment, and concentration, and accounts for 65 percent of all cases of dementia. Like many other dementias, the initial signs are subtle, beginning as early as 40 years of age. Clients observe changes such as forgetfulness and inability to concentrate, which can result in frustration and depression. In the early stages, there may be denial of symptoms. Family members and the client may notice these changes and attribute them to fatigue, stress, or the normal aging process. Early nursing assessment occurs in the community setting, and care is provided by the client, the family, and the nurse.

B. Stage 1 is characterized by mild-to-moderate cognitive loss. The clinical signs include absent-mindedness, lack of concentration, carelessness, and some emotional instability. In the early stages, the family members and the client require emotional support, informational counseling, and plans and goals for long-term care. Traditional family roles may change as the disease progresses. Families and clients require information about the progressive symptoms and community resources that are available for both respite care and group meetings.

C. In stage 2, the client usually exhibits signs of progressive dementia. There may be considerable disorientation, lack of comprehension, and restlessness at night. As the disease progresses, it can put stress on family functioning. The client may have difficulty recognizing his or her own face (mirror sign). Inability to read and write (agraphia) or to carry out skills and purposeful movements (apraxia) also occurs. These symptoms may be coupled with increasing physical incapacity, such as decreased muscle tone and an unsteady gait. Even in these later stages, care may be provided by family members (typically the spouse). This is the preferred situation; however, it does put a major burden on family members. Nursing interventions must focus on the care of family members as they may be limited by their own health problems or by trying to balance other responsibilities such as child rearing or working outside the home (in the case of the children). Community support services such as respite care and daily care programs can help alleviate stress and social isolation.

D. The third stage is the most incapacitated stage and requires long-term institutionalization. There is increased irritability, low frustration, and aggressive behavior. There may be such signs and symptoms as bulimia, visual agnosia, agnosia, aphasia, and apraxia. Symptoms vary according to the extent and degree of the pathologic lesions. The focus continues to be support of family with ongoing education and interpretation of the disease progression. It can be very difficult for family members to accept the total incapacity of the patient. It is important at this time to make family members aware of power of attorney and possibly the use of a public trustee. Although the long-range outlook is not hopeful, the quality of life for both the individual and the family can be improved through informed and caring professional interventions.

References

Deppel R, Hutton J. Caring for the Alzheimer patient: practical guide. Buffalo: Prometheus Books, 1988.

Dewis M, Baumann A. Alzheimer disease: the silent epidemic. Can Nurse 1982; 78:32–35.

Edelson J, Lyons W. Institutional care of the mentally impaired elderly. New York: Van Nostrand Reinhold, 1985.

Kelly W, ed. Alzheimer disease and related disorders: research and management. Springfield, IL: Charles C Thomas, 1984.

More N, Rabins D. The 36-hour day. Baltimore: The Johns Hopkins University Press, 1981.

Powell L, Courtier K. Alzheimer's disease: a guide for families. Reading, MA: Addison Wesley, 1983.

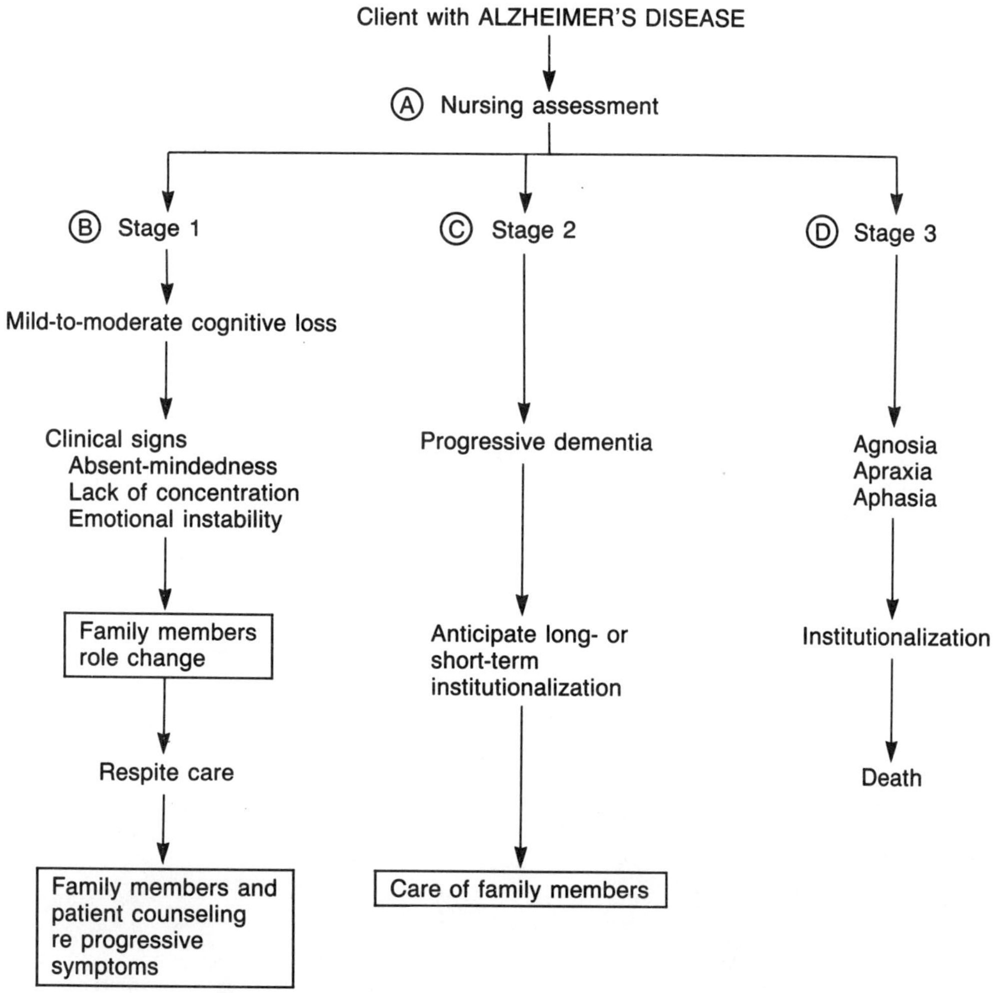
Client with ALZHEIMER'S DISEASE
(A) Nursing assessment
(B) Stage 1
(C) Stage 2
(D) Stage 3
Mild-to-moderate cognitive loss
Clinical signs
Absent-mindedness
Lack of concentration
Emotional instability
Family members role change
Respite care
Family members and patient counseling re progressive symptoms
Progressive dementia
Anticipate long- or short-term institutionalization
Care of family members
Agnosia
Apraxia
Aphasia
Institutionalization
Death

III NURSING THERAPEUTICS

GROUPS

THE THERAPEUTIC RELATIONSHIP

Nancy E. Johnston

A. The primary emphasis in therapeutic interviews is on the development of a supportive relationship. This relationship allows the client to identify and work through personal issues, concerns, and problems. Although the main purpose of the relationship is to help the client, it is important to recognize that both the nurse and the client bring perceptions, values, judgments, and expectations to the relationship. The degree to which the nurse is effective in establishing a relationship that is truly therapeutic depends on her own self-awareness, the extent to which she has clarified her own values, and the expertise with which she approaches the situation.

B. During the early phase of the relationship it is important to establish a warm tone and a comfortable climate. This can be facilitated by conveying to the client that the nurse is empathic and able to view the world from the client's particular frame of reference. Rapport is strengthened by congruence between what the client is attempting to convey and the nurse's correct understanding of the message. The nurse's accurate perception is then reflected back to the client. During this relationship-building phase all judgment is suspended and unconditional positive regard is emphasized.

C. As the client begins to relax, more information is offered. How the client thinks and behaves in relation to people and situations becomes evident from both what is said and what is not said. Careful observation of client's verbal and nonverbal behavior provides the nurse with extensive data on conflicts that the client may be neither aware of nor able to articulate. Shifting eye-contact, vocal qualities, and body posture provide clues as to the comfort level with which the client is able to discuss various subjects. Changing topics of discussion, selective focus, and the use of key words are other observations the nurse may use to discover underlying messages and hidden conflicts. It is essential to ask the client a number of questions in order to clarify the nature of the problem and the request for help. It is, however, important to avoid overusing closed questions that tend to make the client feel interrogated. Encouragement, paraphrasing, and summarizing allow further exploration of certain issues. The accurate reflection of feeling and meaning allow the client to be explicit about feelings that may have remained hidden or only partially revealed. The reflection of meaning helps to facilitate the interpretation of the client's own values, goals, and experience.

D. As the client gains greater confidence in pursuing the deeper meanings of various feelings and experiences, a strong working alliance between the nurse and the client emerges. The client trusts the nurse to attend to the technical details of facilitating insight, while the client pursues the exploration of issues that heretofore had been elusive or overwhelming.

E. In order to facilitate better self-understanding on the part of the client, it is necessary that the nurse enable the client to be specific rather than vague when describing problematic feelings or situations. Abstract generalities are to be avoided, and concrete examples are elicited in order to pave the way to seeking definite change. As the necessity for change becomes more apparent, the client may experience stronger resistance. The genuineness and immediacy of the nurse are emphasized in order to decrease resistance and promote a heightened sense of authenticity, closeness, and deep valuing. Within this intensely meaningful context the client is often able to grieve, thereby achieving catharsis. Catharsis then frees energy that can be channeled toward positive change.

F. As the client begins to take tentative and cautious steps toward change it may be helpful to use a number of more directive skills. Caution must be exercised to ensure that the client has given permission to the nurse to use these skills; otherwise the client may feel manipulated and will become resistant. Pointing out the logical consequences of certain actions, reframing the client's interpretation, and providing feedback are some of the ways the nurse can actively influence the client to find a focus for change.

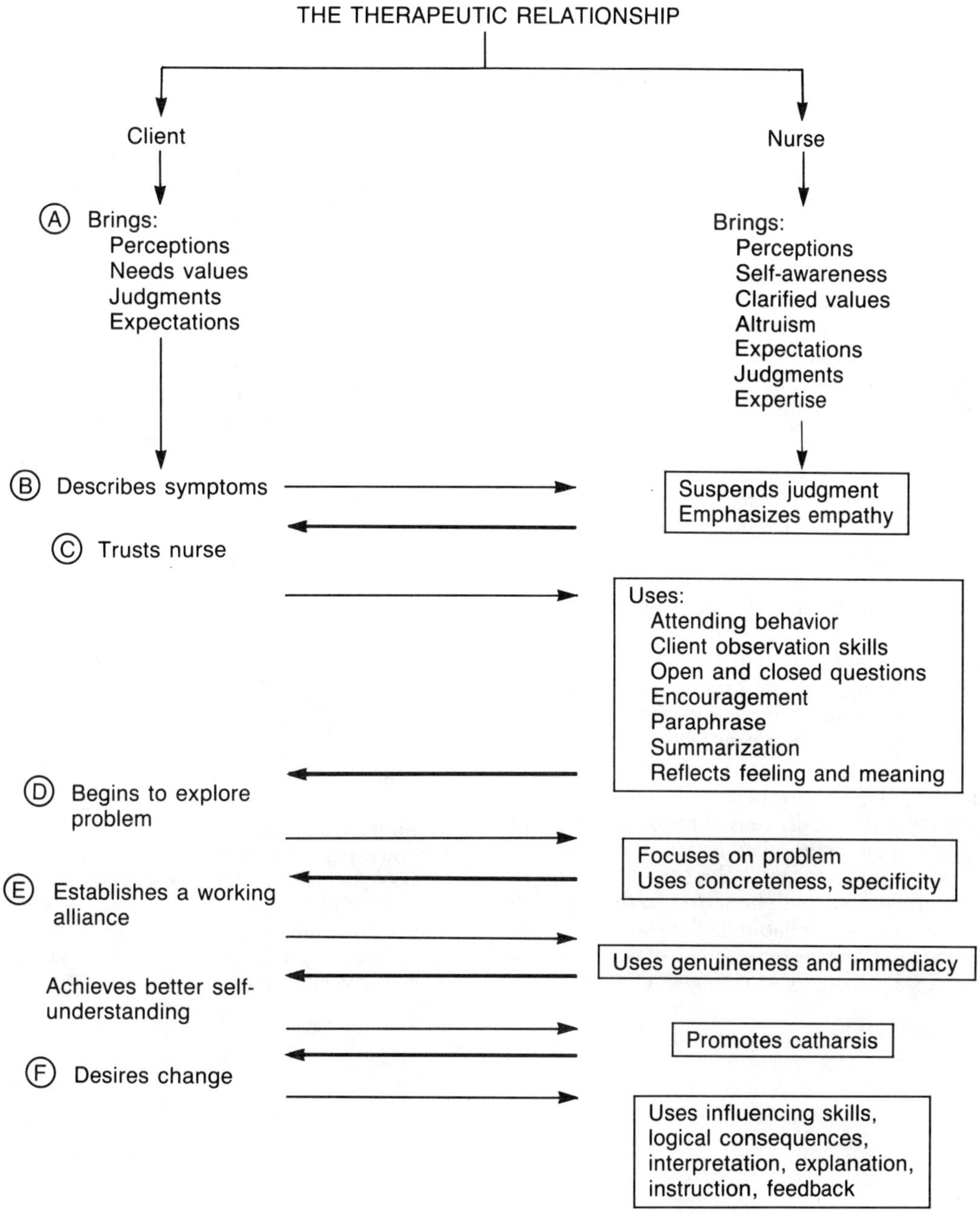

Cont'd on p 101

G. Defining a goal is the pivotal point of the therapeutic relationship. Notwithstanding the nurse's perception of the problem and her expertise, it is necessary for the client rather than the nurse to assume the responsibility for goal definition. Once the goal has been defined, the nurse uses the skill of confrontation to identify mixed messages and incongruities between the client's goals and behaviors. Once the incongruities and discrepancies are identified, they must be communicated to the client.

H. Once the goal has been defined it may become obvious that there are several ways to meet the goal. Confusion related to the choice of the most desirable alternative may ensue. Role playing various alternatives may be a helpful method of selecting one. Frequently the pain and uncertainty associated with giving up a nonadaptive behavior and learning a new one elicits strong transference and countertransference issues (p 114). The resistance of the client or a strong countertransference reaction from the nurse may result in a therapeutic impasse that has to be resolved before further progress can occur.

I. As the client regains a feeling of security within the therapeutic relationship, confidence is restored and the client begins to take more appropriate action or direction. It becomes extremely important at this stage for the nurse to reinforce and reward these behaviors so that they become consolidated and reliable methods of coping. As the nurse and the client become confident that the client is able to sustain these new changes, the subject of closure is raised. The nurse summarizes the issues that have been dealt with and reviews remaining issues to be resolved outside of the therapeutic relationship.

J. The client is content with the changes that have occurred but fears "going it alone." Sadness is also experienced in relation to the termination of the therapeutic relationship. As these issues are worked through, positive coping is generalized to everyday life. The client understands that termination does not mean the end of personal growth. Rather the strength and knowledge acquired through the therapeutic relationship are used in the continuing process of achieving positive gains.

References

Coad-Chapman A. Therapeutic superficiality and intimacy. In: Longo DC, Williams RA, eds. Clinical practice in psychosocial nursing. 2nd ed. Norwalk, CT: Appleton-Century-Crofts, 1986:23–46.

Cormier LS, Cormier WH, Weisser RJ. Interviewing and helping skills for health professionals. Monterey, CA: Wadsworth, 1984.

Ivey AE. Intentional interviewing and counseling. Monterey, CA: Brooks/Cole, 1982.

Northouse PG, Northouse LL. Health communication: a handbook for health professionals. Englewood Cliffs, NJ: Prentice-Hall, 1985.

Smith S. Communications in nursing, communicating assertively and responsibly in nursing: a guidebook. Toronto: McGraw-Hill Ryerson, 1986.

Cont'd from p 99

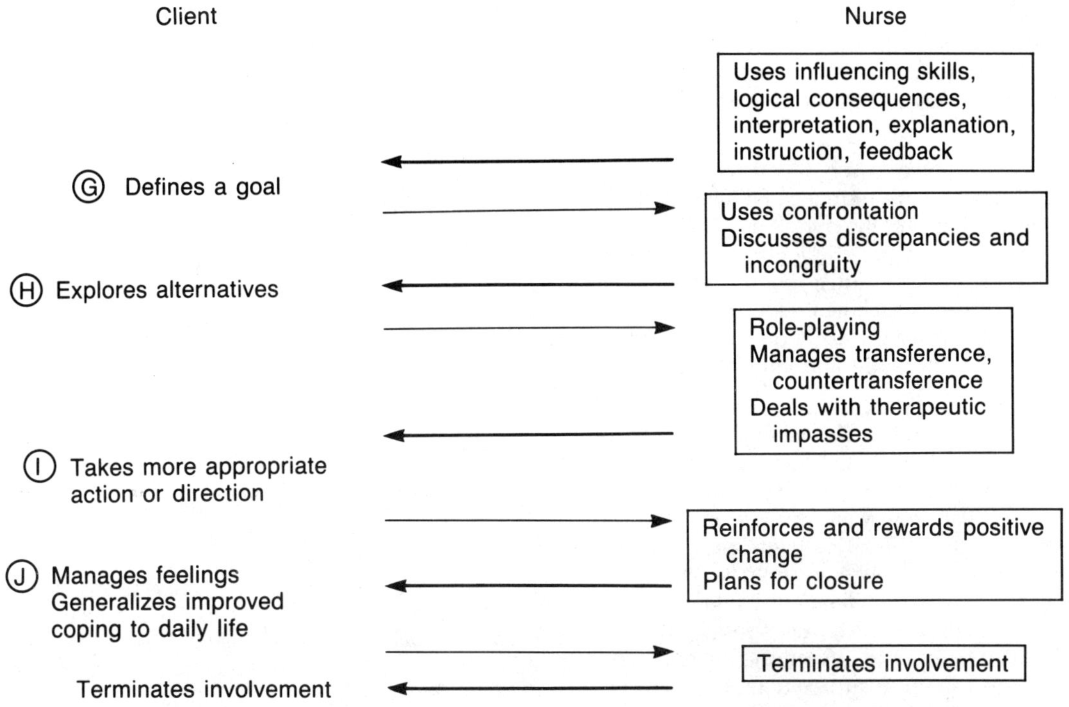

THERAPEUTIC USE OF SELF

Jan Westwell
Cheryl Forchuk

A. Both the client and nurse bring themselves, their history, and their values to an interaction. This combination creates unique interactions and relationships. Each encounter evokes feelings and thoughts within both the nurse and client.

B. Clinical supervision and/or psychotherapy promotes the exploration of perceptions, thoughts, feelings, and behaviors. Understanding how the nurse's personal dynamics are enacted within nurse-client interactions is essential, because unconscious, poorly understood material will be played out. Clinical supervision and psychotherapy for the nurse are usually provided by someone with advanced education and clinical expertise.

C. Feelings, thoughts, and behaviors arise from a variety of sources. They provide a sense of what might be happening with the nurse, the client, and their interaction. The nurse reflects upon all thoughts, feelings, and behaviors, as these may facilitate self-awareness and insight. The nurse differentiates the feelings, thoughts, and behaviors that result from the client's behavior, from those feelings and thoughts that emerge from the nurse's internal world. These are not mutually exclusive categories. By identifying the probable sources and influences, the nurse can identify: (1) when work needs to be done on his or her own issues, (2) what thoughts and feelings originating from client behavior might mean about the client (and his or her relationships with others), and (3) when issues can be worked on within the nurse-client relationship.

D. Being aware of thoughts, feelings, and behaviors is not enough. Part of being clinically competent is to make sense of the myriad of feelings, thoughts, and behaviors. Making sense of these allows the nurse to know how and when to use or act on them. The more self-understanding the nurse has, the more available she or he will be to focus on the client. What happens within the nurse, the nurse-client interactions, and the nurse-client relationship become the focus of clinical supervision. Psychotherapy enhances the nurse's self-understanding.

References

Cross PW. Intellectualizing about the value of the unconscious. Perspect Psychiatr Care 1976; 14(3):130–132.

Gauthier M. Countertransference and supervision: a discussion of some dynamics from the point of view of the supervisee. Can J Psychiatry 1984; 29:513–519.

Gregg DE, Bregg EA, Spring FE. Individual supervision: a method of teaching psychiatric concepts in nursing education. Perspect Psychiatr Care 1976; 14(3):115–129.

Peplau HE. Interpersonal constructs for nursing practice. Nurse Educ Today 1987; 7:201–208.

Riemen DJ. Noncaring and caring in the clinical setting: patients' descriptions. Top Clin Nurs 1986; 8(2):30–36.

Searles HF. The informational value of the supervisor's emotional experiences. Psychiatry 1955; 18:135–146.

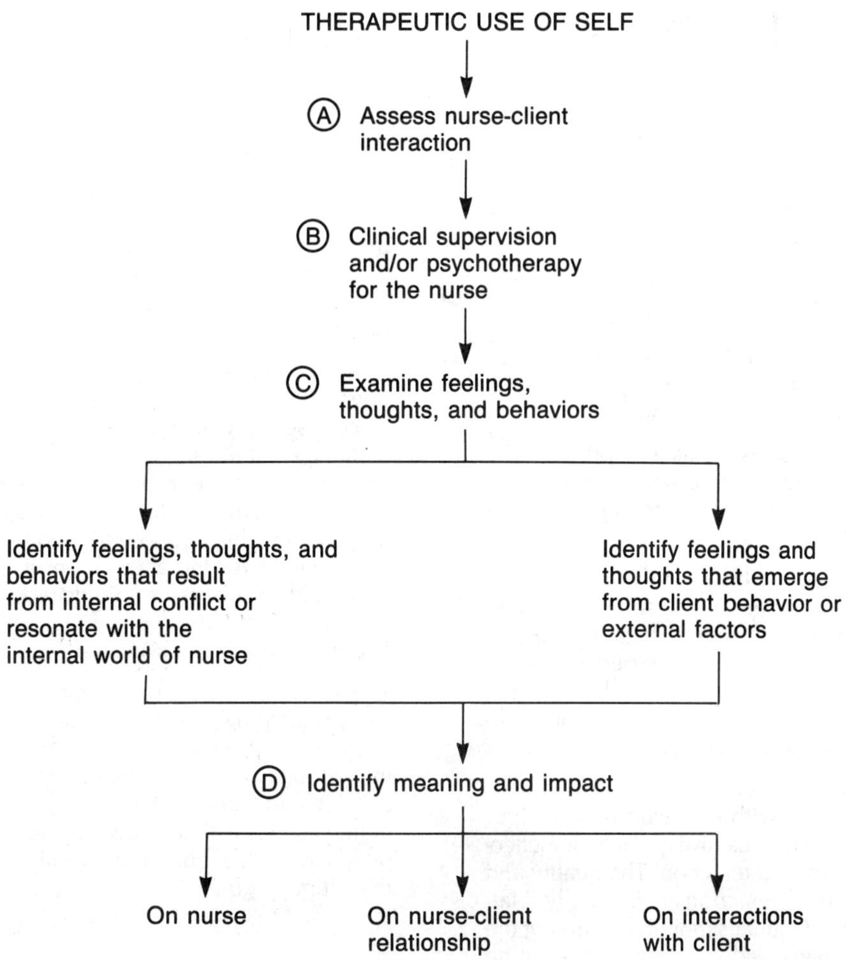
THERAPEUTIC USE OF SELF
(A) Assess nurse-client interaction
(B) Clinical supervision and/or psychotherapy for the nurse
(C) Examine feelings, thoughts, and behaviors
Identify feelings, thoughts, and behaviors that result from internal conflict or resonate with the internal world of nurse
Identify feelings and thoughts that emerge from client behavior or external factors
(D) Identify meaning and impact
On nurse
On nurse-client relationship
On interactions with client

IMPAIRED INTERPERSONAL INTERACTION

Mary-Lou Martin
Jan Westwell

Interpersonal interaction refers to a pattern of relating (i.e., not one single interaction) between at least two individuals. All persons in the interaction contribute to the process. Interpersonal interaction is a dynamic process that requires awareness of the relationship and the social context. Each interaction is a unique multidimensional experience that includes both verbal and nonverbal communication.

A. Learning to interact with others is a lifelong process. The establishment and maintenance of satisfying interpersonal interactions is critical to most individuals' sense of self.

B. When a client identifies dissatisfaction with his or her pattern of interaction, impaired interpersonal interaction is likely present. Clients with mental health problems may have more difficulty with their interpersonal interactions, depending upon the age of onset and the severity of their illness. These factors influence the client's ability to acquire the knowledge and skills required for interpersonal interaction.

C. The client's dissatisfaction with interactions may occur because of an insufficient or excessive quantity or ineffective quality of interpersonal interaction. The quality and quantity of interpersonal interaction are integrally related. For example, one individual's monopolization of the conversation may be perceived by another as affecting the quality of their interactions. Three areas to assess in interaction are communication factors, interpersonal factors, and intrapersonal factors. Communication factors include listening abilities, speech content, and amount of talking. Interpersonal factors include cultural fit, interpersonal attractiveness, and interpersonal skills. Intrapersonal factors include values and beliefs, comfort, and self-concept.

D. All individuals (e.g., the nurse and client) play a part in the process and outcome of any interaction. Each participant's perception of that interaction may be different. Through a therapeutic relationship, the nurse and client seek to understand the meaning of the client's interpersonal interactions. The nurse's understanding of the interaction process can be assisted by the examination of the nurse's personal experience and participation in the interaction with the client. Clinical supervision and self-awareness can assist the nurse in this endeavor. Discussions with others may also provide the nurse with a more complete picture of the client's interactional style. One individual may have specific problems in an interaction; however, the interaction is not a reflection of only one individual.

E. A variety of therapeutic modalities can be used to influence the interaction process. Individual psychotherapy or counseling will provide a nurturing relationship in which the client can identify the subjective experience, relate events in order to make sense of the experience, and explore ways of interacting. Group therapy is another modality in which the client's understanding of self and others facilitates the acquisition of increased interpersonal skills. Social skills training provides education and opportunities for the client to practice relating to others. A pluralistic approach is often the most effective.

F. The ability to interact satisfactorily with others is a continuous learning process. Evaluation involves assessment of the client's awareness of his or her participation in interactions and the ability to be cognizant of the relationship and context. Others' observations and responses to interactions with the client are also an important component of evaluation. Mutually satisfying interactions are the ultimate goal.

References

Brady JP. Social skills training for psychiatric patients. I: Concepts, methods and clinical results. Am J Psychiatry 1984; 141:333–340.

Brady JP. Social skills training for psychiatric patients. II: Clinical outcome studies. Am J Psychiatry 1984; 141:491–498.

Breier A, Strauss JS. The role of social relationships in the recovery from psychotic disorders. Am J Psychiatry 1984; 14:949–955.

Liberman RP. Assessment of social skills. Schizophrenia Bulletin 1982; 8(1):62–64.

Manderino MA, Bzdek VM. Social skill building with chronic patients. J Psychosoc Nurs 1987; 25(9):18–22.

Methven D, Schlotfeldt RM. The social interaction inventory. Nurs Res 1962; 11(2):83–88.

Westwell J, Martin M-L. Impaired social interaction. In: McFarland GK, Thomas MD, eds. Psychiatric mental health nursing: nursing diagnosis and process. Philadelphia: JB Lippincott, in press.

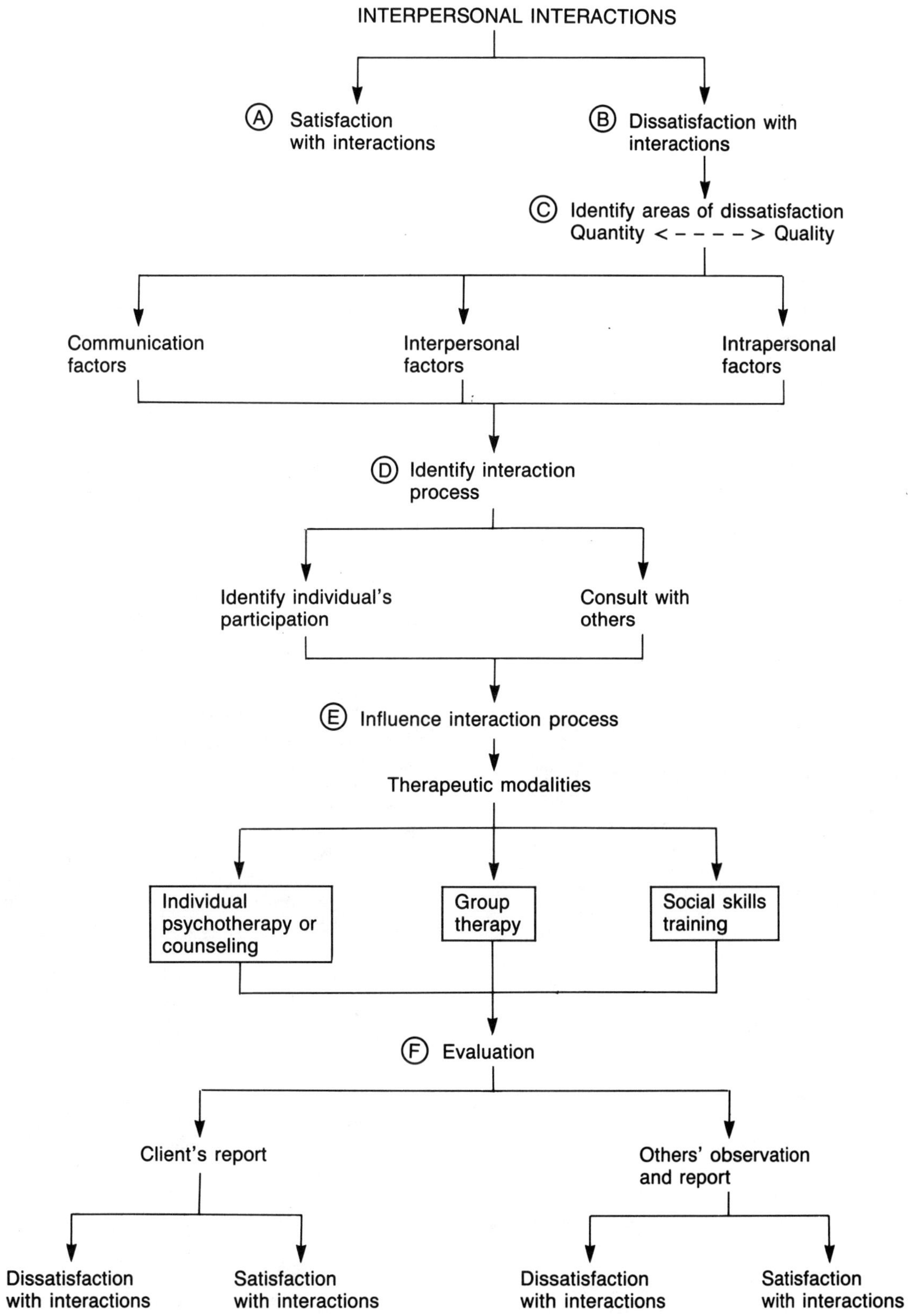
INTERPERSONAL INTERACTIONS
(A) Satisfaction with interactions
(B) Dissatisfaction with interactions
(C) Identify areas of dissatisfaction
Quantity < - - - - - > Quality
Communication factors
Interpersonal factors
Intrapersonal factors
(D) Identify interaction process
Identify individual's participation
Consult with others
(E) Influence interaction process
Therapeutic modalities
Individual psychotherapy or counseling
Group therapy
Social skills training
(F) Evaluation
Client's report
Others' observation and report
Dissatisfaction with interactions
Satisfaction with interactions
Dissatisfaction with interactions
Satisfaction with interactions

PROBLEM SOLVING

Gulrosebegum N. Jiwani

The problem-solving approach is a common psychotherapeutic technique used by nurses to assist clients to cope more effectively with identified problem areas. Its efficacy is seen when clients experience successful outcomes and exhibit improved coping skills and problem-solving competence.

A. Suitability for problem solving requires possession of intact cognitive capabilities as noted in the mental processes of reality testing, reasoning, comprehension, problem-solving, judgment, memory, and abstraction.

B. Clients unsuitable for problem solving include those who (1) are acutely ill and unable to think logically; (2) have compromised intellectual capabilities (e.g., mental retardation, delirium, and organic mental disorders); (3) are experiencing conditions that interfere with concentration and thought patterns (e.g., schizophrenia, delusional [paranoid] disorder, acute psychotic states, anxiety disorders); and (4) are under the influence of mind-altering substances. Extreme use of ego defense mechanisms also renders the client unsuitable, since defense mechanisms produce denial, misinterpretation, or distortion of reality. Coping skills provide valuable information about the client's past and present attempts to deal with problems.

C. Receptiveness to problem solving depends on past experience related to the immediate problem as well as individual personality characteristics. These characteristics are: (1) **value system**—the client's values, beliefs including cultural orientation give direction and meaning to the client situation, and direct priority-setting; (2) **self-concept**—acceptance of the client's worth will influence the client's confidence and ability to deal successfully with complex problems; (3) **ambiguity tolerance**—the nurse encourages the client to weigh the costs and rewards of several alternatives and gather adequate information before making a decision; (4) **risk taking**—the nurse gently explores the client's fears and uncertainties about various alternatives; the nurse's ongoing availability and support facilitates client commitment to a decision; (5) **locus of control**—clients with an internal locus of control will be more receptive to problem solving and assume responsibility for outcomes, whereas those with external loci of control will have difficulty exerting influence on attaining specific outcomes. The nurse's self-awareness is critical, since the nurse's own locus of control directly affects the nurse-client relationship. The nurse with an external locus of control may allow clients to blame others for life's problems and foster unhealthy dependence. The nurse with an internal locus of control will redirect clients to devote energy to themselves and to problem solving. Internality is preferred in both participants for effective problem solving, and can be fostered in the client by increasing client involvement in the plan of care; (6) **motivation for change**—clients experiencing low desire for alleviation of an intolerable situation, low disparity between hoped-for and actual situation, and low internal and external demands for change, including high payoff in existing circumstances, are unlikely to engage in effective problem solving. The nurse needs to address issues related to the client's motivation to change before engaging in the problem-solving process.

D. Problem identification involves four areas: (1) client's definition of present problems—the nurse helps the client describe and specify problems; (2) significance of the problem—the nurse asks about the onset of the problem and what contributes to its continuation; (3) past and future influences—the nurse helps the client describe values and beliefs influencing the client's definition of the problem; and (4) prioritizing problems—immediacy and relevancy of the problems to the client is considered paramount, with problems being ranked as to their degree of importance to the client.

E. Focus on one problem at a time so that the client does not feel overwhelmed. The problem-solving process involves six steps. First, **identifying past attempted solutions**. The nurse listens, observes, encourages, and evaluates, as the client verbalizes the specifics of past attempts, how they were implemented, and what occurred as a result. Second, **listing alternative ways of solving the problem**. Brainstorming sessions are helpful since they increase creativity in problem solving. Third, **predicting probable consequences of each alternative**. Fourth, **choosing an alternative**. Care is taken not to make the decision for the client. The nurse conveys extreme sensitivity, and respects the client's right to make his or her decisions and eventually accept responsibility for the consequences of those decisions. Specific, measurable outcomes are then formulated. The fifth step requires **implementing the proposed solution** in either a practice or real situation. Care is taken not to rescue the client from mistakes, since such action conveys that the client is incapable of taking charge of his or her life. The final step in the problem-solving process involves **evaluation**, whereby outcomes are reviewed and a determination of success or failure of each is done.

F. Failing to achieve an outcome requires that the nurse and the client analyze how and in what way the solution was ineffective. Particular attention is given not to blame the client or the nurse for the ineffectiveness of the solution. This exploration is followed by selection of a new solution or modification of the old solution.

G. The nurse can improve problem-solving competence in clients by providing opportunities for role playing with corrective feedback and by supporting the client's efforts at practicing problem-solving skills in a variety of life situations.

References

American Psychiatric Association. Diagnostic and statistical manual of mental disorders. 3rd ed. Washington, DC: American Psychiatric Association, 1987.

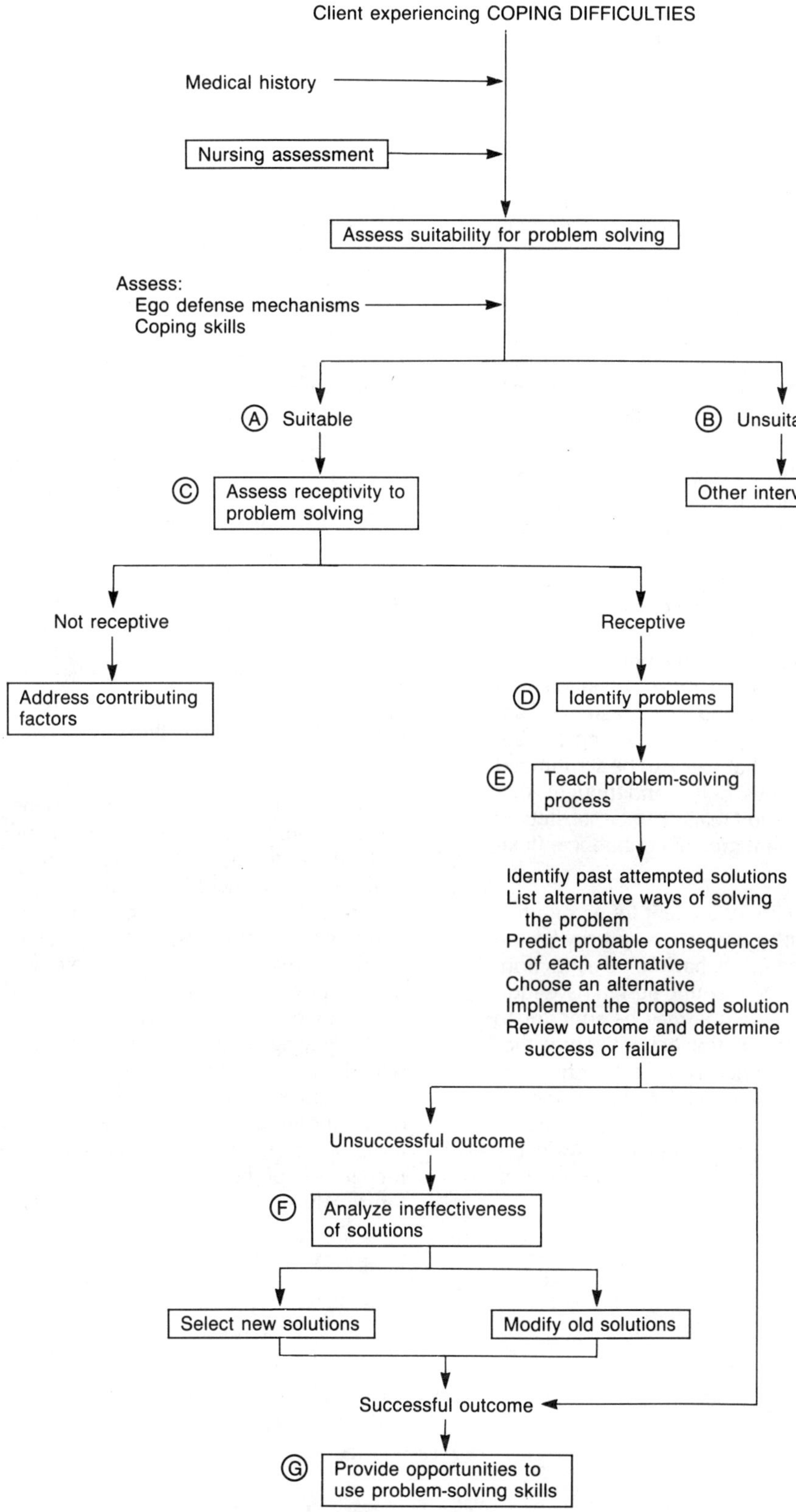

Burnett CN, Pierson FM. Developing problem-solving skills in the classroom. Phys Ther 1988; 68:1381–1385.

Cook JS, Fontaine KL. Essentials of mental health nursing. Menlo Park, CA: Addison-Wesley, 1987.

Pasquali EA, Arnold HM, DeBasio N, Alesi EG. Mental health nursing: a holistic approach. 2nd ed. St. Louis: CV Mosby, 1985.

COGNITIVE THERAPY

Nancy E. Johnston

The idea that thinking patterns can profoundly influence moods and behaviors has been in evidence for the past 2500 years. Recently the rationale and procedures have received their impetus from Aaron Beck's work with depressed clients. Despite the fact that descriptions and applications of cognitive approaches have been most detailed in relation to depressed clients, cognitive therapy has been successfully used to treat clients who experience anxiety states, inflexibility, perfectionism, negativism, chronic anger, and social inhibition.

A. The establishment of a therapeutic relationship allows the nurse to assess the suitability of this approach for a given client (p 98). The principal predictors of success are the persistent willingness on the part of the client to help him- or herself and the capacity of the nurse to establish a working alliance with the client. One of the hallmarks of cognitive therapy is the establishment of a working alliance that is based on collaborative empiricism. This concept requires the nurse to enable the client, through an accepting and nonthreatening approach, to bring into awareness beliefs regarding the self, the world, and the future so that they can be scrutinized for accuracy and validity. Thus, beliefs and thoughts that misrepresent, conceal, or distort reality can be substituted for those that allow the client greater confidence, flexibility, and integration.

B. When judging the suitability of a client for a cognitive approach, it is important to assess the severity of the symptoms or the degree of behavioral dysfunction. Although studies of rigorous scientific design have indicated that cognitive therapy alone may be superior to chemotherapy alone, a combination of both approaches is most effective to treat clients who are experiencing the more severe forms of depression. For clients who are experiencing behavioral dysfunctions of more extreme proportions, an approach that is directed toward behavioral as well as cognitive change may be most effective.

C. In focusing on the client's beliefs, the nurse assesses three broad categories: (1) expectations—the client's view of what will happen or characteristically happens in the course of everyday life; (2) evaluations or ascriptions—the client's judgments about the value of his or her accomplishments relative to the success of others in the client's reference group; (3) attributions of causality or responsibility, or in other words who can be held responsible for a particular event or phenomenon.

D. Since clients have had a lifetime to develop negative patterns of thought that they view as realistic, they are likely to resist any attempt that directly challenges the validity of these thoughts. Consequently, it is strategically imperative to enlist the client's willingness to approach these beliefs as hypotheses. As in any empirical investigation, hypotheses are tested and some are found to be reliable and valid. Others are found to lack appropriate substantiation. Accordingly, invalid hypotheses may either be modified to render them more useful in explaining and predicting a given reality or they may be abandonned entirely.

E. Provided that the client is able to benefit from further specification, the nurse may elect to familiarize the client with 10 commonly encountered forms of cognitive distortions. These include: all or nothing thinking, overgeneralization, mental filter, disqualifying the positive, jumping to conclusions, magnification or minimization, emotional reasoning, "should" statements, labeling and mislabeling, and personalization (for a description and examples of these cognitive distortions refer to Burns, 1980). Having acquainted the client at a theoretical level with the various forms of cognitive distortions, the nurse then enables the client to apply the information to his or her individual situation. The nurse, being careful to monitor the client's receptivity, begins to promote client recognition of the cognitive distortions that are characteristically used.

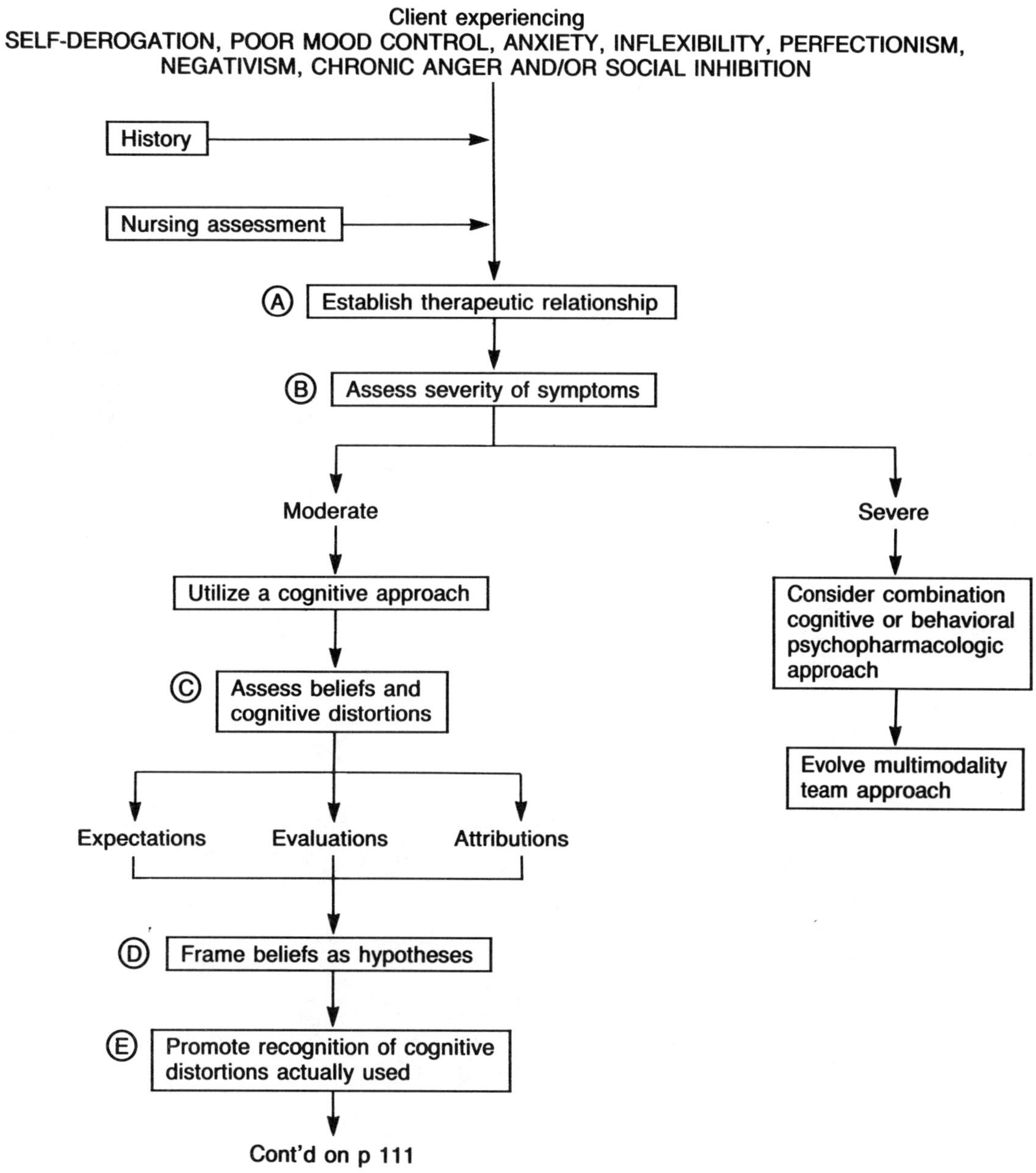
Client experiencing
SELF-DEROGATION, POOR MOOD CONTROL, ANXIETY, INFLEXIBILITY, PERFECTIONISM, NEGATIVISM, CHRONIC ANGER AND/OR SOCIAL INHIBITION
History
Nursing assessment
Ⓐ Establish therapeutic relationship
Ⓑ Assess severity of symptoms
Moderate
Severe
Utilize a cognitive approach
Consider combination cognitive or behavioral psychopharmacologic approach
Ⓒ Assess beliefs and cognitive distortions
Evolve multimodality team approach
Expectations
Evaluations
Attributions
Ⓓ Frame beliefs as hypotheses
Ⓔ Promote recognition of cognitive distortions actually used
Cont'd on p 111

F. The client's collaboration in noting and categorizing cognitive distortions is strengthened by enabling the perception of the interrelationships among thinking negatively, feeling dispirited, and behaving maladaptively. Assuming the client's objective is to feel better or to enjoy more satisfactory relationships, he or she can be encouraged to achieve these objectives by beginning to change the nature of his or her thoughts.

G. Clients are encouraged to achieve a level of distancing and objectification in relation to their beliefs by using the "daily record of dysfunctional thoughts," a format developed by Beck. Clients are encouraged to keep a daily diary that records descriptions of actual events that lead to unpleasant emotions, specify the resultant emotions, and rate the degree of intensity of these emotions. Automatic thoughts that accompany the emotion are documented, and the cognitive distortions involved in each automatic thought are identified. Finally, rational responses are developed to rebut the automatic thoughts and another rating of the intensity of emotions experienced following completion of the process is obtained.

H. Many clients find that this process, when closely adhered to, results in remarkable changes in thought, affect, and behavior. Thus, they are satisfied to continue to apply this approach without pursuing some of the deeper issues that have to do with why and how they came to have these beliefs. For clients searching for a greater understanding of the origins of these beliefs, it may be advisable to consider exploring early childhood experiences, particularly in relation to the influence of parental sanctions on the development of negative self-models. The client is then encouraged to evolve self-models that are not constrained by obsolete imperatives.

References

Beck AT. Cognitive therapy and emotional disorders. New York: New American Library, 1979.

Bulechek GM, McCloskey JC. Nursing interventions: treatments for nursing diagnoses. Philadelphia: WB Saunders, 1985.

Burns DD. Feeling good: the new mood therapy. New York: New American Library, 1980.

Guidano VF. A systems, process-oriented approach to cognitive therapy. In: Dobson KS, ed. Handbook of cognitive-behavioral therapies. New York: Guilford, 1988.

Sideleau BF. Irrational beliefs and intervention. J Psychosoc Nurs 1987; 25(3):18–24.

Cont'd from p 109

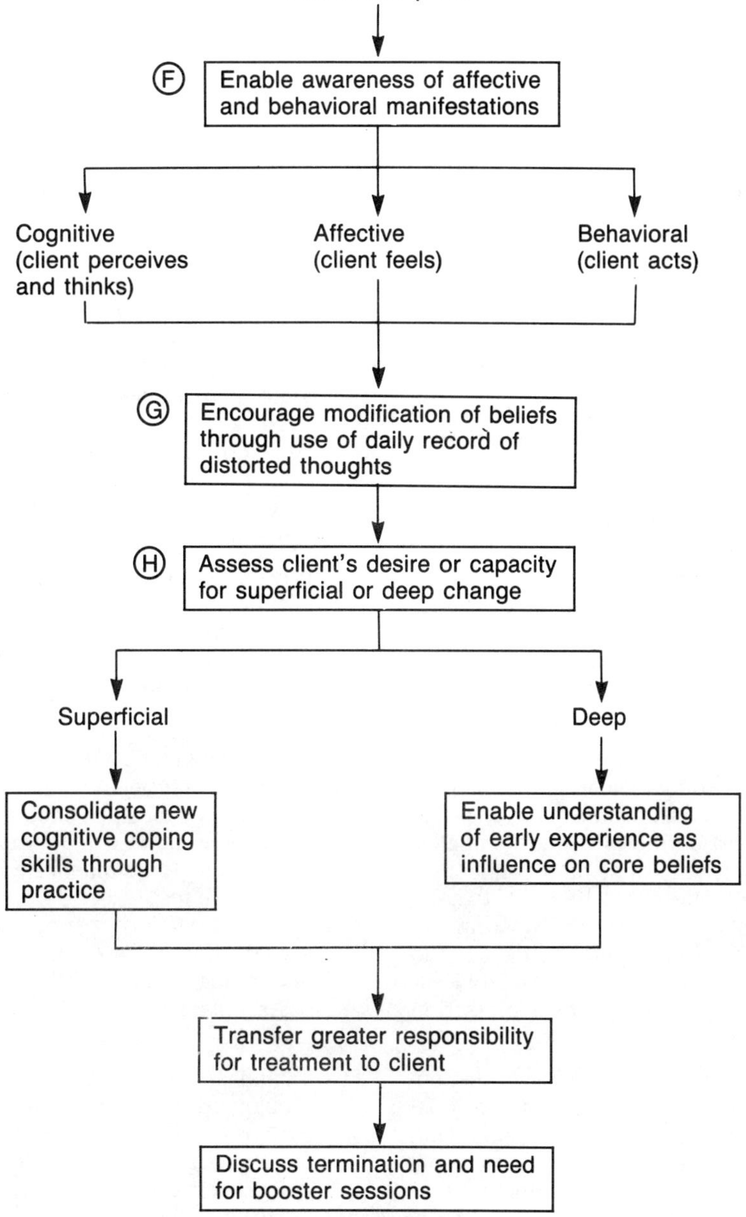

SHORT-TERM PSYCHOTHERAPY

Nancy E. Johnston

A. The trend toward short-term psychotherapy has been influenced by greater consumer demand, the prohibitive cost of longer-term modalities, and the impressive results of short-term approaches. Careful assessment is considered a crucial step in effective brief psychotherapy. Clients who may be excluded fall into three categories: (1) clients who cannot attend to the process of active verbal interaction (e.g., those suffering mental retardation, delirium, dementia, and active psychotic states); (2) clients with diagnoses for which other treatment modalities take precedence (i.e., schizophreniform disorders, major affective disorders, specific phobias, and panic states); (3) clients with a characterologic style that precludes the likelihood of enduring through the psychological work (i.e., repeated suicide attempts, alcohol or substance abuse, chronic obsessive or phobic patterns, and severe personality disorders). Inclusion criteria are motivation for change, ability to form meaningful relationships, psychological mindedness, ability to state the major complaint, and evidence of ego strength.

B. Two dimensions comprise the therapeutic alliance: the helping alliance and the working alliance. The helping alliance is engendered by the admixture of therapist and client qualities. Therapist attributes include empathy, warmth, respect, genuineness, hope, and confidence. The most important client attribute is the ability to enter into a relationship with the therapist. The working alliance refers to the ability of the client and therapist to collaborate in the exploration of the client's problems and to determine the core conflicts to be addressed in subsequent therapy sessions.

C. The recent research on short-term psychotherapy demonstrates a shift from an intrapsychic to an interpersonal focus. Identifying accurately the focus for therapy and establishing a time frame are procedures that are especially critical in short-term therapy. Various methods for determining a focus have been described by Strupp, Luborsky, M. Horowitz, Budman, Klerman, and L. Horowitz. Opinions differ among mental health professionals as to the length of time the client needs to spend in therapy. These differences tend to reflect theoretical biases and preferences. The range of time for brief psychotherapy suggested in the literature is 12 to 25 sessions. With the exception of Mann, the majority of short-term psychotherapists approach the issue of time-limiting in a flexible manner, with some specifying the termination date in advance and others being less particular about therapy duration.

D. Short-term psychotherapeutic activity, which is more active and structured than more lengthy modalities of psychotherapy, is directed toward the simultaneous accomplishment of three goals: (1) maintaining a sharp focus on the central issues or core conflicts, (2) perpetuating the therapeutic alliance, and (3) encouraging the client to begin to generalize the gains made during the psychotherapeutic process to everyday life.

E. If the client does not respond favorably to this therapeutic modality, it is imperative that his or her suitability be reassessed. Was the therapist's initial assessment superficial and inaccurate? During the assessment process, did the client withhold critical information which, if known, would have resulted in disqualification? Was the therapist overly zealous? Is the client's motivation for change insufficient? If the answers to these questions are affirmative, it is wise to consider termination of the therapy and/or referral for a type of treatment that is more appropriate.

F. If reassessment confirms the client's suitability, assess whether the central issue has really been accurately identified. Has the client succeeded in deflecting attention from the most painful issue by consciously or unconsciously introducing red herrings into the explorative process?

G. Provided that the focus is correct, it becomes necessary to address transference and countertransference issues (p 114). Is the therapist unable to maintain a therapeutic alliance? Is there a tendency for countertransference phenomena to be manifested in a subtle blaming attitude? Have resistances developed in reaction to relentless interpretations that have pushed the client too far too fast? Careful and objective scrutiny by the therapist may frequently uncover the cause of the therapeutic impasse, but it is usually advisable to seek the observations and suggestions of an impartial colleague or supervisor.

H. Should a reassessment of the nature of the client's problem reveal that it has been misdiagnosed, two options are possible. One possibility includes referring the client. Referral is certainly preferable in situations where the therapist lacks suitable resources or expertise to treat the client. Frequently however, the therapist may effect moderate changes in focus and technique that render the psychotherapeutic process more relevant, immediate, and productive.

References

Bauer GP, Kobos JC. Brief therapy: short-term psychodynamic intervention. Northvale, NJ: Aronson, 1987.

Bevis EH. Short-term psychotherapy. In: Beck CM, Rawlins RP, Williams SR, eds. Mental health—psychiatric nursing. St. Louis: CV Mosby, 1984.

Garfield SL, Bergin AE, eds. Handbook of psychotherapy and behavior change. 3rd ed. New York: Wiley, 1986.

Horowitz MJ. States of mind. 2nd ed. New York: Plenum, 1987.

Mackenzie KR. Recent developments in brief psychotherapy. Hosp Commun Psychiatry 1988; 39:742–752.

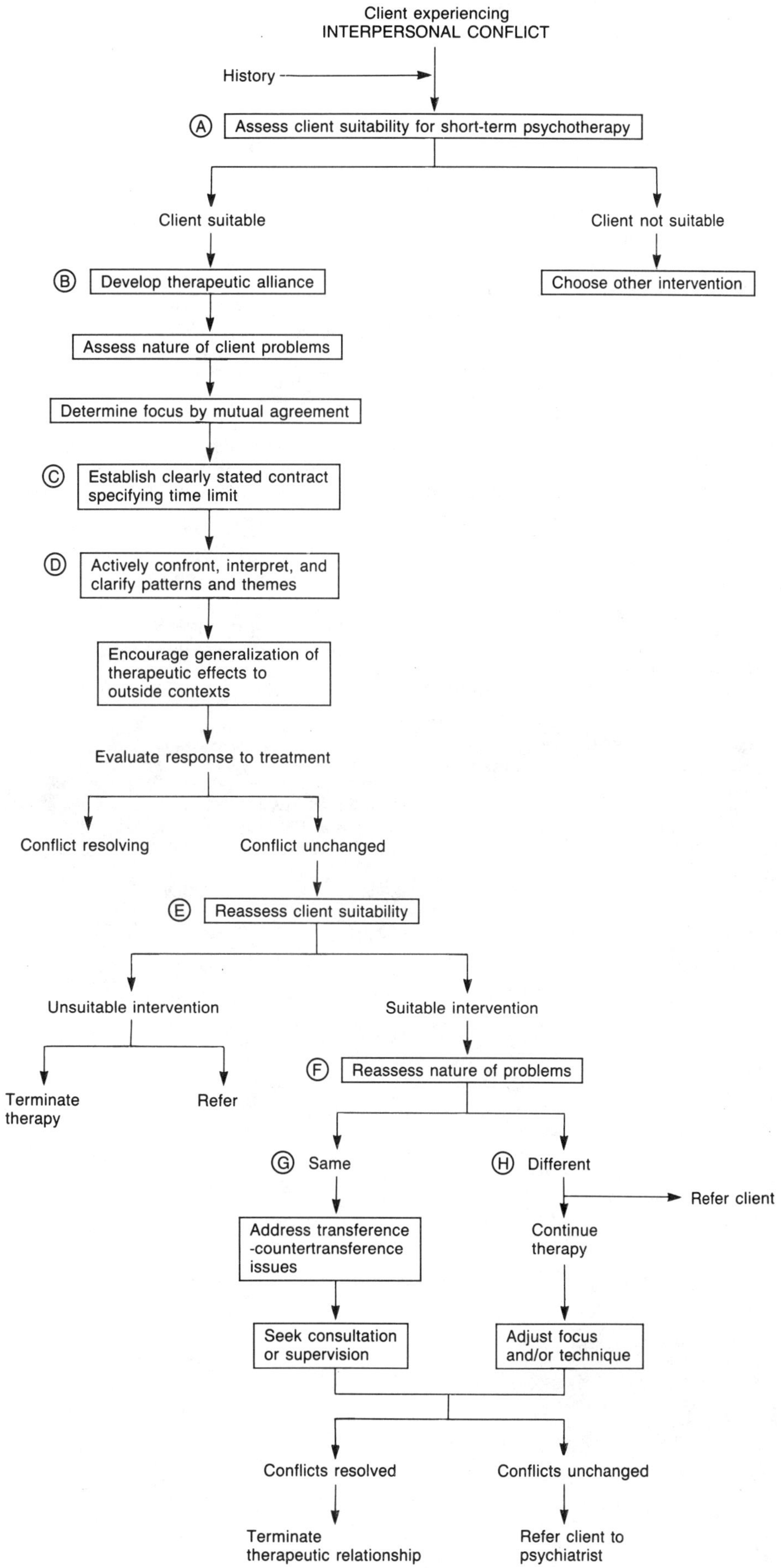
Client experiencing
INTERPERSONAL CONFLICT
History
Ⓐ Assess client suitability for short-term psychotherapy
Client suitable
Client not suitable
Ⓑ Develop therapeutic alliance
Choose other intervention
Assess nature of client problems
Determine focus by mutual agreement
Ⓒ Establish clearly stated contract specifying time limit
Ⓓ Actively confront, interpret, and clarify patterns and themes
Encourage generalization of therapeutic effects to outside contexts
Evaluate response to treatment
Conflict resolving
Conflict unchanged
Ⓔ Reassess client suitability
Unsuitable intervention
Suitable intervention
Terminate therapy
Refer
Ⓕ Reassess nature of problems
Ⓖ Same
Ⓗ Different
Refer client
Address transference -countertransference issues
Continue therapy
Seek consultation or supervision
Adjust focus and/or technique
Conflicts resolved
Conflicts unchanged
Terminate therapeutic relationship
Refer client to psychiatrist

TRANSFERENCE AND COUNTERTRANSFERENCE

Deborah Antai-Otong

Transference is a situation in psychotherapy in which the client reacts toward the therapist with feelings, attitudes, and behaviors similar to those they have experienced with significant others in the past. Countertransference refers to an emotional reaction by the therapist toward the client because the client has mannerisms or behaviors of a significant other that evoke reactions in the therapist.

A. In transference, the client may react in a positive or negative manner. An example of transference in a relationship can be seen in the following situation. The client may form a relationship with his female therapist, perceiving her as a mother figure and have related feelings such as excessive warmth and attachment. When the therapist does not respond in this manner, the client becomes hostile and angry and expresses feelings of rejection. It is essential that the client be made aware of this faulty perception and recognize that the therapist is just that and not his mother, even though she is warm and caring.

B. Clients should be encouraged to interpret the meaning of these reactions and recognize displacement. Interpretation of these reactions facilitates insight into and resolution of earlier conflicts. The nurse should assist the client to recognize the reasons for seeking treatment and resolving relationships.

C. "Working through" is a later stage of psychotherapy that allows the client to gain a healthier insight into unresolved conflicts that facilitate adaptive behavioral patterns, which often result in anxiety.

D. The therapist may respond to countertransference by being overprotective or by making the client feel rejected. An example of countertransference can be seen in the following situation. The therapist who has an irresponsible and manipulative father encounters a client who seems unmotivated and unwilling to work in therapy. Each time she works with the client she becomes angry and "lectures" him. The therapist does not recognize the source of her anger and fails to build a therapeutic relationship with the client because of her failure to recognize unresolved conflict with her father.

E. Professional supervision enables the therapist to deal with her own unresolved conflicts more appropriately and minimize "contaminating" her relationship with her client, thus facilitating a therapeutic relationship. Supervision also provides support and affirms techniques and feelings that are generated in therapy.

References

Basch MF. Doing psychotherapy. New York: Basic Books, 1980.

Johnson BS. Psychiatric mental health nursing: adaptation and growth. 2nd ed. Philadelphia: JB Lippincott, 1989.

TRANSFERENCE AND COUNTERTRANSFERENCE

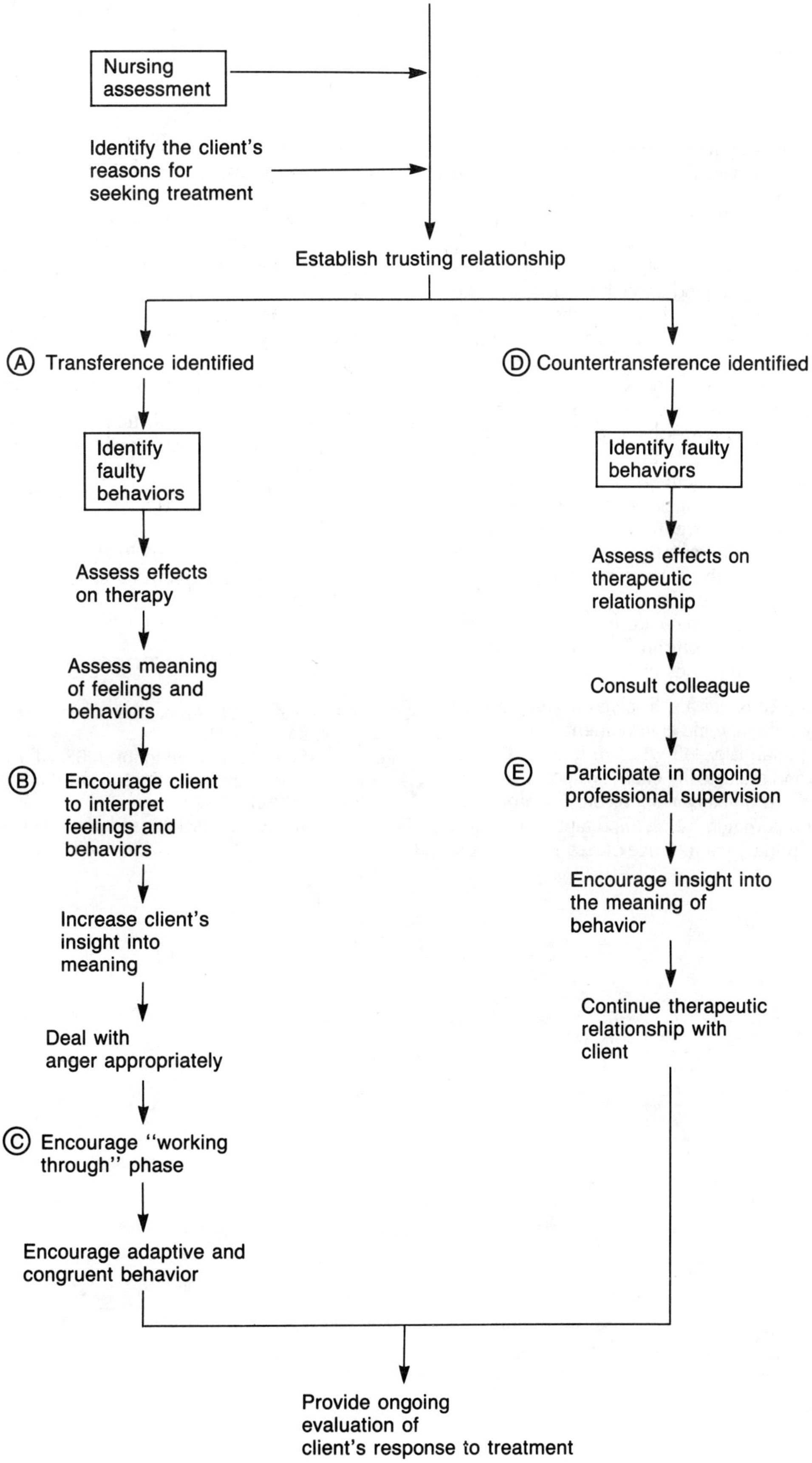

MILIEU THERAPY

Deborah Antai-Otong

Milieu therapy refers to an environment that facilitates psychological restoration and maintains physical integrity. Milieu therapy is based on several basic assumptions. The first is that the client has inner strengths and potential that will respond to a therapeutic environment. The second is that clients are motivated to participate in treatment, and the third is that severely mentally ill clients depend upon the expertise of the health-care system and professionals to help them. Characteristics of this environment include individualized treatment plans that address the needs of each client and allow each client to be an active participant. Activities encourage independence and prevent regression, while promoting self-esteem and enhancing problem-solving and social skills. Clients are encouraged to interact with staff and other clients in both inpatient and outpatient settings to test new skills and reinforce adaptive behavioral changes. Clients are encouraged to identify the meaning of current stressors and ways to minimize future crises. Family members are included in the treatment process and are actively involved in the teaching throughout hospitalization of the family member, and their feedback is used as valuable data during the evaluation process. Clients are linked to community resources during hospitalization by weekend passes and outings.

A. Many administrative issues are involved in maintaining and developing a therapeutic environment. Patient care involves having adequate staff who are qualified to assess, intervene, and evaluate the client's response to treatment. Nurses are ultimately responsible for providing 24-hour care and communicating important information to the interdisciplinary team. Since nurses are the most accessible members of the treatment team, they are ultimately responsible for creating and managing a therapeutic environment, and are actively involved in discharge planning. Throughout hospitalization they provide numerous teaching strategies to assist clients in improving their self-esteem, problem-solving, and communication skills. Teaching opportunities include relaxation and stress reduction training, cognitive therapy, and values clarification. Adaptive and improved behavioral changes are reinforced, and constructive feedback is used to deal with maladaptive behaviors.

B. Assess clients from a holistic perspective and focus on biophysiologic and psychosocial issues. Provide ongoing evaluation and documentation of the client's response to treatment and maintain physical and psychological integrity.

C. Provide safety and security to all clients by setting limits and monitoring and minimizing dangerous and destructive behaviors.

References

Chitty KK, Maynard CK. Managing manipulation. J Psychosoc Nurs 1986; 24:9–13.

Greene JA. Milieu therapy. In: Johnson BS, ed. Psychiatric nursing: adaptation and growth. 2nd ed. Philadelphia: JB Lippincott, 1989:171–182.

Stuart GW, Sundeen SJ. Principles and practice of psychiatric nursing. St. Louis: CV Mosby, 1983:580–591.

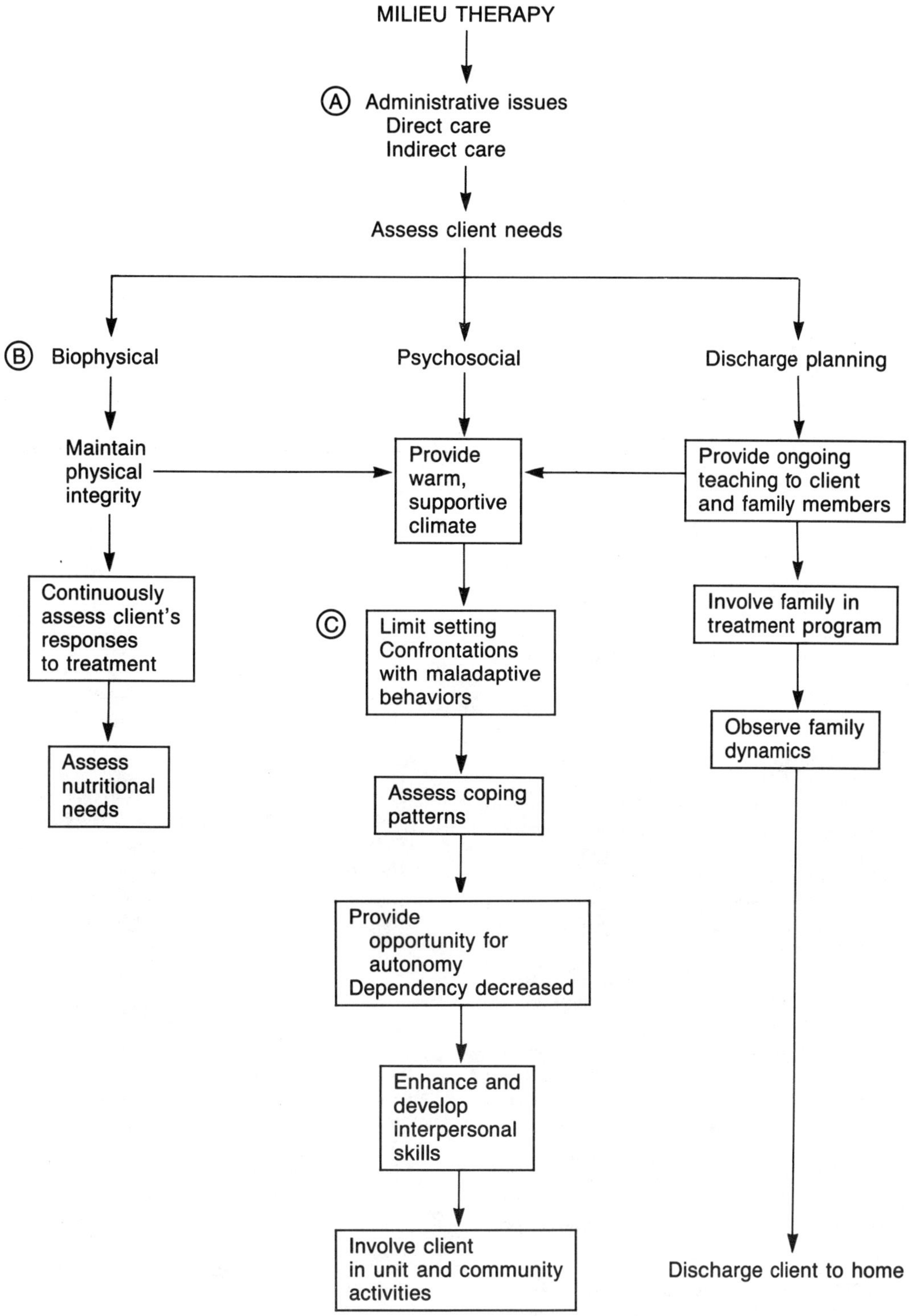
MILIEU THERAPY
(A) Administrative issues
Direct care
Indirect care
Assess client needs
(B) Biophysical
Psychosocial
Discharge planning
Maintain physical integrity
Provide warm, supportive climate
Provide ongoing teaching to client and family members
Continuously assess client's responses to treatment
(C) Limit setting
Confrontations with maladaptive behaviors
Involve family in treatment program
Assess nutritional needs
Observe family dynamics
Assess coping patterns
Provide opportunity for autonomy
Dependency decreased
Enhance and develop interpersonal skills
Involve client in unit and community activities
Discharge client to home

PROGRESSIVE RELAXATION

Magda Bishai

Progressive relaxation has been found to increase the client's ability to cope with various stressful situations such as pain, chronic illness, medical and nursing procedures, surgery, childbirth, difficulty with sleep, and problematic situations that precipitate anger, criticism, fear, and anxiety.

A. Progressive relaxation is a technique developed by Edmunt Jacobson in 1929. This technique is based on empirical evidence of the physiologic impossibility of being relaxed and emotionally tense at the same time. The aim of this approach is to equip clients with a technique that enables them to feel comfortable and aware of their internal and external environments. The client is taught to create tension in the muscle group, making the muscles as tight as possible without causing pain or cramps. This tightness is held for about 5 seconds during which the client concentrates on how the tension feels. The client then relaxes the muscles, letting them become completely loose. This procedure is repeated twice for each group of muscles. The major groups of muscles are:

1. Hands, forearms and biceps: To tighten this group, the client is asked to make a fist with the right hand, followed by bending in tightly the right elbow.
2. Head, neck and shoulders: The client is instructed to squint the eyes, wrinkle the brows, clench the jaw, press the tongue against the roof of the mouth, purse the lips into an O, press the head back as far as possible, roll it slowly and bring it forward by pressing the chin against the chest, shrug the shoulders up and hunch the head down in between them.
3. Chest, stomach and lower back: The client is instructed to breathe in deeply and slowly, and to tighten the stomach and arch the back without straining it.
4. Thighs, buttocks, calves and feet: The client is instructed to tighten the buttocks and thighs by pressing down the heels, and then pointing the toes backward and forward.

B. Consultation with the attending physician is recommended when considering clients with neurologic conditions, since it is possible to cause or worsen rigidity by tensing the muscles.

C. Common problems in achieving relaxation include:

1. Movement of body parts: The client must assume a comfortable position by sitting or lying down, so that every part of the body is supported. If assuming such a position disrupts relaxation, reviewing the effectiveness of the technique becomes essential.
2. Muscle cramps: To avoid this problem, ask the client to decrease the tension and apply it more slowly while shortening the period of time.
3. Noise: Initially, a quiet room is ideal. Gradually, the client needs to learn to relax in a noisier environment.
4. Sleep: Falling asleep decreases the effectiveness of the relaxation especially when this technique is practiced at bedtime, unless this is the desired outcome. Modulating pitch and volume of the voice may correct this problem. Selecting a time for practicing the technique when the client is not fatigued may also be useful.
5. Sense of losing control: To avoid this potential problem, ensure that the client understands the objectives of the relaxation and that the exercise is introduced gradually.
6. Annoying or distressing words and phrases: Be attuned to the words and phrases that might increase the tension of the client and ensure that these are avoided.

D. It is impossible to teach the client how to relax when the nurse is tense. Therefore, ensure that you can successfully utilize this technique yourself before attempting to teach it to clients. Relaxation is an acquired skill that becomes more highly developed with regular practice. Therefore, pushing the client too quickly to relax can have an opposite effect.

References

Carpenito LJ. Nursing diagnosis. Philadelphia: JB Lippincott, 1987.

Fanning P. Visualization for change. Oakland, CA: New Harbinger, 1988.

McKay M, Davies M, Fanning P. Thoughts and feelings. Oakland, CA: New Harbinger, 1983.

Murray RB, Huelskoetter MW. Psychiatric/mental health nursing. Norwalk, CT: Appleton & Lange, 1987.

Stuart GW, Sundeen SJ. Principles and practice of psychiatric nursing. St. Louis: CV Mosby, 1983.

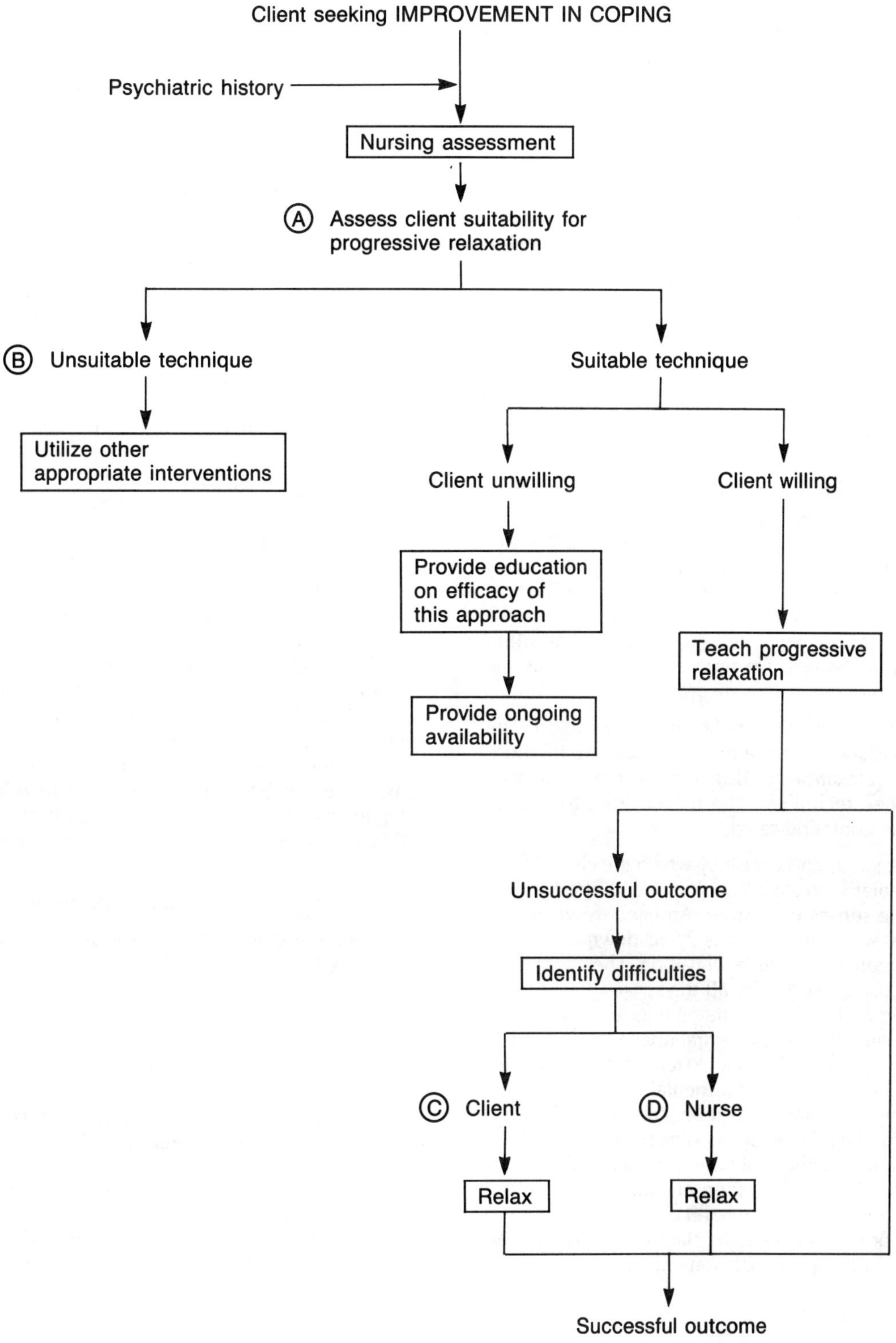
Client seeking IMPROVEMENT IN COPING
Psychiatric history
Nursing assessment
Ⓐ Assess client suitability for progressive relaxation
Ⓑ Unsuitable technique
Suitable technique
Utilize other appropriate interventions
Client unwilling
Client willing
Provide education on efficacy of this approach
Provide ongoing availability
Teach progressive relaxation
Unsuccessful outcome
Identify difficulties
Ⓒ Client
Ⓓ Nurse
Relax
Relax
Successful outcome

VISUALIZATION AND GUIDED IMAGERY

Magda Bishai

A. Visualization is the conscious programming for change in behavior through positive and creative mental images. It is a natural and automatic mental activity that humans use while daydreaming, thinking of someone, or recalling a past experience. The aim of this technique is to teach the client how to use and improve his or her already existing power of visualization for better functioning in life.

B. The technique of visualization is not recommended for psychotic patients, because it might precipitate or aggravate hallucinations and/or delusions.

C. The application of visualization has been found effective with clients seeking (1) self-improvement (e.g., weight-control, habit-breaking, problem-solving, and improvement of performance in sports and learning in general), (2) therapy (e.g., reducing stress, improving self-esteem, overcoming insomnia, shyness, depression, anxiety, and controlling anger), (3) healing and controlling pain (e.g., from injuries, infectious and noninfectious diseases, and immune system disorders).

D. Relaxation is the first step for effective visualization. The client is encouraged to use his or her favorite method. Progressive relaxation (p 118) may be the chosen or recommended technique. The use of drugs to induce relaxation is contraindicated.

E. Guided imagery is an exercise by which the client learns how to mentally create a specific and desired scene, using all the senses if possible. An effective visualization occurs when the client is lying down with eyes closed in a state of complete relaxation. The client is instructed to use and intensify all the senses. Resistances are explored and affirmative statements are repeated in order to create the desired mental image. Visualization can be used as a helpful adjunct to relaxation techniques. The client creates or recalls a mental image of a place where enjoyment and relaxation can occur. Tension headache can be relieved by assisting the client to create a mental picture of the headache (e.g., a metal band or tight clamp). The client is then encouraged to picture this symbol relaxing (i.e., the band becomes a soft crown of feathers or flowers, the tight clamp becomes loose). To facilitate healing, a cancer patient may visualize the body as a beautiful garden, the cancer cells as ugly weeds, and the chemotherapeutic agent as a weed killer. He or she then imagines the weeds being killed and disappearing. Research is beginning to show that cancer patients who effectively practice visualization to fight the illness tend to have fewer symptoms and less pain than patients who view themselves as helpless.

F. Communication with an inner guide is a more structured and advanced technique. The client is instructed to create an inner guide that may tell or insinuate an answer to the problem. The inner guide could be a person, animal, object, or even an event. This technique is preceded by the various steps mentioned above.

G. The ability to imagine is essential. Although visualization is a natural mental activity, some individuals have more difficulty developing images than others. To overcome this, the nurse assists the client to create an image in a step-by-step fashion beginning with basic elements of the image and gradually developing the complexity. Incorporating the five senses to develop an image that includes sound, touch, smell, taste, and sight enables the client to develop a powerful and vivid image. Use of aids such as cassettes may help to develop this ability. A client with low self-esteem will have difficulty learning to visualize. However, some practitioners have used this technique successfully in assisting clients to build self-esteem.

H. A definite and realistic goal is essential.

I. Practicing two to three times a day for a period of 20 minutes is recommended.

References

Carpenito LJ. Nursing diagnosis. Philadelphia: JB Lippincott, 1987.

Fanning P. Visualization for change. Oakland, CA: New Harbinger, 1988.

McKay M, Davies M, Fanning P. Thoughts and feelings. Oakland, CA: New Harbinger, 1983.

Murray RB, Huelskoetter MW. Psychiatric/mental health nursing. Norwalk, CT: Appleton & Lange, 1987.

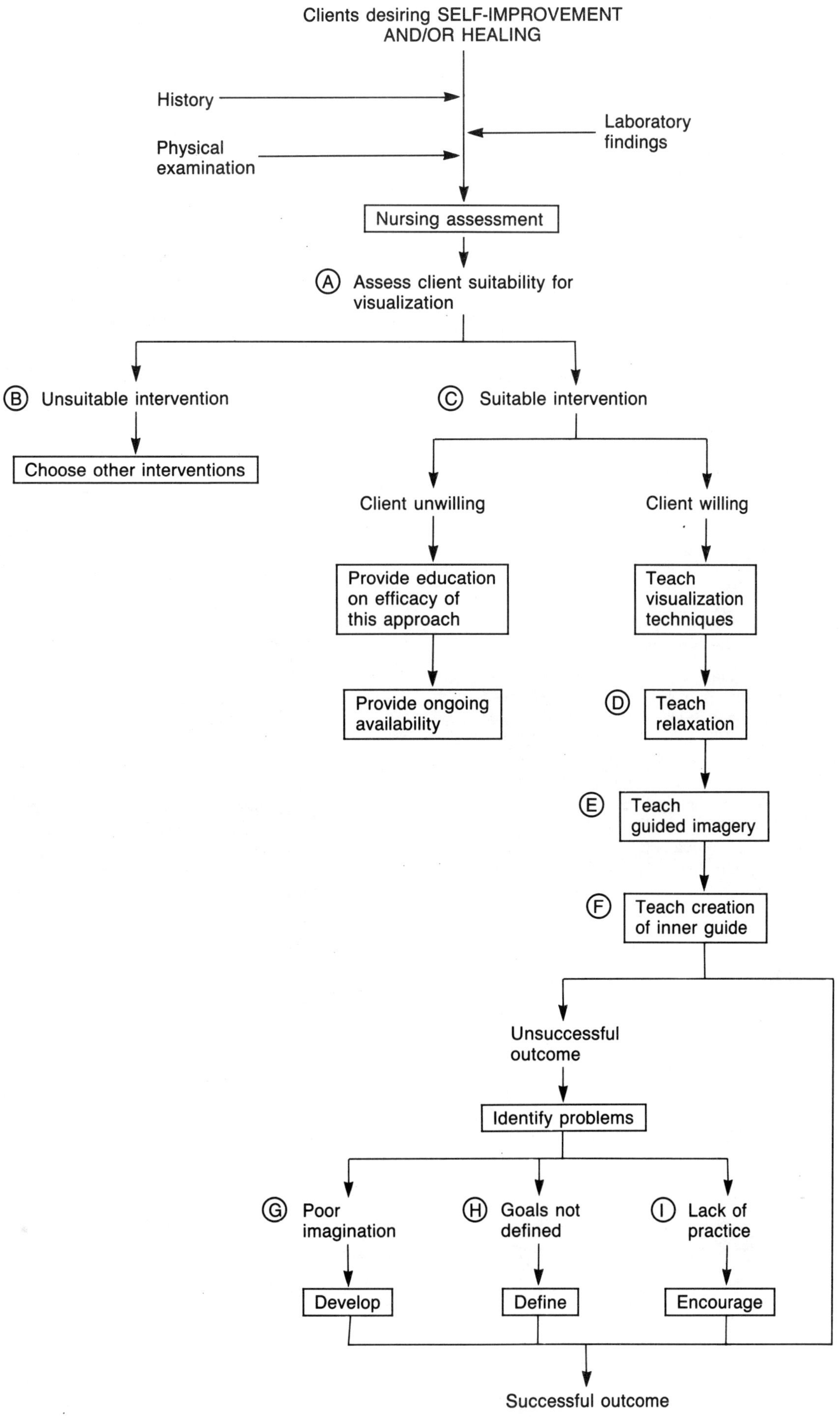
Clients desiring SELF-IMPROVEMENT AND/OR HEALING
History
Physical examination
Laboratory findings
Nursing assessment
(A) Assess client suitability for visualization
(B) Unsuitable intervention
Choose other interventions
(C) Suitable intervention
Client unwilling
Provide education on efficacy of this approach
Provide ongoing availability
Client willing
Teach visualization techniques
(D) Teach relaxation
(E) Teach guided imagery
(F) Teach creation of inner guide
Unsuccessful outcome
Identify problems
(G) Poor imagination
Develop
(H) Goals not defined
Define
(I) Lack of practice
Encourage
Successful outcome

MODELING AND ROLE PLAYING

Magda Bishai

A. Modeling has proven to be effective in assisting the client, directly or indirectly, to change or acquire a new pattern of behavior in interpersonal communication and emotional expressiveness. It is done by imitating the behavior of others.

B. Care should be taken to ensure that this technique is suitable for the client. Individuals who are acutely ill or experiencing significant levels of anxiety or pain are not appropriate candidates until these factors can be sufficiently controlled. Consultation with other members of the health-care team is recommended when making decisions on suitability.

C. Covert modeling is a technique developed by Joseph Cautela in 1971. This technique was designed to enable the client to identify, refine, and role-play the desired behavior.

D. Relaxation is the first step in covert modeling. The client is encouraged to use his or her favorite method of relaxation. Progressive relaxation (p 118) may be the technique chosen or recommended.

E. Visualization (p 120), the ability to imagine scenes using different senses, is the next technique to learn.

F. The steps for covert modeling are (1) identifying and writing out the problem behavior in sequence of occurrence; (2) writing the desired behavior in sequence of occurrence (start with step 2 when client is seeking to learn a new behavior); (3) practicing imagining the context in which the problem or new behavior occurs; (4) visualizing a very different person in age, sex, and attire performing the desired behavior successfully; the scene is held for 15 seconds and repeated twice; (5) visualizing a similar person performing the desired behavior, first while having difficulty, then successfully; the scene is held for 15 seconds and repeated twice; (6) visualizing self performing the desired behavior in the same manner as was stated in step 5; (7) role-playing the desired behavior, which could be practiced in front of a mirror, or by videotaping oneself performing, playing back the tape and repeating until the desired behavior is obtained; this could also be done with the nurse or in a group setting (this step is optional); (8) preparing some coping statements—short positive statements to use while preparing for the situation, confronting it, and reinforcing the success (also an optional step); and (9) performing the desired behavior in real life. Evaluating and acknowledging the gradual change is then recommended.

G. An unsuccessful modeling attempt could be due to the client's difficulty in relaxing and/or visualizing.

H. The nurse must be aware of her own behavior and impact on the client. In order to be effective in her role, the nurse must be willing to be genuine, show warmth, and imply a level of enthusiasm and involvement. She will also attempt to inspire clients to develop their potential fully by providing examples of desirable behavior. Sensitivity in attending and responding not only to what is said, but also to the hidden messages, is essential.

References

Corey G. Theory and practice of group counseling. Belmont, CA: Wadsworth, 1985.

Corsini RJ. Current psychotherapies. Itasca, IL: FE Peacock, 1983.

McKay M, Davies M, Fanning P. Thoughts and feelings. Oakland, CA: New Harbinger, 1983.

Murray RB, Huelskoetter MW. Psychiatric/mental health nursing. Norwalk, CT: Appleton & Lange, 1987.

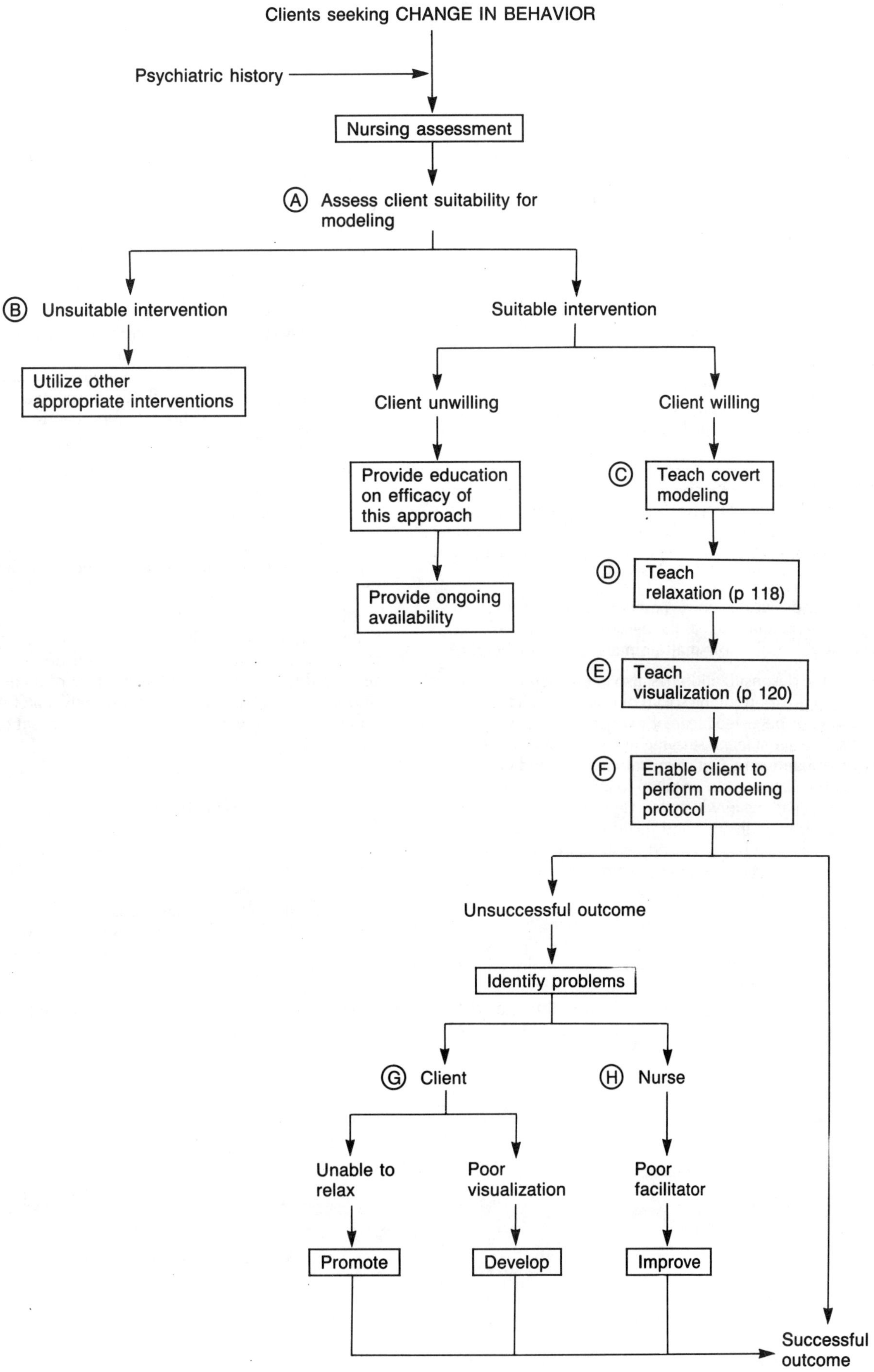
Clients seeking CHANGE IN BEHAVIOR
Psychiatric history
Nursing assessment
(A) Assess client suitability for modeling
(B) Unsuitable intervention
Utilize other appropriate interventions
Suitable intervention
Client unwilling
Provide education on efficacy of this approach
Provide ongoing availability
Client willing
(C) Teach covert modeling
(D) Teach relaxation (p 118)
(E) Teach visualization (p 120)
(F) Enable client to perform modeling protocol
Unsuccessful outcome
Identify problems
(G) Client
(H) Nurse
Unable to relax
Poor visualization
Poor facilitator
Promote
Develop
Improve
Successful outcome

SYSTEMATIC DESENSITIZATION

Magda Bishai

Systematic desensitization, introduced by Wolpe in 1958, is a technique by which certain anxieties may be reduced using a counter-conditioning method that employs progressive relaxation. The approach is based on a rationale that acknowledges the physiologic and psychological impossibility of maintaining concurrently a relaxed condition and an anxious emotional state.

A. This technique has been found particularly useful for clients with simple and social phobias. As for agoraphobic and other types of anxieties, systematic desensitization can also be useful, especially if the underlying elements of the anxieties have been disclosed or understood. If the client cannot use or is not suited to an approach involving visual imagery, desensitization "in vivo" might be effective (i.e., the client, while accompanied, is exposed to the real situation in which he or she experiences fear or panic). The nurse must assess the client's condition in order to decide whether desensitization is best accomplished using a "systematic" (constructed hierarchy) or "in vivo" (actual exposure) approach.

B. Systematic desensitization is particularly effective in treating simple phobias such as the persistent fear of an object or situation or fear of small animals, water, or height.

C. Systematic desensitization has also been useful in treating persons experiencing social phobias, which typically involve a persistent fear of exposure or scrutiny by others. The client fears behaving in a way that is humiliating or embarrassing. Criticism, "aloneness," and ridicule are feared. Care should be taken to assess the difference between situations in which the client could benefit from more assertive behavior and those in which an actual phobic response has occurred. Systematic desensitization and assertiveness training (p 126) cannot be considered interchangeable strategies.

D. When determining the suitability of clients for an approach involving systematic desensitization, it is wise to confer with the consulting psychiatrist. Generally, clients who are not acutely ill, have some insight into their condition, are able to comprehend and follow through with the protocol, and have strong motivation to overcome their anxieties are those who will benefit most from this approach.

E. In teaching a client how to follow a systematic desensitization protocol, the nurse encourages the client to develop a fear inventory by listing all anxiety-producing situations. Following this, the client groups items on the list into their common themes. A specific fear is selected from one theme, and a hierarchy of threatening situations is developed from the least to the most disturbing. A successful desensitization will occur, and anxiety is eliminated when the client is able to relax and at the same time visualize, with all the senses, the least disturbing situations. The client then proceeds to the next item on the hierarchy until all situations are exhausted.

F. To achieve a completely relaxed state the client must relax all four major muscle groups. For a more complete treatment of progressive relaxation, see p 118.

G. Problems in visualization can often be overcome by using special exercises to gain experience in utilizing all the senses. See p 120.

H. A misconstructed hierarchy, in which an item eliciting higher anxiety mistakenly precedes a lesser anxiety item, reduces the possibility of a successful desensitization since it does not facilitate the mastery of anxiety in a smoothly gradated manner. Accordingly, careful attention should be given to the correct placement of items on the hierarchy.

References

American Psychiatric Association. Diagnostic and statistical manual of mental disorders. 3rd ed. Washington, DC: American Psychiatric Association, 1987.

Corvini RJ. Current psychotherapies. Itasca, IL: FE Peacock, 1979.

McKay M, Davies M, Fenning P. Thoughts and feelings. Richmond, CA: New Harbinger Publications, 1981.

Pender NJ. Health promotion in nursing practice. Norwalk, CT: Appleton & Lange, 1987.

Stuart CW, Sundeen S. Principles and practice of psychiatric nursing. St. Louis: CV Mosby, 1983.

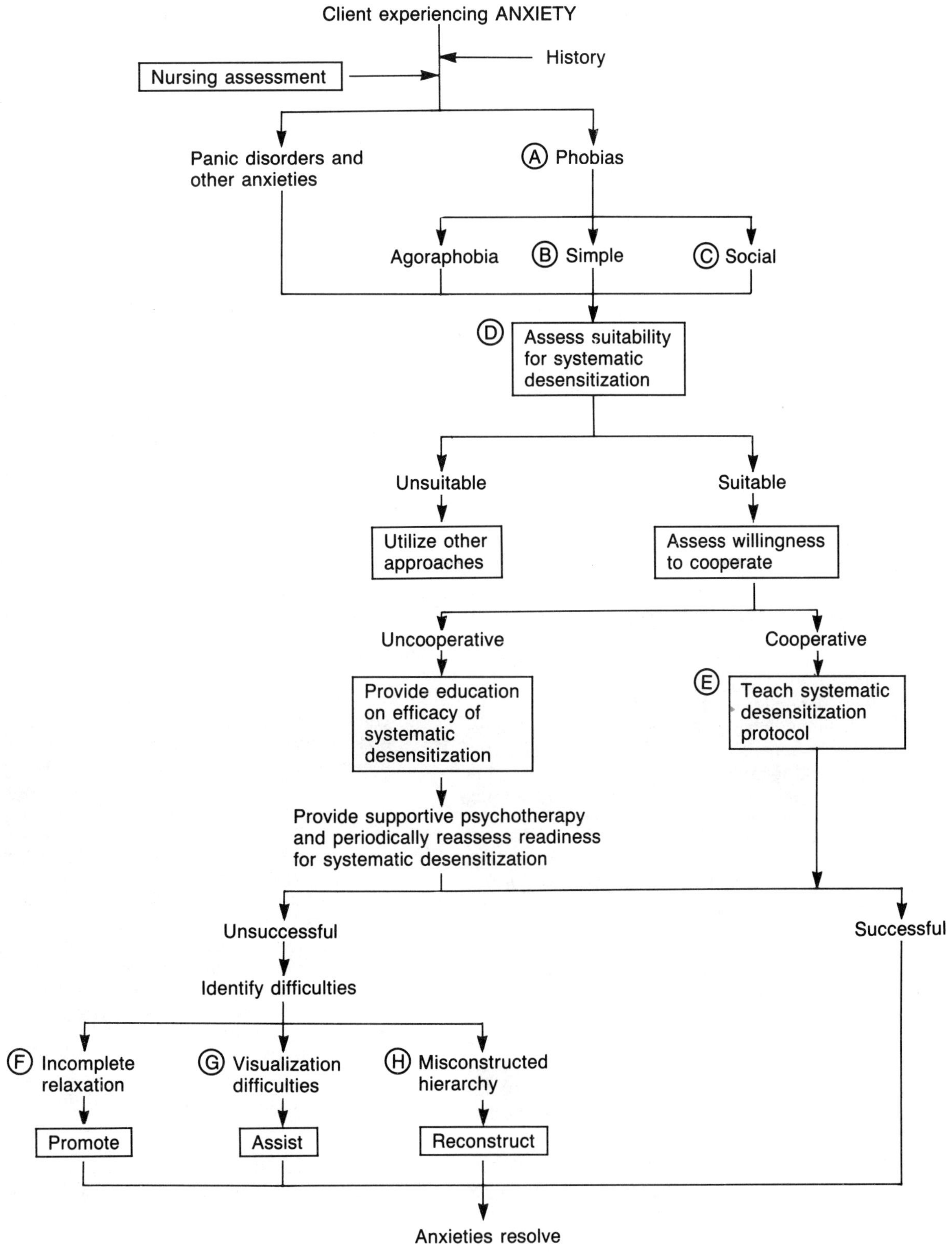
Client experiencing ANXIETY
History
Nursing assessment
Panic disorders and other anxieties
(A) Phobias
Agoraphobia
(B) Simple
(C) Social
(D) Assess suitability for systematic desensitization
Unsuitable
Suitable
Utilize other approaches
Assess willingness to cooperate
Uncooperative
Cooperative
Provide education on efficacy of systematic desensitization
(E) Teach systematic desensitization protocol
Provide supportive psychotherapy and periodically reassess readiness for systematic desensitization
Unsuccessful
Successful
Identify difficulties
(F) Incomplete relaxation
(G) Visualization difficulties
(H) Misconstructed hierarchy
Promote
Assist
Reconstruct
Anxieties resolve

ASSERTIVENESS TRAINING

Diane T. Brisson

Many psychiatric clients seldom manifest truly assertive behaviors. Their capacity to express their feelings, thoughts, desires, and rights openly, precisely, and constructively is too often restrained by inner fears of displeasing and hurting others, of being rejected and ridiculed, and of feeling worthless and powerless (p 184) to change the events of their lives. Several factors including benefits of the status quo, poor verbal ability, and a history of psychosocial problems add to their reluctance to assert themselves.

A. Before endeavoring to provide assertiveness training to others, the nurse clinican should have had training in cognitive and behavioral approaches at both the individual and group level and should be a model of assertiveness. In consultation with the multidisciplinary team members, the nurse selects candidates for assertiveness therapy. Highly medicated and acutely dysfunctional people and those who are cognitively impaired are not usually suitable candidates. When selecting clients for assertiveness training, cultural orientations must also be taken into consideration, since self-expression is often regulated by sociocultural parameters. Furthermore, selected candidates must display an ability to control aggressive behaviors, especially in a group setting. The nurse's decision to work with a client individually, rather than in a group, depends on the client's capacity to tolerate group situations. Highly anxious and overly sensitive people might benefit from systematic desensitization (see p 124) and relaxation training (see p 118) in addition to individual assertiveness sessions before joining a group. In contradistinction to traditional insight-oriented therapy, assertiveness therapy does not focus on the "whys," but is only directly concerned with the "hows," the "whats," and the "whens." Preferably led by two animators, an assertiveness group ideally meets once or twice weekly for 1 to 1½ hours for 8 weeks; it has an average of 10 members of both sexes and can function on an inpatient or outpatient basis. A microcosm of society where mutual confidence and togetherness can be enhanced and reinforced, the group becomes an effective real-life laboratory where assertiveness skills are learned, discussed, and practiced by a variety of persons who can serve as models to each other and partners for role playing, behavioral rehearsal, problem solving, and feedback.

B. Each member is introduced and informed about the goals of these group sessions, which seek mainly to modify self-defeating attitudes and negative thoughts and beliefs about oneself. The nurse teaches the basic assumptions of assertiveness therapy, which include the following: (1) inhibition, fears, irrational beliefs, self-doubt, and anxiety are learned during early life and can be corrected by cognitive restructuring; (2) the learning of effective assertiveness skills reduces and even prevents excessive anxiety and/or anger from interfering with self-expression; and (3) assertiveness is about better understanding of self and being able to stand up for one's rights without being aggressive, while acknowledging other people's rights and freedoms.

C. In order to change unassertive behaviors, clients should state accurately their problem behaviors. Questions such as "What happens when you feel that way?", "What do you have difficulty with?", or "In which situations do you have more difficulty expressing yourself?" help the client to pinpoint problematic behaviors. Assertiveness self-assessment questionnaires are useful and are good indicators of the client's present level of assertiveness; they can also facilitate group discussion and are useful for measuring the progress at the end of the training.

D. Participants are advised to keep weekly records or a diary about what they did and didn't do, their feelings, thoughts, accomplishments or failures, and significant interpersonal relationships. Furthermore, each group member is instructed to perform specific assignments with spouses, children, colleagues, friends, or other people, in which assertiveness behaviors are practiced. Beginning with easier tasks, the client gradually progresses to more demanding tasks.

E. The therapists encourage successful performance, challenge the clients' false beliefs or unsound excuses, and explain the connections between defeating inner dialogues and lack of assertiveness (see also "Cognitive Therapy," p 108). Using cases drawn from weekly records and assigned performances, positive behaviors are reinforced by a variety of approaches. Role playing, role modeling, behavior rehearsals, coaching, performance feedback, and group problem solving are all used to facilitate learning. Initially, the nurse can anticipate the reluctance of introverted, shy, or anxious clients to become involved in these activities. For these clients, systematic relaxation techniques can facilitate the reduction of tension. Although clients should not be coerced to participate in these activities, the therapist may query feeble participation and question whether it is in fact another symptom of unassertiveness. Group discussions may focus on not only the advantages of assertion but also the repercussions that the new assertiveness can have for significant others and/or colleagues who have tended to reinforce nonassertive behavior. In this type of situation, role playing or behavior rehearsal can enable the client to deal effectively with negative reactions that occur in relation to new forms of self-expression.

F. At the end of the recommended 8-week training period, participants evaluate their progress. Comments reporting higher self-confidence, self-esteem, and good feelings are noted and openly supported. Changes in the client's nonverbal communication, such as more direct eye contact and firmer tone of voice, and improved frequency, clarity, and timing of self-expression are also

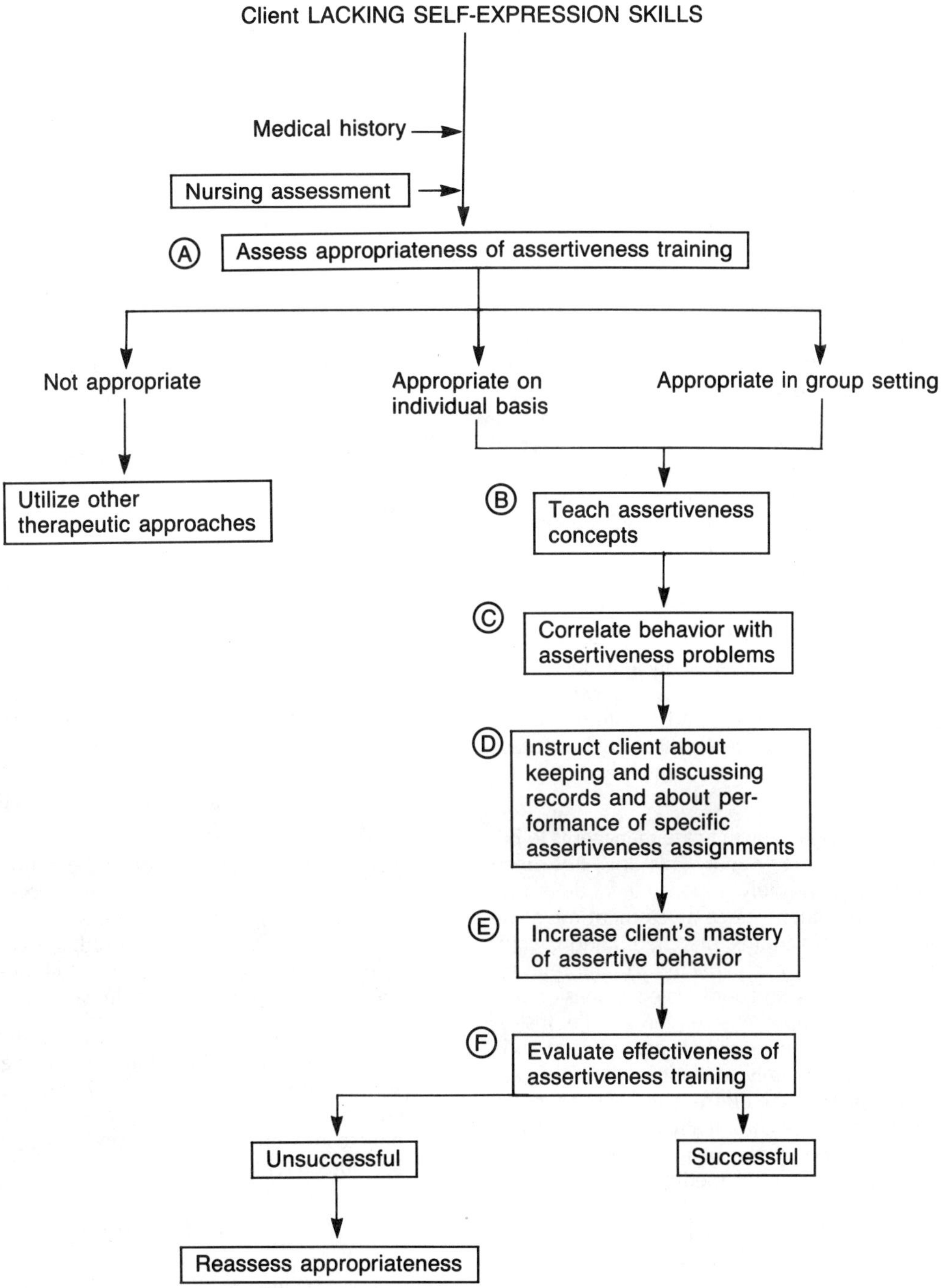

acknowledged. Results of self-assessment questionnaires can also be compared to those completed at the start of treatment.

References

Alberti RE, Emmons ML. Your perfect right: guide to assertive behavior. San Luis Obispo, CA: Impact Publishers, 1974.

Bowman Sister C, Spadoni AJ. Assertion therapy: the nurse and the psychiatric patient in an acute, short-term hospital setting. J Psychiatr Nurs Mental Health Serv 1981; 19(6):7–20.

Jakubowski P, Lange AJ. The assertive option: your rights and responsibilities. Champaign, IL: Research Press, 1978.

Rathus SA, Nevid JS. Bt, behavior therapy: strategies for solving problems in living. New York: Doubleday, 1977.

CASE MANAGEMENT FOR CHRONICALLY MENTALLY DISABLED CLIENTS

Nancy E. Johnston
Lynn Cochrane

The process of deinstitutionalization, begun in the early 1960s, and the emphasis on reducing the average length of stay in acute treatment facilities has resulted in steadily increasing numbers of psychiatrically disabled persons living in the community. Insufficient or fragmented services have frequently prevented clients from achieving their full potential for participation in community life and have resulted in high rates of recidivism, commonly referred to as the revolving door syndrome. Clients experiencing severe mental illness, such as those whose diagnoses may be schizophrenia, major affective disorder, organic brain syndrome, and paranoid or other psychoses, and who experience significant levels of disability are among those most handicapped to confront complex, duplicative, and uncoordinated services.

A. Case management has gained popularity as a mechanism for improving continuity of care. It is directed toward enhancing comprehensiveness and coordination of services. Other objectives frequently associated with case management are accessibility, accountability, and efficiency.

B. The most basic role played by the case manager is to become aware of the client's needs. This does not mean that the case manager is solely responsible for determining the needs of the client, since assessment might be done by a discharge-planning or rehabilitation team. Rather, the case manager is expected to take relevant recommendations and, with appropriate supervision and support, develop a comprehensive plan of care. Just as case managers are not necessarily expected to provide assessment functions entirely on their own, neither are they required to provide the entire range of services required by the client. Since chronically mentally disabled clients have many needs, it may be realistic to anticipate that referrals will be made for medicotherapeutic care (medication administration and brief counseling), family support, financial assistance, recreational planning, life-skills training, and vocational programming.

C. Among the functions that a case manager typically assumes is the provision of direct care. The unique educational and clinical experience of nurses prepare them to provide a number of direct services. These may include the monitoring of chemotherapeutic approaches, including the early identification and amelioration of symptoms associated with the long-term use of major tranquilizers and antiparkinsonian agents. Nurses are also prepared to offer individual counseling, perform family assessments, and facilitate improved family functioning. Community assessment and client advocacy are additional skills commonly taught in baccalaureate programs of nursing. Specialized training in psychiatric rehabilitation is frequently available by special arrangement between local mental health agencies and university programs.

D. The case manager also acts as a client advocate. Accordingly, the nurse-case manager determines when advocacy needs to occur on behalf of the client at an individual level and when advocacy is more effectively directed toward the systems level. Clients frequently lack the knowledge, perseverance, and assertiveness to pursue their options and rights in the course of daily living. Being careful not to take on tasks that could be reasonably accomplished by the client, the nurse may offer support in the form of articulating and interpreting the needs and rights of the client to others in the client's immediate environment. Clients frequently experience difficulty in gaining access to essential services. In such situations it becomes the nurse-caseworker's role to advocate on the client's behalf for services to which the client is entitled.

E. The caseworker's role involves the continuous monitoring of all services to ensure that optimal mix, balance, and sequencing occurs. Since ideal conditions of service coordination are seldom achieved, it becomes the nurse's role to identify and subsequently to lobby for additional programs to reduce inevitable gaps in service delivery.

F. Finally, the nurse reevaluates the overall treatment plan to assess when objectives have been met and when some services are no longer needed. The nurse-caseworker in collaboration with other members of the multidisciplinary team then updates and modifies treatment and service objectives.

References

Anthony WA, Cohen M, Cohen B. The philosophy, treatment process and principles of the psychiatric rehabilitation approach. New Directions Mental Health 1983; 17:67–69.

Intagliata J. Improving the quality of community care for the chronically mentally disabled: the role of case management. Schizophrenia Bull 1982; 8:655–674.

Rogers ES, Barry F, Cohen KS, Danley DH, William AA. Training mental health workers in psychiatric rehabilitation. Schizophrenia Bull 1986; 12:709–719.

Wasylenki DA, Goering PN, Lancer WJ, Ballantyne R, Farkas M. Impact of a case manager program on psychiatric aftercare. J Nerv Ment Dis 1985; 173:303–308.

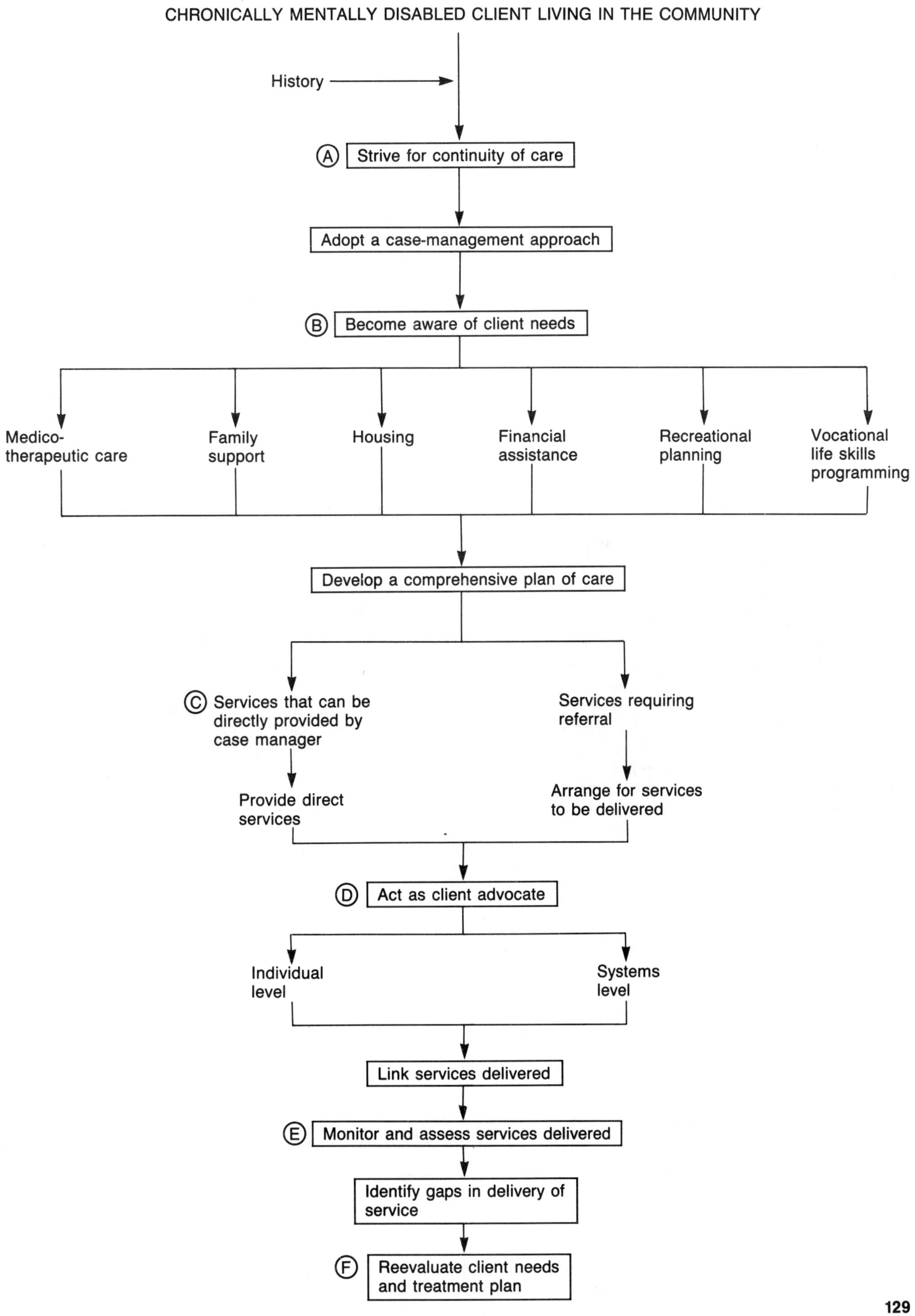
CHRONICALLY MENTALLY DISABLED CLIENT LIVING IN THE COMMUNITY
History
(A) Strive for continuity of care
Adopt a case-management approach
(B) Become aware of client needs
Medico-therapeutic care
Family support
Housing
Financial assistance
Recreational planning
Vocational life skills programming
Develop a comprehensive plan of care
(C) Services that can be directly provided by case manager
Services requiring referral
Provide direct services
Arrange for services to be delivered
(D) Act as client advocate
Individual level
Systems level
Link services delivered
(E) Monitor and assess services delivered
Identify gaps in delivery of service
(F) Reevaluate client needs and treatment plan

CLIENT CONTRACTING

Nancy E. Johnston

Client contracting is defined as a mutually agreed upon process that brings the nurse and client together, with the client's goal to attain a desired or targeted new behavior and the nurse's to assist in the process. Since the contract is usually written, it serves the purpose of maintaining a sharp focus for nurse-client interactions. When carried out in a collaborative rather than coercive manner, it allows the client greater responsibility and control over his or her health outcomes.

A. This strategy is predicated on the ability of the nurse to establish a caring relationship. If the caring aspect of the relationship is not felt by the client, the contracting process may be experienced as an impersonal business transaction, a manipulation, a coercive ploy, or an empty and meaningless exercise.

B. Contracting is not suitable for some clients. Clients who are experiencing severe distortions in thought processes such that they are unable to comprehend or follow through on the requirements of the contracting process, acutely psychotic individuals, or persons experiencing toxic or organic brain syndromes should be considered ineligible. Moreover, contracting should be used only with utmost discretion for the suicidal client, since the desire to terminate a subjective experience characterized by overwhelming despair and futility may preclude the ability to honor the terms of a contract. Clients seeking an insight-oriented therapy may find the contracting approach too behaviorally oriented or unnecessarily explicit.

C. The nurse meets clients with varying degrees of competence for self-care. For those seeking to enhance an already superior level of functioning, approaches that are intensely supportive are usually unnecessary; a role that reinforces motivation and commitment to self-care by providing suggestions and appropriate resources such as reading materials, tapes, films, and charts often receives the most positive response.

D. Clients whose competence for self-management is judged to fall within the medium category are those who may be experiencing severe situational crises and whose usual coping mechanisms are compromised. Clients suffering from mental or physical conditions from which recovery is expected, or for whom disablement is moderate, will benefit from an enabling approach that seeks to support the reestablishment of capability for self-care. Although some regression may act to conserve energy for subsequent and renewed efforts to cope effectively, the tendency to perpetuate a downward spiral of continued deterioration should be guarded against.

E. Clients whose competence for self-care is judged to be low include those who suffer chronic and severely disabling conditions, individuals who have experienced multiple and prolonged hospitalizations and whose social and occupational roles demonstrate severe disengagement and decay. Restore confidence in the ability to attain an improved level of self-care by expressing belief in the individual's potential, reducing influences that reinforce dependence, and encouraging the client to select more assertive options.

F. Once it can be established that the client has some motivation for self-care, encourage further discussion and elaboration on the nature of the problems. Free-flowing discussion is gradually transformed into an exploration of the relationship of problem resolution to the need for behavioral change. For some clients this relationship will be obvious, while for others this insight will be developed as a result of unfolding awareness. It is important

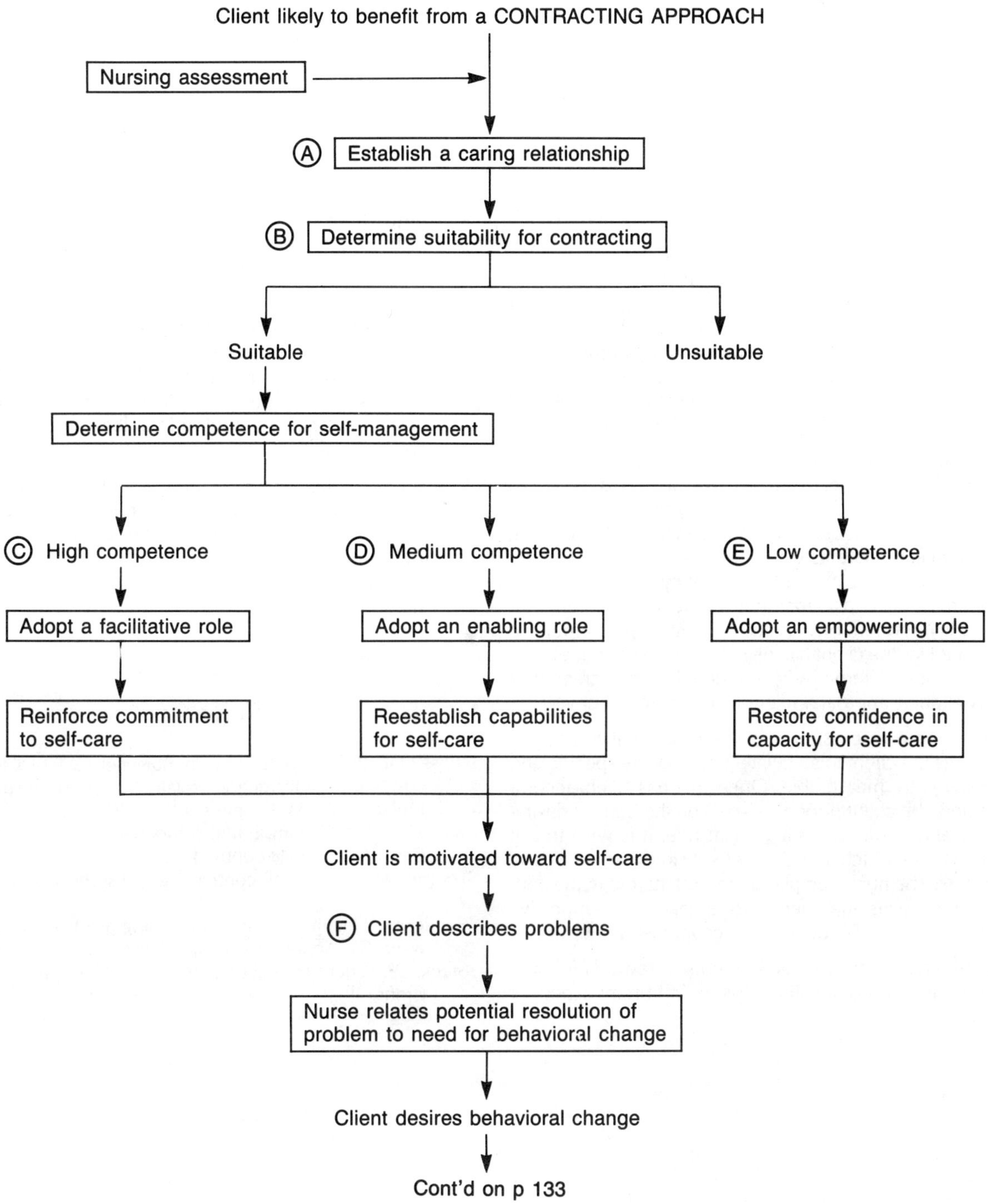
Client likely to benefit from a CONTRACTING APPROACH
Nursing assessment
Ⓐ Establish a caring relationship
Ⓑ Determine suitability for contracting
Suitable
Unsuitable
Determine competence for self-management
Ⓒ High competence
Ⓓ Medium competence
Ⓔ Low competence
Adopt a facilitative role
Adopt an enabling role
Adopt an empowering role
Reinforce commitment to self-care
Reestablish capabilities for self-care
Restore confidence in capacity for self-care
Client is motivated toward self-care
Ⓕ Client describes problems
Nurse relates potential resolution of problem to need for behavioral change
Client desires behavioral change
Cont'd on p 133

that the client develop strong insight into the rationale for behavioral change so that the process of undertaking change involves active commitment.

G. Introduce the idea of developing a contract as a method of assisting the client to make the changes he or she has already agreed are necessary and/or desirable. Encourage the client to think of the contract as a self-authored and flexible document that will help to maintain motivation by specifying the manner in which the changes will occur and the rewards for successful accomplishment.

H. Despite assurances of the advantages of contracting, some clients may resist further commitment. Rather than pressing the client, it is more useful to explore thoroughly any concerns, doubts, and fears, thereby diminishing resistance. For clients who continue to resist, it may be appropriate to reconsider the suitability of this approach. Also meriting consideration is the nurse-client relationship. Is it too tenuous to make contracting an attractive option? Has the client had negative past experiences with contracting? Alternatively, is a more informal gradual or less explicit approach likely to be more effective?

I. Following a discussion of goals in general terms, encourage the client to articulate goals that are specific and behaviorally measurable. Once this has been accomplished, the client prioritizes goals on the basis of desirability and difficulty. As a general rule, it is wise to opt for goals for which the client is likely to experience early success. The nurse can play an important role in the contracting process by offering to engage in a supportive activity that will further goal accomplishment.

J. Identifying effective reinforcements or rewards for successful goal accomplishment is an important aspect of the contracting process. In the case of highly autonomous individuals, these may be provided by the client him- or herself. Other clients may require more obvious and concrete reinforcements, some of which may be provided by themselves and others by the nurse.

K. Barriers or roadblocks to behavioral change are discussed so that the client can anticipate in advance the difficulties of following through with the desired activities. In cases where the barriers appear likely to create major obstacles it may be advisable at least initially, to work on easier goals.

L. The final phase in developing a contract involves establishing a time frame for implementation and checking to ensure that the contract is practical. One way of reviewing the contract is to use the SMART check list. Is the contract *s*pecific, *m*easurable, *a*cceptable, *r*ealistic, and *t*ruthful?

References

Jensen DB. Patient contracting. In: Bulechek GM, McCloskey JC, eds. Nursing interventions: treatments for nursing diagnoses. Philadelphia: WB Saunders, 1985:92–98.

Kort M. Support: an important component of health promotion. Can J Nurs 1984; 80(4):24–26.

Loomis ME. Levels of contracting. J Psychosoc Nurs 1985; 23(3):9–14.

Pender NJ. Health promotion in nursing practice. 2nd ed. Norwalk, CT: Appleton & Lange, 1987:229–252.

Steckl SB. Patient contracting. Norwalk, CT: Appleton-Century-Crofts, 1982.

Cont'd from p 131

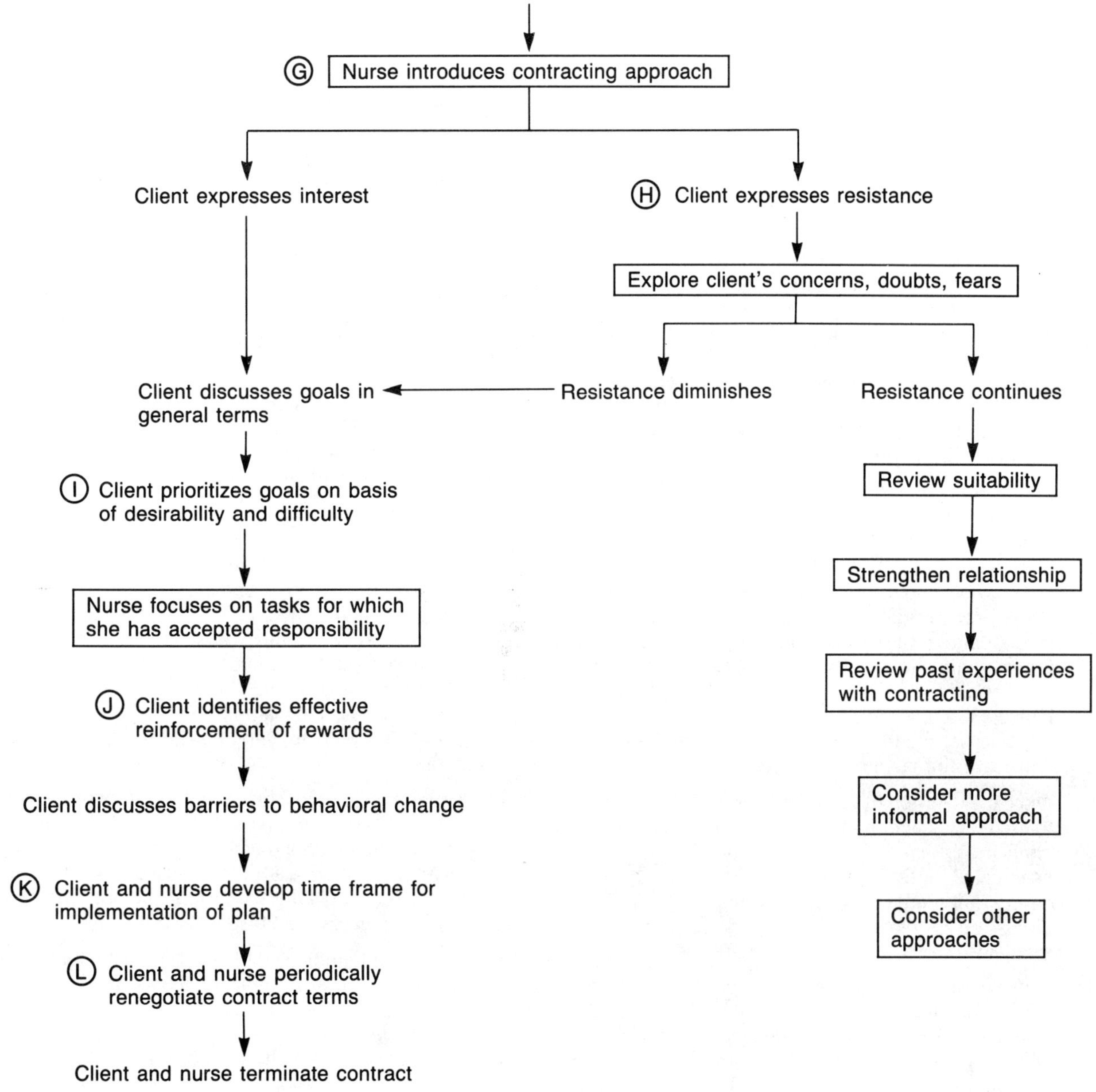

ELECTROCONVULSIVE THERAPY

Brenda Ingram

A. Electroconvulsive therapy (ECT), the use of unilateral or bilateral electrodes to pass approximately 15 to 35 joules of electricity through the brain in order to induce a grand mal seizure, has been used since 1937 to treat schizophrenic and severely depressed clients. Initially ECT was administered "straight," without using anesthesia and muscle relaxants. Today only modified ECT is recommended. Clients are anesthetized with fast-acting, short half-life general anesthetics and muscle relaxants. This change has made this form of therapy more acceptable because it has minimized the incidence of severe muscle spasms and fractures.

B. Clients for whom ECT is indicated include those who have a history of severe depression that has not responded to one or more trials of antidepressants and those who have responded well to ECT in the past. Others for whom ECT may be helpful are (1) severely depressed clients who are actively suicidal or who are not suicidal but who have not responded to one or more trials of antidepressants; (2) catatonic clients who are in danger of malnutrition or dehydration because of their lack of or inadequate oral intake; (3) manic clients who are on the verge of physical collapse; and (4) clients with schizoaffective disorders who have not responded to alternative treatments.

C. Once the decision has been made by the treatment team to use ECT, clear documentation of the rationale for and clinical appropriateness of this form of treatment is essential. A signed informed consent form is needed to ensure that the client's rights are protected. For further discussion of informed consent, see the chapter "The Law and Informed Consent" (p 230).

D. Nurses working as team members on the inpatient unit are actively involved in the medical work-up to facilitate clearing clients for ECT. Nursing responsibilities include alleviating the client's anxieties about ECT and patient teaching both before and after ECT. The nurse informs clients of the necessary work-up procedures done by cardiology (electrocardiogram), orthopaedics (spinal radiographs), general medicine (complete physical examination), neurology (a computed tomographic scan of the head or electroencephalogram may be required), and anesthesiology. The nurse also informs the client and family that the client will not be allowed to drink or eat on the morning of treatment, that voiding prior to the procedure will be required, and that jewelry and dentures will be removed and a hospital gown will be worn. Laboratory work includes SMA-18, urinalysis, serology, and thyroid function studies. All of these procedures depend upon each institution's protocol for ECT.

E. Inform the client that general anesthesia will be used and that he or she will need to be NPO at least 4 hours before the procedure. A consent form for anesthesia is required. Briefly describe the ECT process to the client and family and stress that the client's safety will be maintained at all times. Clients are usually confused and disoriented for approximately an hour after the procedure. Tell the client and family that this is temporary.

F. The Hamilton Rating Scale for Depression can be used to assess the client's level of depression. It may be helpful to have clients complete this scale before ECT and once a week after treatment begins. Comparing these scores is an objective way to assess the client's response to treatment.

G. Post-ECT care includes monitoring the client closely, including checking vital signs every 15 minutes for at least 1 hour or until stable and monitoring the intravenous line, which will probably be discontinued when the client is able to eat or take oral fluids.

H. One of the main aftereffects of ECT is memory impairment, which may range from mild forgetfulness to severe confusion. This memory impairment may persist for weeks or months after ECT. Assure the client and family that this is temporary. Most clients show a positive response to ECT after five treatments. This can be evaluated by comparing the client's baseline (pre-ECT) level of functioning and Hamilton Rating Scale score with the post-ECT level of functioning and Hamilton Rating Scale score.

I. Once the client reaches premorbid functioning, follow-up care can be implemented, including maintenance antidepressant drug therapy and individual and/or group psychotherapy. For additional discussion of group therapy see the chapters "Group Therapy" (p 136) and "Major Depressive Episodes" (p 46).

J. ECT is contraindicated in clients with the following conditions: (1) elevated intracranial pressure related to brain tumors or hemorrhage; (2) a history of myocardial infarction within 6 weeks prior to treatment; (3) a cerebrovascular accident within 3 months prior to treatment; or (4) a documented history of pseudocholinesterase deficiency or myasthenia gravis (the rationale for these contraindications is that they require special anesthetic techniques); (5) less than 2 weeks post partum; or (6) large aneurysms. When ECT is contraindicated, alternative forms of treatment should be explored by the treatment team. Client teaching and follow-up care should be based on the treatment modality and the needs and goals of the client.

References

Cochran C. A change of mind about ECT. Am J Nurs 1984; 84:1004–1005.

Crossfield T. Curse or cure? Nurs Times 1988; 84:66–67.

Fine M, Jenike MA. Electroshock: exploding the myths. RN 1985; 48:59–66.

Mawson D. Shock waves. Nurs Times 1985; 81:42–44.

National Institute of Mental Health. Consensus development conference statement. Vol 5, No 11. Washington, DC: U.S. Department of Health and Human Services, 1985.

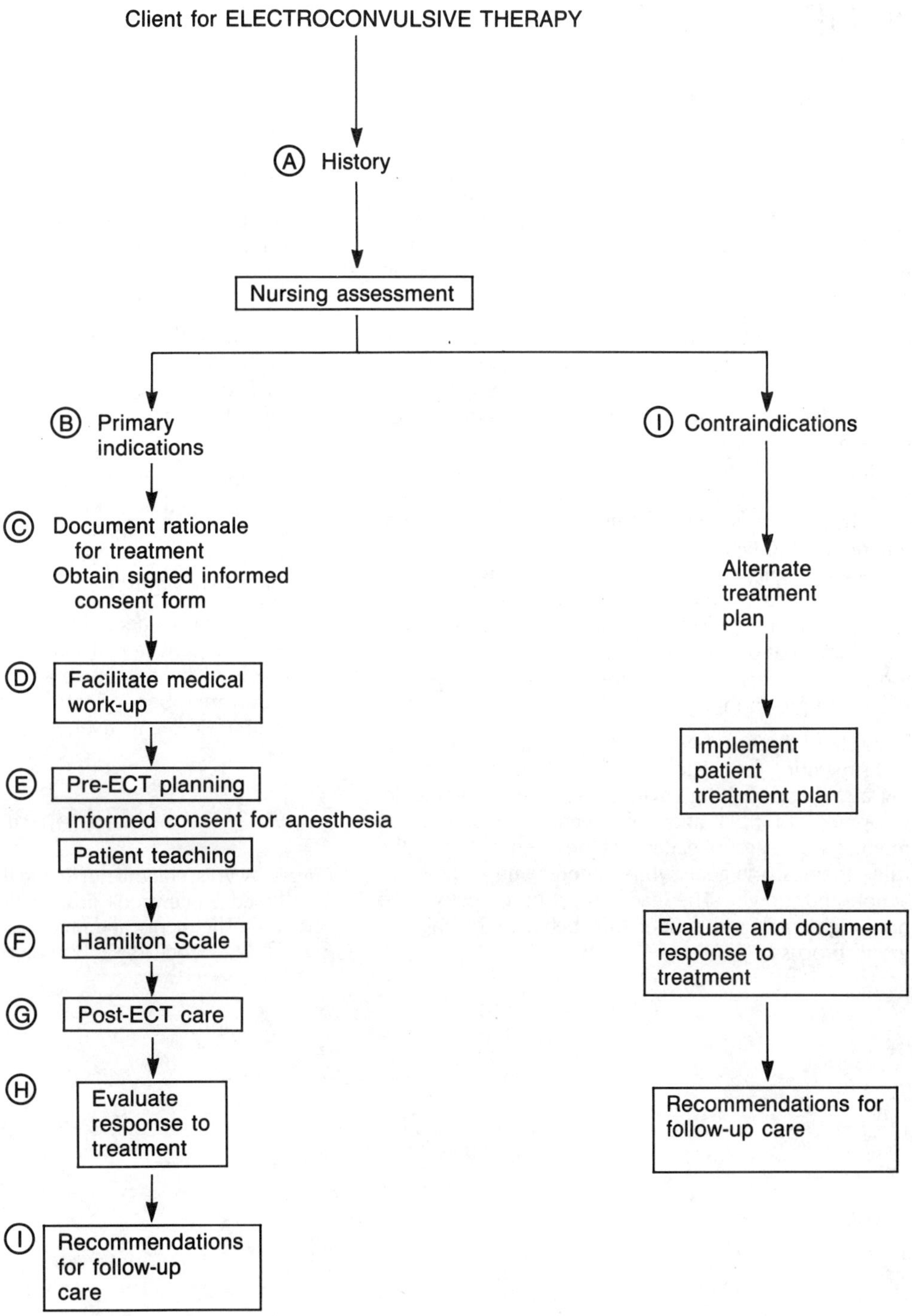
Client for ELECTROCONVULSIVE THERAPY
(A) History
Nursing assessment
(B) Primary indications
(C) Document rationale for treatment
Obtain signed informed consent form
(D) Facilitate medical work-up
(E) Pre-ECT planning
Informed consent for anesthesia
Patient teaching
(F) Hamilton Scale
(G) Post-ECT care
(H) Evaluate response to treatment
(I) Recommendations for follow-up care
(I) Contraindications
Alternate treatment plan
Implement patient treatment plan
Evaluate and document response to treatment
Recommendations for follow-up care

GROUP THERAPY

Deborah Antai-Otong

A. The nursing assessment should include current and past psychiatric treatment, reasons for treatment, type of treatment (i.e., individual or family therapy), and response to treatment. Clients seeking group therapy need to identify reasons for seeking treatment and their expectations.

B. Group selection should be determined by group goals, target symptoms, the client's level of function, and ego function. Clients selected for psychodynamic groups should be self-motivated and willing to experience personal growth and maturity. They must be capable of working with others and forming interpersonal relationships. The therapist must be able to work constructively with the group members. Clients who should be excluded from psychodynamic groups include those with emotional and cognitive impairments (i.e., actively psychotic, delusional, and those with organic disorders), and those exhibiting poor impulse control and dangerous behaviors (i.e., homicidal or suicidal). These clients have difficulty forming interpersonal relationships and are often disruptive in group therapy.

C. The role of the nurse-group therapist includes creating and structuring the group. This can be facilitated by creating a safe and trusting environment that facilitates development of trust and cohesiveness among group members. The group leader provides members with the rules, themes, and goals while encouraging group interaction and growth. The leader must be objective and nonjudgmental and model this behavior during the group process.

D. Assessing the individual needs of the group members can be facilitated by asking members what they expect from group therapy and encouraging them to identify group and individual goals. Assisting the members to meet these goals is the primary objective.

E. The nurse therapist must establish themes and agendas that encourage group members to actively interact with each other while allowing those who wish to remain quiet to do so.

F. Group members must feel physically and emotionally safe in group settings, and they must be assured that the therapist will intervene when appropriate to maintain a safe setting. The initial group rules and expectations must include discussions about safety and confidentiality, and these issues must be maintained throughout treatment.

G. Encouraging clients to evaluate their progress throughout treatment can be facilitated by constructive feedback provided by the nurse and group members. Use the group members' identified goals and expectations to evaluate the effectiveness of group therapy.

References

Burgess AW. Psychiatric nursing in the hospital and community. 4th ed. Englewood Cliffs, NJ: Prentice-Hall, 1985:835–849.

Yalom ID. The theory and practice of group psychotherapy. 3rd ed. New York: Basic Books, 1985.

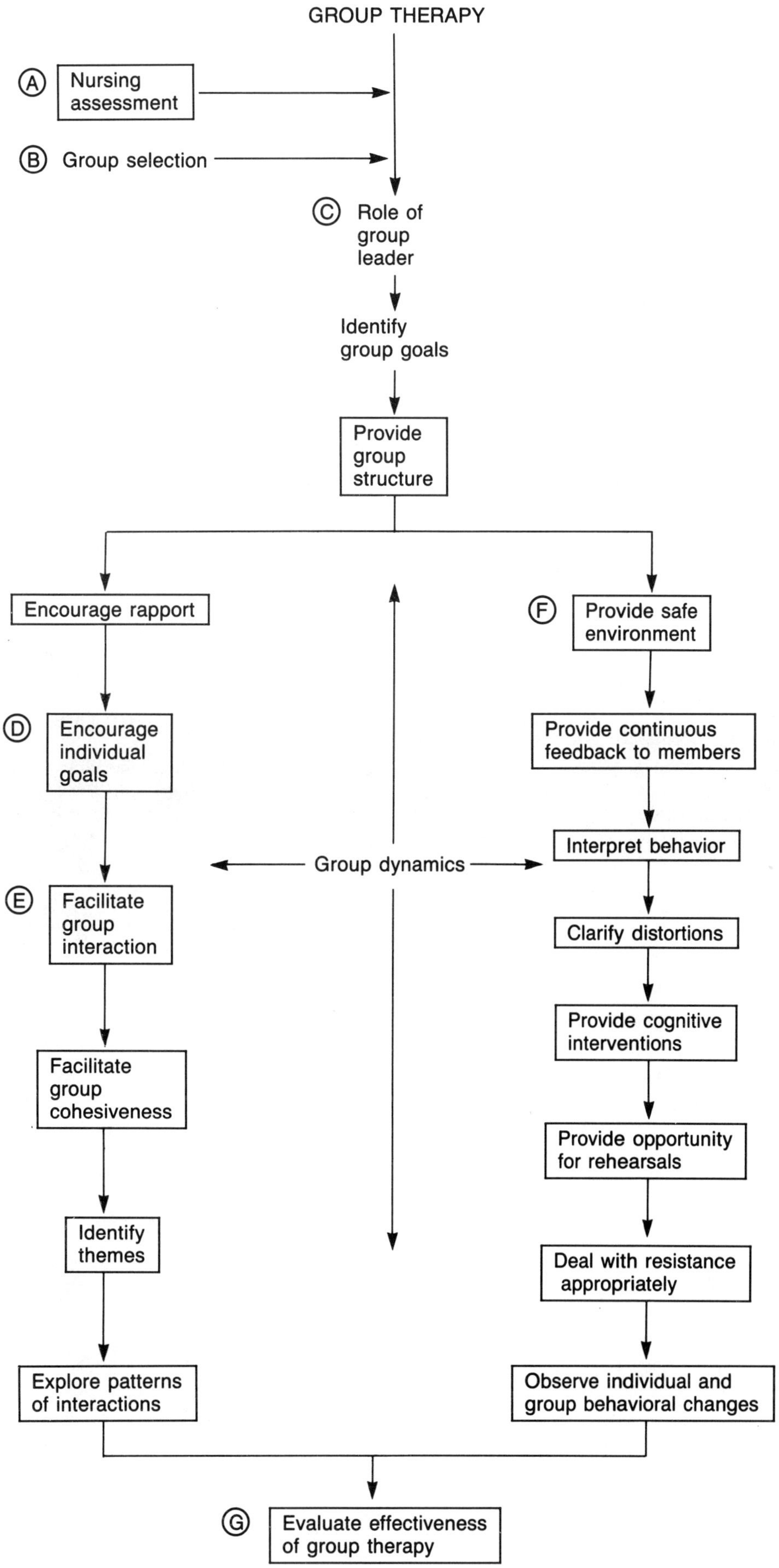
GROUP THERAPY
A Nursing assessment
B Group selection
C Role of group leader
Identify group goals
Provide group structure
Encourage rapport
D Encourage individual goals
E Facilitate group interaction
Facilitate group cohesiveness
Identify themes
Explore patterns of interactions
Group dynamics
F Provide safe environment
Provide continuous feedback to members
Interpret behavior
Clarify distortions
Provide cognitive interventions
Provide opportunity for rehearsals
Deal with resistance appropriately
Observe individual and group behavioral changes
G Evaluate effectiveness of group therapy

SUPPORT AND LIFE SKILLS GROUPS

Deborah Antai-Otong

A. Support and life skills groups provide opportunities for clients to improve their social and interpersonal skills. They also facilitate improvement in occupational skills. Clients feel encouraged and supported emotionally in these groups. Support groups increase the client's social interaction and decrease feelings of alienation. The nurse assists clients to recognize their strengths and accept their shortcomings. The nonthreatening atmosphere assists clients to develop basic social and interpersonal skills. They learn how to express feelings and understand their meaning. The themes of support and life skills groups may vary from improving social skills to mobilizing support systems. Other themes may revolve around medication compliance issues. Members must be self-directed and competent. The nurse must initially obtain the history from each group member (including past and present psychiatric treatment, medical status, and current medications) and determine the client's level of functioning over the past year. This information assists the nurse in making the group selection.

B. The nursing assessment for group selection must include assessing each member's mental status, coping patterns, and problem-solving capabilities. Individual goals and expectations must be considered and used to make the group selection. Clients must be assessed for suicidal and homicidal potential (see "Suicide Attempt" [p 42]). The client must be physically able and willing to attend the group sessions. Certain clients should be excluded from groups, such as those who are actively psychotic, suicidal, or homicidal, those who are not willing to participate in groups, those with severe delusional disorders, and those with histories of assaultive, aggressive behaviors and poor impulse control. For further discussion of group therapy and group dynamics, see page 136.

C. These groups provide a safe, structured group setting that allows the nurse to provide reality orientation, development of adaptive social skills, and opportunities to enhance interpersonal and problem-solving skills. Support and life skills therapy evokes minimal anxiety and stress while mobilizing support systems.

D. Values clarification allows the nurse to help clients analyze their feelings and behaviors in a safe setting. This process encourages self-examination, personal growth, and self-gratification. It fosters awareness of personal values and how they influence decision making and behaviors.

References

Brady JP. Social skills training for psychiatric patients. II: Clinical outcome studies. Am J Psychiatry, 1984; 141:491–408.

Steele SM, Harmon VM. Values clarification in nursing. 2nd ed. Norwalk, CT: Appleton-Century-Crofts, 1983.

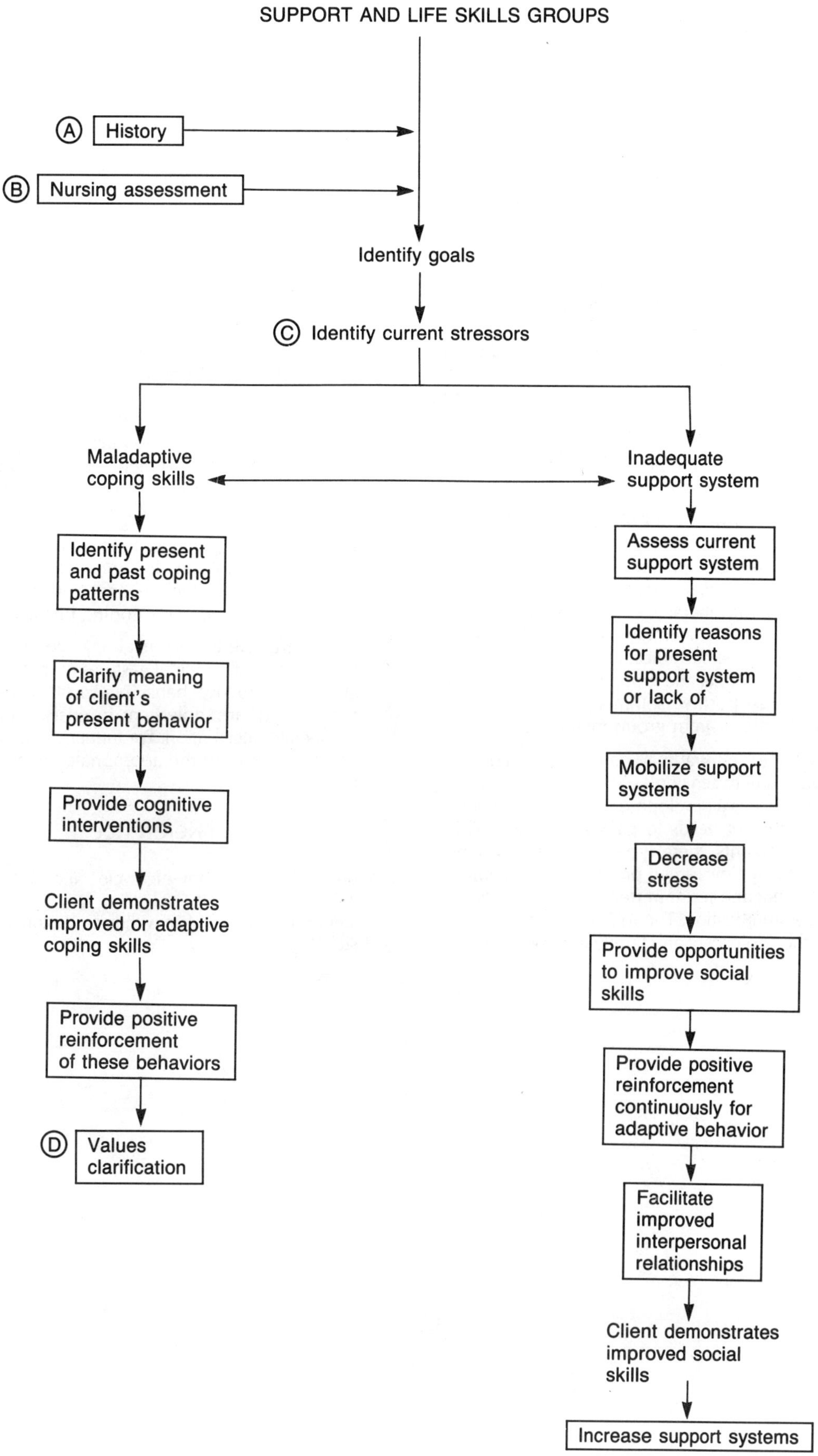
SUPPORT AND LIFE SKILLS GROUPS
(A) History
(B) Nursing assessment
Identify goals
(C) Identify current stressors
Maladaptive coping skills
Inadequate support system
Identify present and past coping patterns
Clarify meaning of client's present behavior
Provide cognitive interventions
Client demonstrates improved or adaptive coping skills
Provide positive reinforcement of these behaviors
(D) Values clarification
Assess current support system
Identify reasons for present support system or lack of
Mobilize support systems
Decrease stress
Provide opportunities to improve social skills
Provide positive reinforcement continuously for adaptive behavior
Facilitate improved interpersonal relationships
Client demonstrates improved social skills
Increase support systems

ADOLESCENT GROUPS

Deborah Antai-Otong

A. For a further discussion on assessing the family system, refer to "Child with Depression" (p 58), "Family Therapy" (p 170), and "Adolescent Suicide Attempt" (p 152).

B. Adolescents referred for treatment often exhibit dysfunction through poor academic performance, and their history reveals an average-to-good academic performance with a sudden drop in grades, apathy, and withdrawal from both school and social activities. Poor academic performance often reflects stress and chaos in the family system. These individuals often suffer a lack of self-confidence and self-esteem. Psychological testing must be performed by a trained administrator (i.e., psychologist) to rule out organic or other factors, such as depression, that may interfere with academic performance.

C. Since adolescence is a time of physical and emotional turmoil, teenagers become easily discouraged and sometimes have low self-esteem. They may easily resort to negative feelings and make negative self-statements in individual and group therapy. Discourage adolescents from making negative statements, encourage them to focus on their positive attributes, and assist them to develop realistic individual and group goals. Provide activities that enhance positive self-image and encourage constructive feedback from group members.

D. Another reason for referral may be ineffective communication patterns between adolescents and their parents. Since adolescence is a developmental period characterized by concomitant needs to gain autonomy and be dependent on parents, these types of conflicts are not uncommon. Many times small problems are magnified by the adolescent and result in frequent arguments and ineffective communication. The role of the nurse centers on helping the adolescent and family members identify these areas and develop more effective communication patterns.

E. Determine the developmental issues in the group and individual members. This information assists assessment of the areas of conflicts and facilitates resolution. Common adolescence issues include those related to identity versus role diffusion and intimacy versus isolation. Adolescents must be encouraged to function independently while understanding that the nurse is available when needed. Be consistent with limit setting, and provide group rules that are realistic and attainable. Recognize that peers are important during this stage of development, and assist members to define their identity while adapting to the enormous emotional and physical changes that occur during this period.

F. Homework assignments that involve practicing these learned behaviors in the home situation with family members to assist the teenager to test them in the real world enhance adaptive coping behaviors.

G. Self-destructive behaviors at any age that express a cry for help include suicidal gestures or threats or substance abuse. Destructive behaviors must be identified as a symptom of an adolescent in crisis, and followed by immediate intervention. For further discussion of specific behaviors, refer to the appropriate chapters (see pp 30 to 42).

References

Erikson E. Identity and the life cycle. New York: WW Norton, 1979.

Minuchin S. Families and family therapy. Boston: Harvard University Press, 1974.

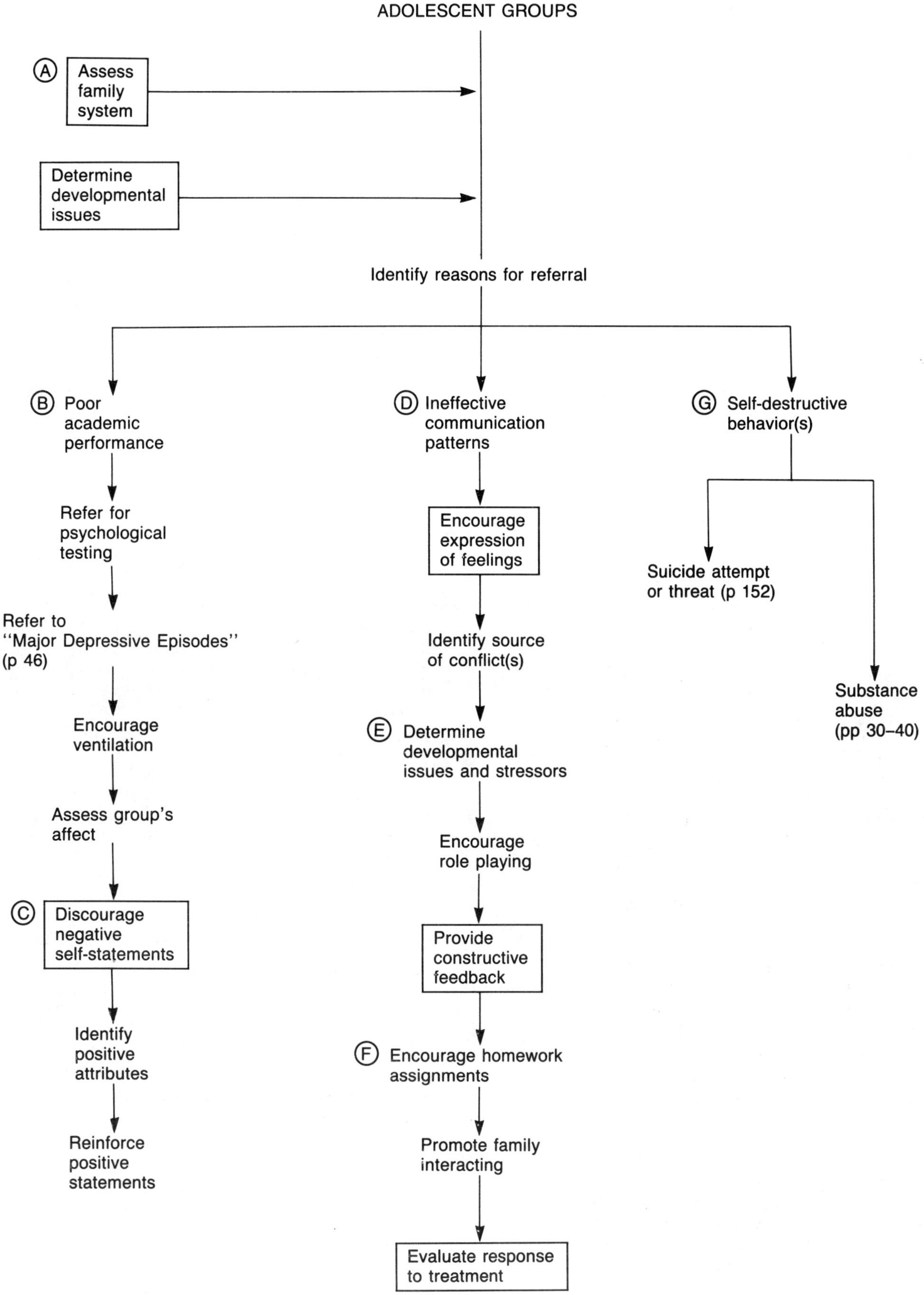
ADOLESCENT GROUPS
A Assess family system
Determine developmental issues
Identify reasons for referral
B Poor academic performance
Refer for psychological testing
Refer to "Major Depressive Episodes" (p 46)
Encourage ventilation
Assess group's affect
C Discourage negative self-statements
Identify positive attributes
Reinforce positive statements
D Ineffective communication patterns
Encourage expression of feelings
Identify source of conflict(s)
E Determine developmental issues and stressors
Encourage role playing
Provide constructive feedback
F Encourage homework assignments
Promote family interacting
Evaluate response to treatment
G Self-destructive behavior(s)
Suicide attempt or threat (p 152)
Substance abuse (pp 30–40)

OUTPATIENT CRISIS GROUP

Kay Burke

A. Obtain an individual history for each client. Approach the client in a manner that reflects concern. Appear calm and in control, since this is reassuring to clients who may feel confused and poorly controlled. The history should include current and past psychiatric treatment, including past and present medication. Determine whether chronic psychiatric disorders exist, whether acute disorders have occurred, and how and when they were treated. Inquire as to drug and alcohol history, since these increase risk potential. Explore past homicidal, suicidal, and impulsive gestures, seeking details and whether alcohol or drugs were involved. Obtain a family psychiatric history, especially noting any homicidal, suicidal, or impulsive behaviors that put the client at higher risk. Seek the family history of alcohol and drug use and whether suicidal, homicidal, or impulsive gestures were related. Obtain a medical history, including major illnesses, treatment, and medications being used. Determine the events that led the client to present for treatment. Use information obtained from significant others for clarification and verification. Determine the functional level that existed prior to these events, how similar situations have been handled in the past, and the meaning the client places on the situation.

B. Complete a psychiatric nursing assessment. An initial physical assessment is ideally done with laboratory testing prior to referral to a psychiatric service. If this has not been done, refer the client for a medical evaluation. The client may require treatment in a medical unit with a psychiatric consultation until physiologic disorders are adequately controlled. Then, the client could be considered for a crisis group. Perform a complete mental status examination. Clients found to be psychotic or actively homicidal or suicidal require hospitalization with appropriate observation and medical intervention. Assess the risk factors carefully for self-destructive or other destructive behavior potential. Clients who display other active psychiatric disorders or severe personality disorders may require therapies other than a crisis group. Clients with significant cognitive or language limitations may not be capable of participation in a crisis group. Active substance abuse or alcohol problems in clients require specialized referrals that also address these addictions.

C. Those clients who are found to be in a crisis uncomplicated by disorders that would hinder participation are referred to an outpatient crisis group. Some typical situations that may lead to a crisis response include death of a spouse, diagnosis of terminal illness, job loss, and home loss by fire. Crises occur when previous means of dealing with such problems are inadequate. Disequilibrium is reflected in a dysfunctional, overwhelmed state with inadequate problem-solving ability. Support systems are inadequate or absent. Consideration is given to differences in culture, language, intellect, maturity, and type of problem when referring to a suitable crisis group. Limit group numbers to about five to eight to allow enough time for all to work, since members attend about four to six meetings, in keeping with the short life of a crisis.

D. Referral is made to a suitable crisis intervention group. The crisis state generates tension for members to work toward problem resolution. Goals for these groups include problem resolution, relief of anxiety, improvement of coping strategies, replacing maladaptive behaviors, decision making, insight gaining, and strengthening or formation of support systems. Growth is accomplished as members help each other to reach these goals.

E. An individual session with each prospective group member promotes understanding of goals that may be accomplished in the group. Role expectations, behavioral limitations, and agreement with this form of treatment are also discussed. Preparation of those who choose to enter the group enables the new member to be more readily introduced and assimilated into the group.

F. The group process is ongoing, with the needs of the participants determining the process direction. Assessment of destructive behavior potential is a continuous requirement because of the intensity of feelings and the disturbances of thought processes. Leaders are more directive than in some other types of groups. A number of issues must be addressed, with care taken to deal with the many issues presented in an organized, meaningful fashion. Bereavement issues are addressed, healthy coping strategies are reinforced, healthy support systems are reinforced or developed, behaviors are carefully observed and appropriate actions taken, active listening is done, decision making is facilitated, and participation is encouraged. Clarification is sought as needed, and reflection is offered to further clarify and summarize. Alternatives for improved coping are explored, with group input encouraged. Cognitive and emotional work of the group is encouraged. A variety of techniques may be utilized in crisis intervention groups to facilitate growth and to accomplish individual and group goals.

G. When a member leaves the group at discharge, leaders and the client may agree that the goals for which he entered the group have been met and that at least the pre-crisis level of functioning has been regained. Unresolved issues that remain at discharge may indicate a need for a therapy follow-up. Other referrals such as support groups may be useful for further growth and support, especially when future adaptation problems are anticipated.

References

Aguilera DC, Messick JM. Crisis intervention theory and methodology. 5th ed. St. Louis: CV Mosby, 1986.

Hoff LA. People in crisis. 2nd ed. Menlo Park, CA: Addison-Wesley, 1984.

Mancini ME. Decision making in emergency nursing. Toronto: BC Decker, 1987.

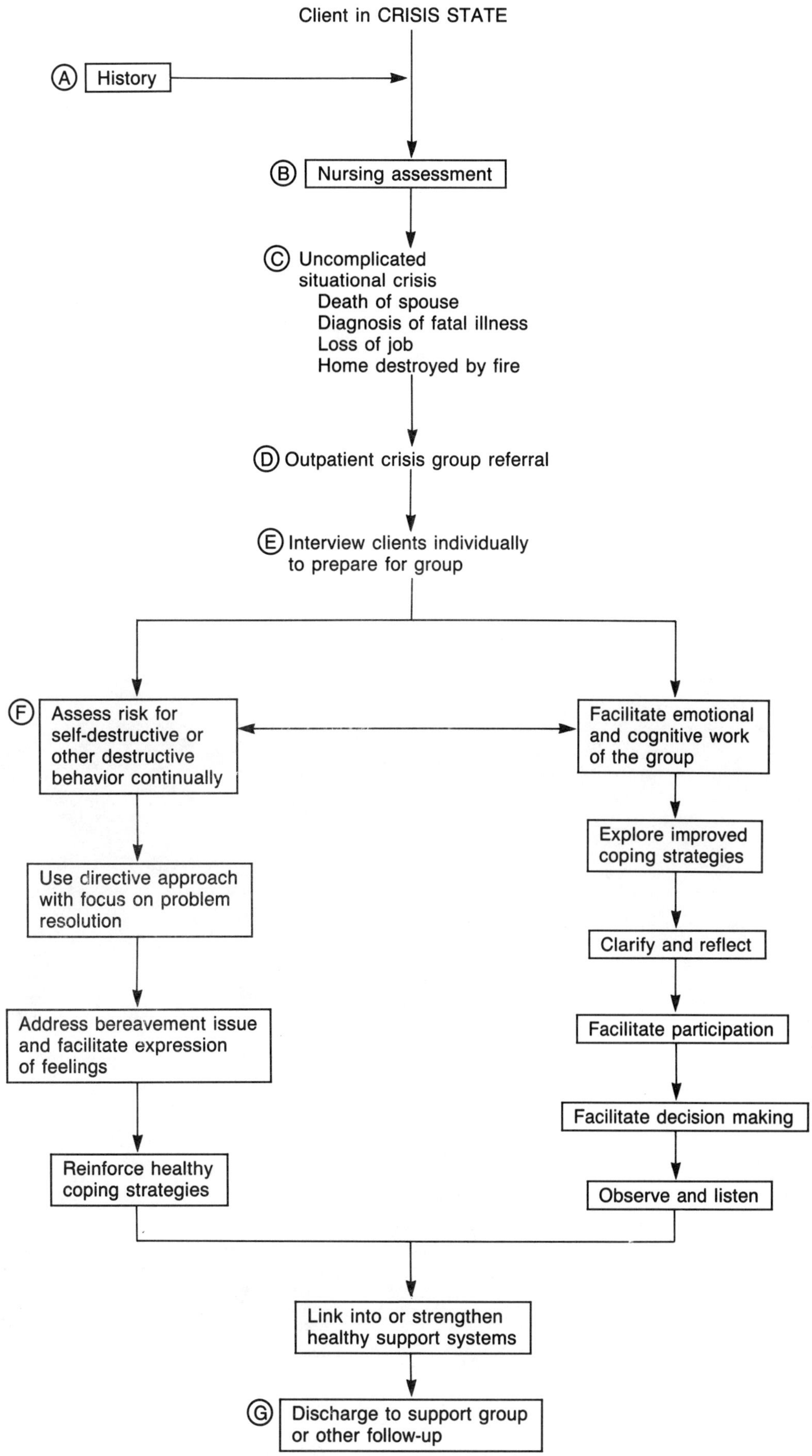

Client in CRISIS STATE
Ⓐ History
Ⓑ Nursing assessment
Ⓒ Uncomplicated situational crisis
Death of spouse
Diagnosis of fatal illness
Loss of job
Home destroyed by fire
Ⓓ Outpatient crisis group referral
Ⓔ Interview clients individually to prepare for group
Ⓕ Assess risk for self-destructive or other destructive behavior continually
Use directive approach with focus on problem resolution
Address bereavement issue and facilitate expression of feelings
Reinforce healthy coping strategies
Facilitate emotional and cognitive work of the group
Explore improved coping strategies
Clarify and reflect
Facilitate participation
Facilitate decision making
Observe and listen
Link into or strengthen healthy support systems
Ⓖ Discharge to support group or other follow-up

IV FAMILY-RELATED CONCEPTS

WOMEN'S HEALTH

Patricia Ellis
Barbara Brown

The concept of health is difficult to define. It is not simply the absence of disease, and it is different from illness. Sandelowski has stated, "Health is a reflection of whatever meaning and value the individual or group attributes to it, a result of the individual's interaction with his/her physical, psychological, and sociocultural environment, and an arbiter of that interaction."

According to McBride, women's health is "the overall experience of women as women, their dis-eases, and not just their diseases or childbearing functions." Women enter the health care system not for cure but to gain control of their health and health of their families.

A. A comprehensive assessment is essential. To discover a woman's personal definition of health, her health status, life goals, roles, and behaviors, Collier suggests that a crucial task is to pay attention to the existence of and interaction between internal and external realities that affect every woman. As an example, women are often labeled as depressed. There is a tendency to focus on the internal situation even though strong evidence exists linking depression, sex roles, and the external environment. Snyder points out that nursing diagnoses are intended to help focus on what nursing can do to assist a client to achieve the chosen health outcomes. Houlden, Saltstein, and Ganley stress the importance of using both wellness-related and health problem–related nursing diagnoses. This allows for a more accurate reflection of the needs and strengths of each client and in turn "to mobilize the health aspect of the client in addition to identifying needs and problems that require nursing intervention." Nursing diagnoses need to be flexible in accepting the chosen health outcomes as those selected by the woman herself and that the internal and external realities of women fluctuate and emerge at different times.

B. Women define health in relation to their situation as well as the physical state of their bodies. Thus, nursing interventions selected for use with women need to be holistic to treat all apsects of a health problem and/or to promote wellness. Mind and body are interrelated. Holistic health practices promote an interaction between the mind and the body, including the spiritual dimension. These interventions encompass more than the western scientific medical model, which is often impersonal and/or physicochemical. Holistic health practices are nonallopathic (not disease-oriented), rebalance human energies, promote a relationship of body structure to environmental forces, and increase self-awareness. For a nursing intervention to be effective, the nurse must possess the quality of caring. Effective nursing is more than technical competence and scientific knowledge. As Benner and Wrubel have stated, "Caring makes the nurse notice which interventions help, and this concern guides subsequent caregivings."

C. Every woman needs her own sense of psychological and emotional power in order to develop and live her life as fully as possible. Assisting the woman to do this by accepting her right as an individual to live however she wishes becomes a goal of nursing. Specific goals that need to be achieved by women in order to gain equality and develop as a human being are as follows: (1) to learn, know, respect, and use her own self-understanding; (2) to expand her choices in behavior and attitudes; (3) to define her health boundaries clearly; (4) to develop new rules and expectations for herself as a "healthy adult" with power over her own life; and (5) to develop new communication styles.

D. In evaluating goal achievement, it is essential to listen to the woman, herself. Through a process of exploration and collaborative work, the nurse and the woman can decide together whether to terminate the therapeutic relationship, to seek further collaboration with each other or other sources of health care, or to refer to a different health care professional.

References

Abrams M. Health care for women. J Obstet Gynecol Neonatal Nurs 1986; 15:250–255.

Benner P, Wrubel J. The primacy of caring: stress and coping in health and illness. Reading, MA: Addison-Wesley, 1989.

Bulechek GM, McCloskey JC. Nursing interventions: treatments for nursing diagnoses. Philadelphia: WB Saunders, 1985.

Collier HV. Counseling women: a guide for therapists. New York: The Free Press, 1982.

Krieger D. Foundations for holistic health nursing practices: the renaissance nurse. Philadelphia: JB Lippincott, 1981.

McBride AB. Women's health: where nursing and feminism converge. In: Griffith-Kenney J, ed. Contemporary women's health: a nursing approach. Reading, MA: Addison-Wesley, 1986:2–10.

Sandelowski M. Women, health, and choice. Toronto: Prentice-Hall of Canada, 1981.

Snyder M. Independent nursing interventions. New York: John Wiley & Sons, 1985.

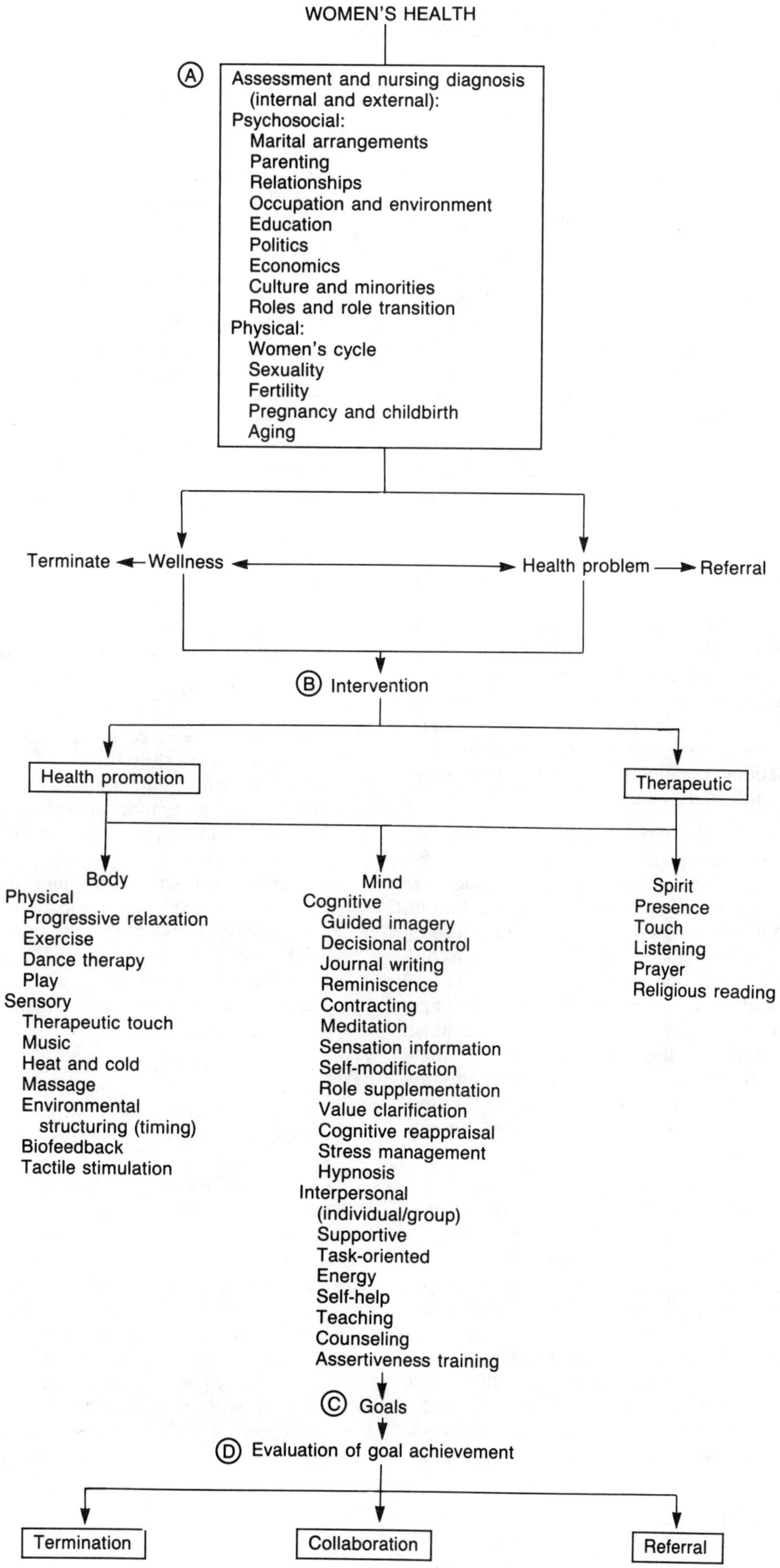
WOMEN'S HEALTH
A
Assessment and nursing diagnosis (internal and external):
Psychosocial:
Marital arrangements
Parenting
Relationships
Occupation and environment
Education
Politics
Economics
Culture and minorities
Roles and role transition
Physical:
Women's cycle
Sexuality
Fertility
Pregnancy and childbirth
Aging
Terminate
Wellness
Health problem
Referral
B Intervention
Health promotion
Therapeutic
Body
Physical
Progressive relaxation
Exercise
Dance therapy
Play
Sensory
Therapeutic touch
Music
Heat and cold
Massage
Environmental structuring (timing)
Biofeedback
Tactile stimulation
Mind
Cognitive
Guided imagery
Decisional control
Journal writing
Reminiscence
Contracting
Meditation
Sensation information
Self-modification
Role supplementation
Value clarification
Cognitive reappraisal
Stress management
Hypnosis
Interpersonal (individual/group)
Supportive
Task-oriented
Energy
Self-help
Teaching
Counseling
Assertiveness training
Spirit
Presence
Touch
Listening
Prayer
Religious reading
C Goals
D Evaluation of goal achievement
Termination
Collaboration
Referral

ATTENTION DEFICIT DISORDER

Sheryl L. Boblin

A. Attention deficit disorder (ADD) is a childhood learning disorder seen by nurses in schools, outpatient departments, and the community. Its essential features are impulsivity and inability to focus attention during problem solving. Because of their short attention span and ready frustration, such children function well below their cognitive ability in school. Impulsivity, temper tantrums, and restlessness can disrupt peer and adult relationships. The biological basis of ADD is unknown. One cause is thought to be lack of neurotransmitter norepinephrine or one of its breakdown products. Thus, CNS stimulants, thought to arouse the CNS inhibitory system and screen out distracting stimuli, are used to treat ADD. Regardless of the etiology, there is currently no cure for learning disabilities.

B. Data should be collected from multiple sources: parents—questionnaires, interviews, and rating scales; the child—self-control rating scales and interview; classroom and physical education teachers—child behavior checklists, intelligence scales, achievement tests, and physical examinations that include vision and hearing screening. Other assessments include evaluations of social and emotional functioning, including self-concept. Masked or unmasked depression, often concurrent with a learning disability, compounds problems with attention, memory, and understanding.

C. Because of many possible types of disabilities with ADD, diagnosis is best done by a team of professionals. A special educator trained in the field of learning disabilities evaluates the existence and types of learning disabilities. The level of intellectual functioning, often not a true indication of the child's abilities, is evaluated by a psychologist. A social worker or nurse assesses the child's development and areas of concern. Speech, language, or hearing problems are assessed by a speech therapist. A physician completes a physical examination, while a developmental or pediatric neurologist evaluates the child's nervous system. Psychological and social functioning are assessed by a psychiatrist or other mental health professional.

D. Parents experience denial, anger, and guilt as they cope with feelings of helplessness. Brothers and sisters, often not informed about their sibling's difficulties, experience anxiety, guilt, and anger at the extra attention given the sibling. Nurses must inform parents of their rights and encourage them to get needed services, coordinate services to reduce fragmented care, and be sensitive to the needs of the family. Parents need guidance, support, positive feedback for efforts, and reassurance that the child's behavior is not willful. They need information on support groups and advice on how to make the home environment conducive to the child's learning and development of self-control.

E. The goal of intervention is the child's acknowledgment of problems, understanding of special needs, and development of appropriate strategies. The appropriate school, including transportation services, may need to be determined. In general, the ADD child can receive three levels of help. If the child is not far behind academically and can handle being in a regular classroom, supplemental instruction might be offered. In this instance, it is crucial that the regular teacher be informed of the child's strengths and weaknesses and work closely with the supplemental teacher. If the child needs more help, a "mainstreaming model" may be recommended: the child receives intensive assistance in a special resource room 2 or more hours a day, spending the rest of the time in carefully selected regular classroom activities. The third level of help is for the child who cannot function in a regular class environment and is placed in a small, structured, self-contained classroom.

F. Social skills training may be needed by the ADD child who has social and interpersonal difficulties. Such training helps the child develop self-control through self-monitoring, self-evaluation, and self-rewarding. It addresses the thoughts, feelings, and behaviors that precede, accompany, and follow social encounters.

G. Interventions require an individualized plan that includes building the child's self-confidence and self-esteem. Maximum benefit of behavioral treatment programs occurs when the child is also on a medication regimen. Cognitive behavioral training increases the ADD child's use of language or inner speech as a means of reducing impulsivity and increasing attention. There are generally three components to cognitive-behavioral training: (1) verbal self-instruction, involving modeling the use of inner speech or self-instruction for the child; (2) response-cost, involving tokens that are removed for inappropriate behavior and are used by the child to "purchase" rewards; and (3) cognitive monitoring, in which the child indicates whether he was paying attention when a bell sounds at irregular intervals.

H. Medications are not treatments in themselves. They must be used along with treatment for the learning disorder. The child should not be on drugs at the beginning of the year so that a baseline of performance and behavior can be obtained. Stimulant medications (Ritalin, Cylert, Dexedrine), the safest of the psychotropic drugs in common use, require medical surveillance. Dosage is adjusted to the child's tolerance. Short-term side-effects include loss of appetite, weight loss, insomnia, headaches, nervous tics, and occasionally irritability as medication wears off. Height may be stunted during the course of the medications. With the correct dose, side-effects are attenuated or disappear for the duration of the drug's action. There has been no indication of withdrawal symptoms, no risk of drug abuse, and no lasting growth retardation if catch-up periods are allowed.

References

Good WV. Behavioral problems in school. In: Dubovsky SL, Feiger AD, Eiseman B, eds. Psychiatric decision making. Toronto: BC Decker, 1984:158–159.

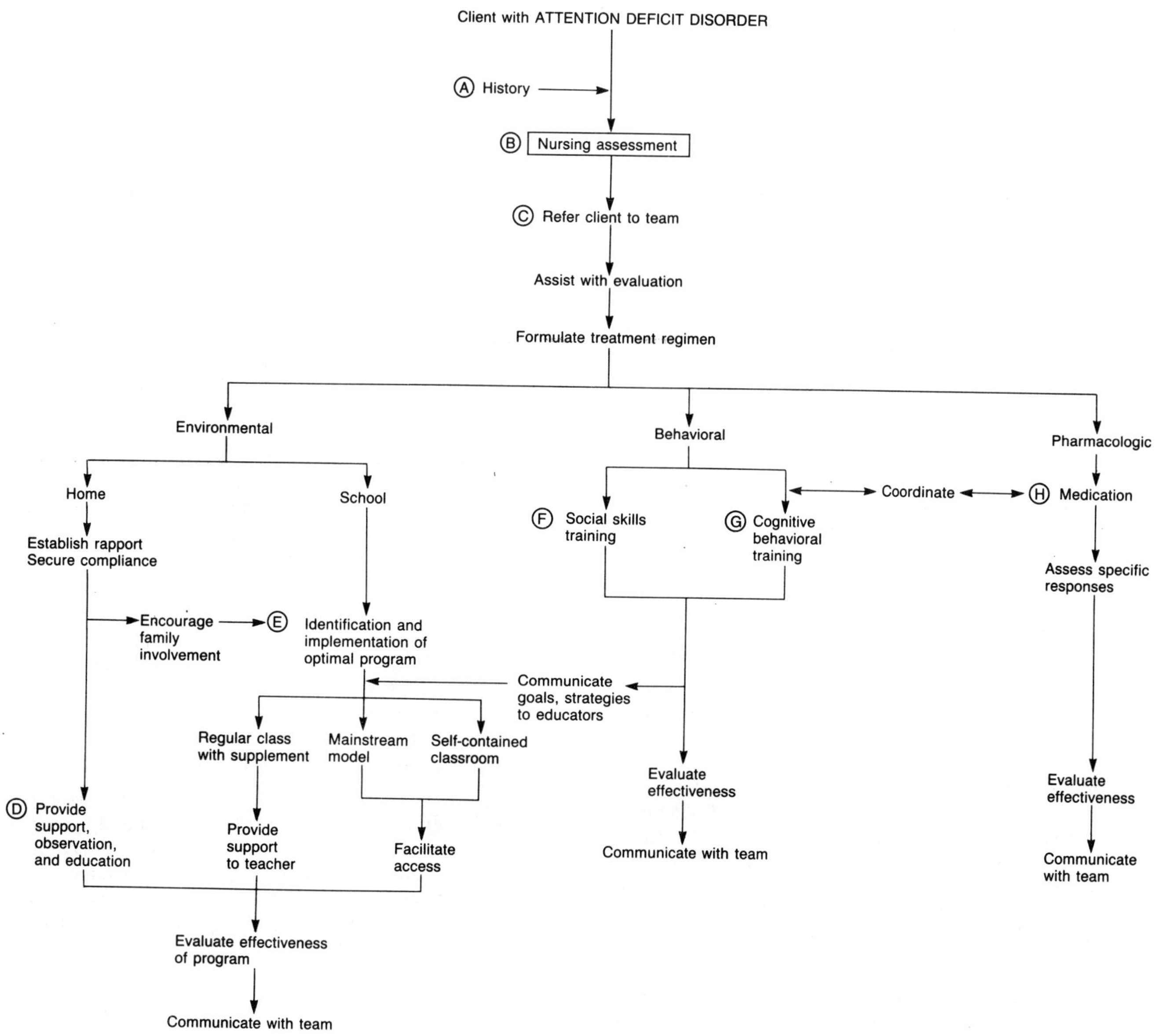

Kirby EA, Grimley LK. Understanding and treating attention deficit disorder. In: Goldstein AP, Krasner L, Garfield SL. Psychology practitioner guidebooks. New York: Pergamon Press, 1986.

Marlow D, Redding BA. Textbook of pediatric nursing. 6th ed. Philadelphia: WB Saunders, 1988.

Porter LS. The what, why and how of hyperkinesis: implications for nursing. J Adv Nurs 1988; 13:229–236.

Selekman J, Goldenthal P, Gordon-Clark K. The learning disabled child: another frontier for nursing. Holistic Nurs Pract 1988:1–10.

Silver LB. Attention deficit disorders. Summit, NJ: CIBA, 1980.

SCHOOL PHOBIA

Sheryl L. Boblin

School phobia is a complex social and emotional disorder. A school phobic child exhibits an extreme reluctance to go to school as a result of severe anxiety or marked fear of some aspect of the school situation. The school or community health nurse is in a position to question the cause of the child's complaints, because school phobic children represent a disproportionate number of visits to the health office. School phobia shows its peak between the ages of 5 and 7 years, when the child first enters school, at the age of 11 years when the child moves from elementary to secondary schools, and again at age 14 years. It increases in severity with the length of time between onset and resolution.

A. The school phobic child is generally brought to a health-care provider for evaluation of somatic complaints such as headache, dizziness, stomachache, lack of appetite, diarrhea, pallor, or fatigue. The first and most important step prior to intervention is the recommendation for a complete physical examination to eliminate any organic cause of the somatic complaints verbalized by the child.

B. The nurse is in an ideal position to coordinate the efforts among the school personnel, the family, and the health team. Such coordination is vital since prompt intervention is important to combat recurrent school phobia. Any decisions regarding the child's attendance should be cooperative among the parents, school personnel, and health-care providers. Parents may require support and assistance with strategies to ensure that the child attends school. It is important that parents be supported and directed without being made to feel in any way to blame.

C. Because of its complex nature, school phobia cannot be treated by one discipline or program. It requires cooperation and communication among the school nurse, classroom teacher, school psychologist, psychiatrist, social worker, occupational therapist, and physician. Together they devise a plan for managing the child.

D. The most crucial factor in the treatment of school phobia is proper identification of the subtype of phobia. There are generally two broad subtypes: an acute subtype and a more chronic form of the disorder. Acute and chronic school phobias are differentiated by the duration of the condition.

E. Seldom is one phobia or anxiety responsible for the child's refusal to go to school. The cause of the resistance to school must be determined before it can be cured. School phobia is the result of a series of small stresses, which are finally triggered by a major stress. Several sources of anxiety can be identified for the school-age child, including separation from a parent, fear of violence or humiliation, fear of bodily exposure (changing for physical education classes), school entrance or transition, difficulty with school work or school failure, or difficulty with a particular teacher or situation.

F. Intervention strategies are geared to the age and symptoms of the individual. Short-term, highly focused interventions have produced some successes in the treatment of acute phobic children. These interventions include avoidance of discussion of somatic complaints, forced school attendance, structured interview with the parents, brief interview with the child, and follow-up. Parents and therapists should use straightforward fear reduction strategies in the early stages of school phobia. With acute phobia, the sooner intervention occurs, the less likelihood the phobia will recur or progress to chronic school phobia.

G. Treatment of the chronic type of school phobia requires a more long-term, intensive approach. Psychotherapy may be necessary to investigate the child's anxieties in greater depth. Because the problem of school phobia is usually only partly the child's, the entire family may require counseling to resolve the issue.

H. Support of the child and family should continue, especially following return to school after holidays, school break, illness, or stressful incident involving the child or family. Friends, the teacher, the school nurse and other members of the health team are all part of the support network necessary to help the child with school phobia attend school regularly.

References

Good WV. School phobia. In: Dubrovsky SL, Feiger AD, Eisman B, eds. Psychiatric decision making. Toronto: BC Decker, 1984:164–165.

McAnanly E. School phobia: the importance of prompt intervention. J School Health 1986; 56:433–436.

Mulvihill D. Coping with school phobia. RNABC News 1987; 19(4):18–20.

Paccione-Dyszlewski MR, Contessa-Kislus MA. School phobia: identification of subtypes as a prerequisite to treatment interventions. Adolescence 1987; 22(86):377–383.

Servonsky J, Opas SR. Nursing management of children. Boston: Jones and Bartlett, 1987.

Turner-Boutle T. School phobia. Nursing Times 1984; 80(33):55–58.

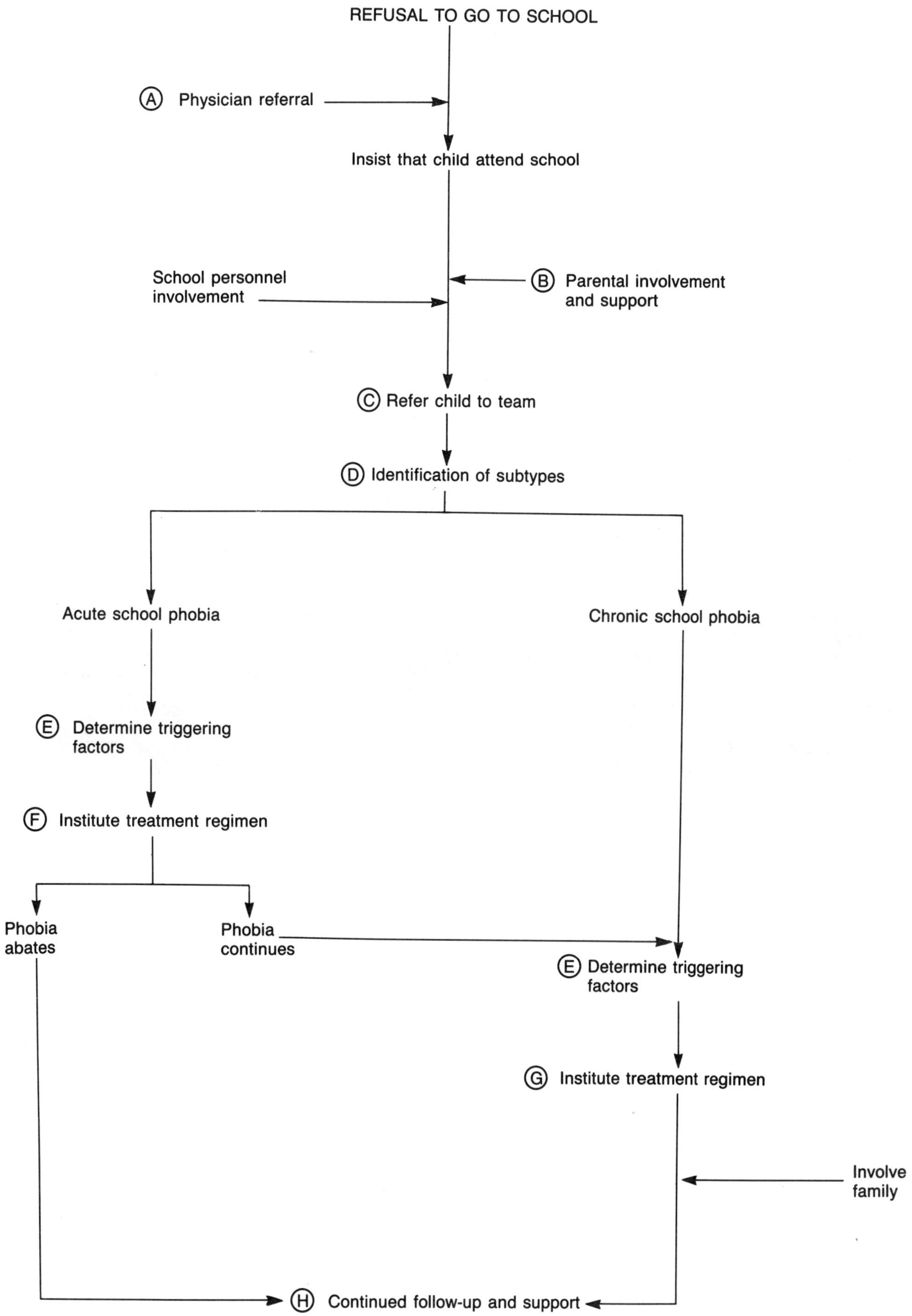
REFUSAL TO GO TO SCHOOL
(A) Physician referral
Insist that child attend school
School personnel involvement
(B) Parental involvement and support
(C) Refer child to team
(D) Identification of subtypes
Acute school phobia
Chronic school phobia
(E) Determine triggering factors
(F) Institute treatment regimen
Phobia abates
Phobia continues
(E) Determine triggering factors
(G) Institute treatment regimen
Involve family
(H) Continued follow-up and support

ADOLESCENT SUICIDE ATTEMPT

Deborah Antai-Otong

A. The suicide rate among adolescents and young adults 15 to 24 years of age in the United States tripled between 1956 and 1977, but the rates decreased between 1978 and 1985 in all age groups except the white 15 to 19 year olds. Research suggests that the increase and decrease in these rates correspond with the fluctuation in the adolescent population in the United States. The major causes of adolescent suicide include poor communication with parents, grief over the death of a parent, child abuse, chaotic families, and dissolution of a meaningful relationship. Depression constitutes a major problem among these youths.

B. The nursing assessment includes developmental level family dynamics, role of the adolescent in the family system, the child's ability to interact with others, including family, peers, and other adults outside the home. Other areas that should be included in the assessment include current stressors, significant changes, coping patterns, performance in school, at work, and at home. Family members should be included during this process. The nurse must assess the adolescent, and family members' feelings about the attempt as well as the failure to commit suicide. See also "Suicide Attempt" (p 42) and other chapters about adolescence (pp 154, 156, 160, and 170).

C. One-to-one observation allows the nursing staff to provide a safe, structured environment as well as constant assessment of the adolescent's behavior and response to treatment. These observations must be documented according to the institution's policy. The environment must be free of potentially dangerous objects and situations.

D. Assess the family dynamics continuously throughout treatment and determine the effects on the adolescent and the recent suicide attempt. Determine whether the family has a history of suicide, attempts, or threats, and assess events around these occurrences and the family's reaction. Family therapy and individual therapy must be available to the adolescent and family members to assess the level of dysfunction in the system. Other issues that must be assessed include family violence, physical abuse, and substance abuse, which increase the incidence of family system dysfunction. For further discussion on family dynamics refer to "Family Therapy" (p 170).

References

Erikson EH. Identity and the life cycle. New York: International Universities, 1959.

Holinger PC, Offer D, Zola MA. A prediction model for suicide among youth. J Nerv Ment Dis 1988; 176:275–279.

Minuchin S. Families and family therapy: a structural approach. Boston: Harvard University Press, 1974.

National Center for Health Statistics. Vital statistics of the United States, mortality, 1977–81. Washington, DC: United States Government Printing Office, 1981–1986.

National Center for Health Statistics. Vital statistics of the United States, mortality, 1978–81. Washington, DC: United States Government Printing Office, 1982–1986.

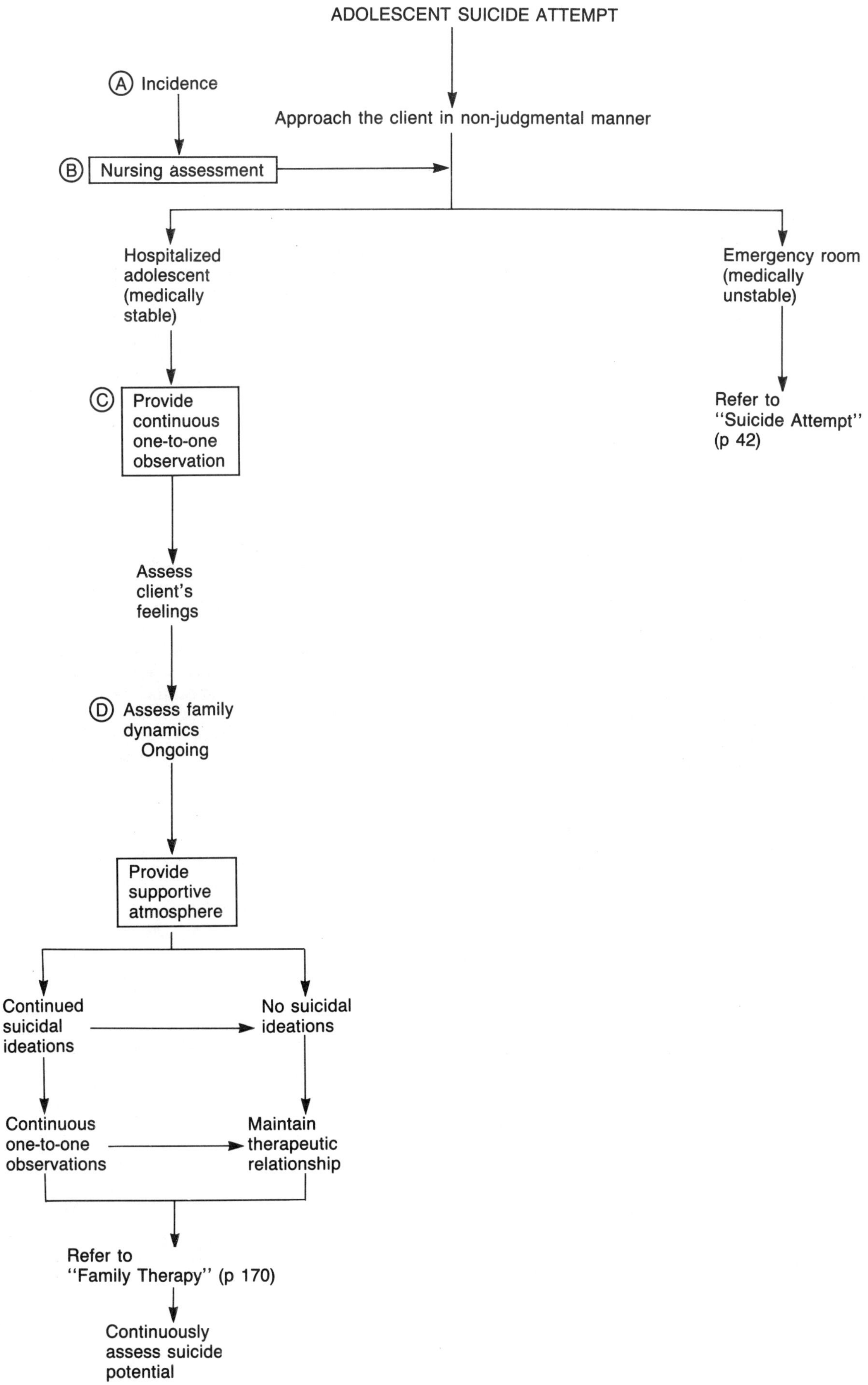
ADOLESCENT SUICIDE ATTEMPT
Approach the client in non-judgmental manner
(A) Incidence
(B) Nursing assessment
Hospitalized adolescent (medically stable)
Emergency room (medically unstable)
Refer to "Suicide Attempt" (p 42)
(C) Provide continuous one-to-one observation
Assess client's feelings
(D) Assess family dynamics Ongoing
Provide supportive atmosphere
Continued suicidal ideations
No suicidal ideations
Continuous one-to-one observations
Maintain therapeutic relationship
Refer to "Family Therapy" (p 170)
Continuously assess suicide potential

ADOLESCENT PRESENTS WITH PROBLEM IN LIVING

S. Taylor Stephens

A. Interview the adolescent, gaining his or her perception of the problem, and determine the contributing factors to the problem. Knowledge of normal adolescent growth, development, and behavior is basic to a thorough assessment of the adolescent. Frequently adolescents state their problem(s) in terms of why they seek treatment of their own volition.

B. Obtain a history of the problem(s) from the parents and/or family of the adolescent. The adolescent's family frequently initiates treatment because his or her misconduct has become increasingly apparent at school and within the community and is brought to their attention by school or police officials.

C. Parents commonly seek treatment for their adolescent because he or she (1) has threatened suicide or made a suicidal gesture; (2) has run away, been truant, failed school, has stolen, is defiant of authority figures, or is sexually promiscuous, generally known as conduct disorders; (3) has suffered a significant loss of body weight due to not eating; (4) has abused drugs or alcohol; and (5) has exhibited withdrawn or bizarre behavior. A supportive, well-organized assessment enables the nurse to evaluate the adolescent's ability to function, develop a set of working diagnoses, and begin to formulate treatment and discharge plans. The assessment should include interviews with the adolescent, and with parents or family members, obtaining their perceptions of the problem(s) and a family assessment, considering the family unit in terms of current stressors, support systems, previously successful coping strategies, and significant events in the family life cycle (e.g., divorce, birth of sibling, recent move). Hospitalization is indicated if the adolescent is suicidal or combative. Obtain insurance coverage information. Psychiatric coverage is frequently minimal.

D. Share information from the assessment with the psychiatrist, assist with the evaluation, and obtain the diagnosis. If immediate hospitalization is recommended, contact the admission office to confirm extent of insurance coverage. Assuming sufficient insurance, the adolescent would be admitted to the hospital. If the adolescent is exhibiting withdrawn or bizarre behavior and is without insurance, prepare to administer medication. If the adolescent exhibits any of the other behaviors and is deemed to be at serious risk, the nurse should be prepared to admit the adolescent and keep him or her hospitalized until stable.

E. Upon discharge, an adolescent whose behavior is problematic should be referred to family or placement with referral to an outpatient mental health peer group. An adolescent with an eating disorder is referred to an outpatient mental health peer group and/or an eating disorders group (see pp 82 and 84). Refer substance abusers to Narcotics Anonymous and/or Alcoholics Anonymous. Schedule the adolescent with withdrawn or bizarre behavior for an appointment with his psychiatrist for medication and periodic evaluation. The adolescent not deemed a serious risk to self or others who is not actively suicidal or has a mild conduct disorder should be discharged to family with a referral to a mental health peer group, community resources, and family therapy. A mild pattern of eating disorders dictates that the adolescent be discharged to family with referral to family therapy, peer group therapy, and an eating disorders group. The substance abuser is discharged to family with referral to Narcotics Anonymous and/or Alcoholics Anonymous (see pp 30 to 40). Patients with mild forms of withdrawn or bizarre behavior are discharged to family with referral to a mental health clinic (for further evaluation of medication regimen by the psychiatrist and the psychiatric nurse and support for compliance with the discharge treatment plan) and to peer group therapy.

References

Feinstein SC, et al. Adolescent psychiatry: developmental and clinical studies. Vol 12. Chicago: University of Chicago Press, 1985.

Haber J, et al. Comprehensive psychiatric nursing. 2nd ed. New York: McGraw-Hill, 1982.

Mirkin M, Koman S. eds. Handbook of adolescents and family therapy. New York: Gardner Press, 1985.

Pasquali E, et al. Mental health nursing: a holistic approach. 2nd ed. St. Louis: CV Mosby, 1985.

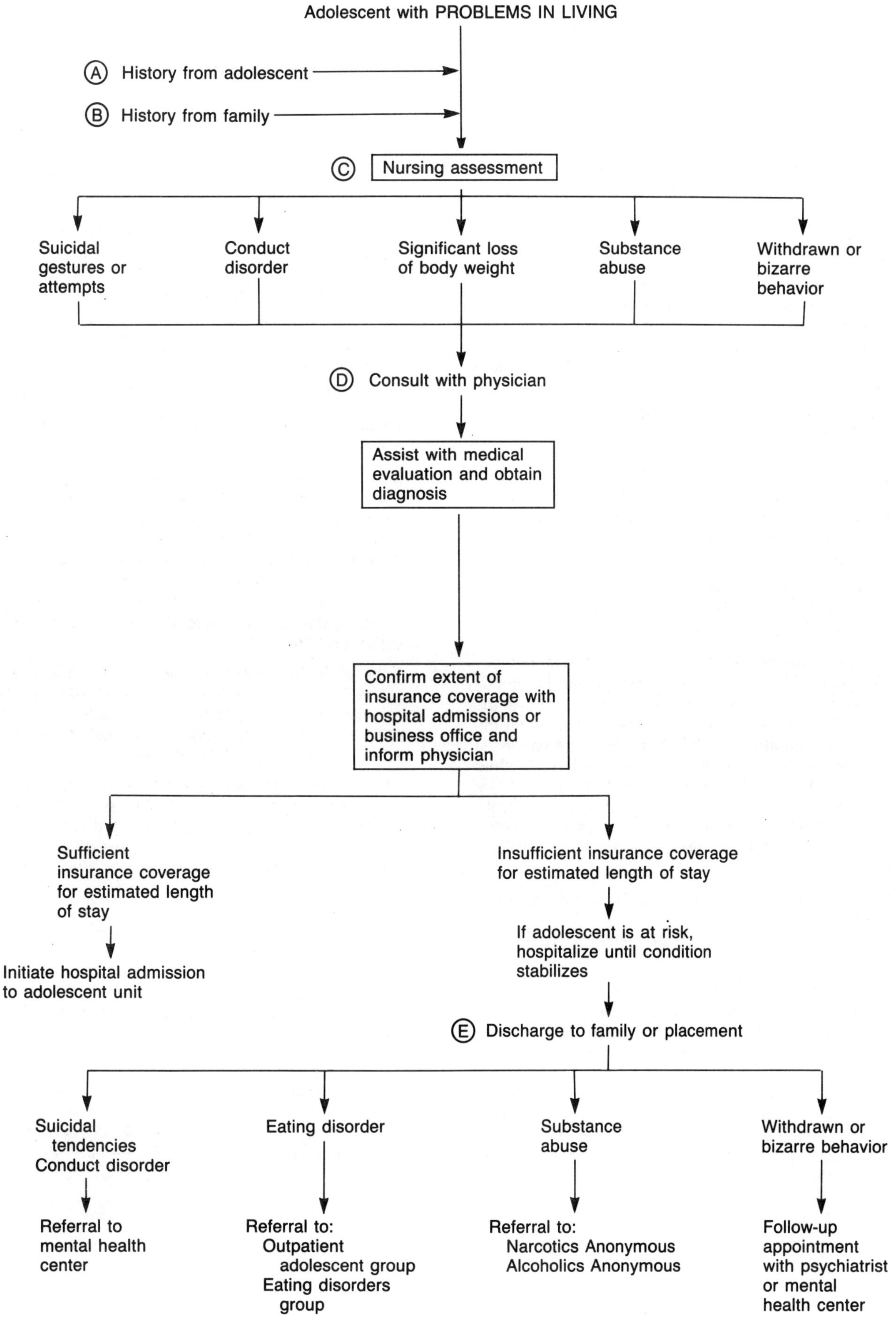
Adolescent with PROBLEMS IN LIVING
A History from adolescent
B History from family
C Nursing assessment
Suicidal gestures or attempts
Conduct disorder
Significant loss of body weight
Substance abuse
Withdrawn or bizarre behavior
D Consult with physician
Assist with medical evaluation and obtain diagnosis
Confirm extent of insurance coverage with hospital admissions or business office and inform physician
Sufficient insurance coverage for estimated length of stay
Initiate hospital admission to adolescent unit
Insufficient insurance coverage for estimated length of stay
If adolescent is at risk, hospitalize until condition stabilizes
E Discharge to family or placement
Suicidal tendencies
Conduct disorder
Referral to mental health center
Eating disorder
Referral to:
Outpatient adolescent group
Eating disorders group
Substance abuse
Referral to:
Narcotics Anonymous
Alcoholics Anonymous
Withdrawn or bizarre behavior
Follow-up appointment with psychiatrist or mental health center

ADOLESCENT PREGNANCY

B. Helen Thomas

A. Assessment of the probability of pregnancy includes obtaining a history of frequency of sexual intercourse, use of a reliable birth control method, and changes in usual menstrual cycle.

B. Pregnant adolescents display a variety of emotions precipitated by the crisis. To establish rapport, nurses need to be nonjudgmental, sensitive, and supportive. The nursing role includes providing accurate information and appropriate referral, support in telling significant others, and assurance of ongoing assistance. It is reassuring for clients to know that a responsible adult is there to help them.

C. Adolescents often require assistance in deciding whom to tell about the pregnancy and when to tell them. The nurse can help the client recognize her need for support at this time and determine who is most likely to provide it. Role playing the act of telling significant others is often helpful. At the client's request, the nurse can be present during the discussion.

D. Prenatal assessment should include the routine examination for pregnancy as well as screening for sexually transmitted disease (STD). Gonorrhea and chlamydia are most common in this age group.

E. This time can be used to explore the client's attitudes towards sexual activity. Reliable birth control methods should be carefully explained. The ways to minimize the risk of STD and acquired immunodeficiency syndrome (AIDS) should also be addressed. The nurse can assist the adolescent in selecting the contraceptive method with which she can most likely comply. Factors to be considered when selecting a method include the client's age, motivation, sense of responsibility, personal preference, probable frequency of sexual intercourse, and number of sexual partners.

F. Regular follow-up (e.g., monthly and bimonthly) has been demonstrated to be effective both for resolving any difficulties encountered with the contraceptive method and also for enhancing compliance.

G. Although about 10 percent of adolescent pregnancies are intended, many of these teenagers are very unrealistic about the future. The nurse's role is to provide a reality base for the client's decision making. Referral to appropriate agencies may be necessary (e.g., social services for financial assistance). The following issues should be addressed in ongoing sessions: planning (pre- and postpartum) living arrangement; assessment of life-style factors that are hazardous during pregnancy (e.g., poor nutrition, smoking, use of "street" drugs) and interventions to alleviate them; compliance with routine prenatal assessments; planning for the infant's arrival (e.g., acquisition of required clothing, furniture); realistic planning for care of the infant and maternal life-style (e.g., returning to school, working, full-time mother) following delivery; attendance at prenatal classes; and assistance in addressing the developmental tasks of normal adolescence.

H. The nurse continues to support the adolescent by providing accurate information about options and assisting the client in decision making and implementation. Depending on the situation, the nurse may intervene as an advocate with the adolescent's family, boyfriend, and/or the health-care system.

I. If an adolescent chooses to continue a pregnancy, the nurse must present the two options facing her and their implications—keeping and parenting the infant, and adoption. Keeping the infant will mean major life-style changes that the client needs to consider carefully. Placing the infant for adoption also means an emotional trauma for most adolescents. In determining the adolescent's decision, the nurse needs to assist her in clarifying her values and life goals.

J. If the adolescent selects abortion as the solution to the problem of pregnancy, the nurse must provide accurate information about legal consent in the province or state, costs involved, and techniques used. Referral to an appropriate health system is necessary.

K. Many adolescents experience a variety of emotional responses after the abortion. The nurse needs to assist the client in identifying and resolving these responses so that she can continue to address the developmental tasks of adolescence in a positive, constructive way.

References

Moore DS, Erickson PI, Wurgel M. Adolescent pregnancy and parenting: the role of the nurse. Top Clin Nurs 1984; 6(3):72–82.

Morrison DM. Adolescent contraceptive behavior: a review. Psych Bull 1985; 98:538–568.

Thomas BH, Mitchell A, Devlin MC. Nursing strategies: pregnancy during adolescence. In: Foster R, Hunsberger M, Anderson J, eds. Family-centered nursing care of children. Philadelphia: WB Saunders, 1989:1144–1160.

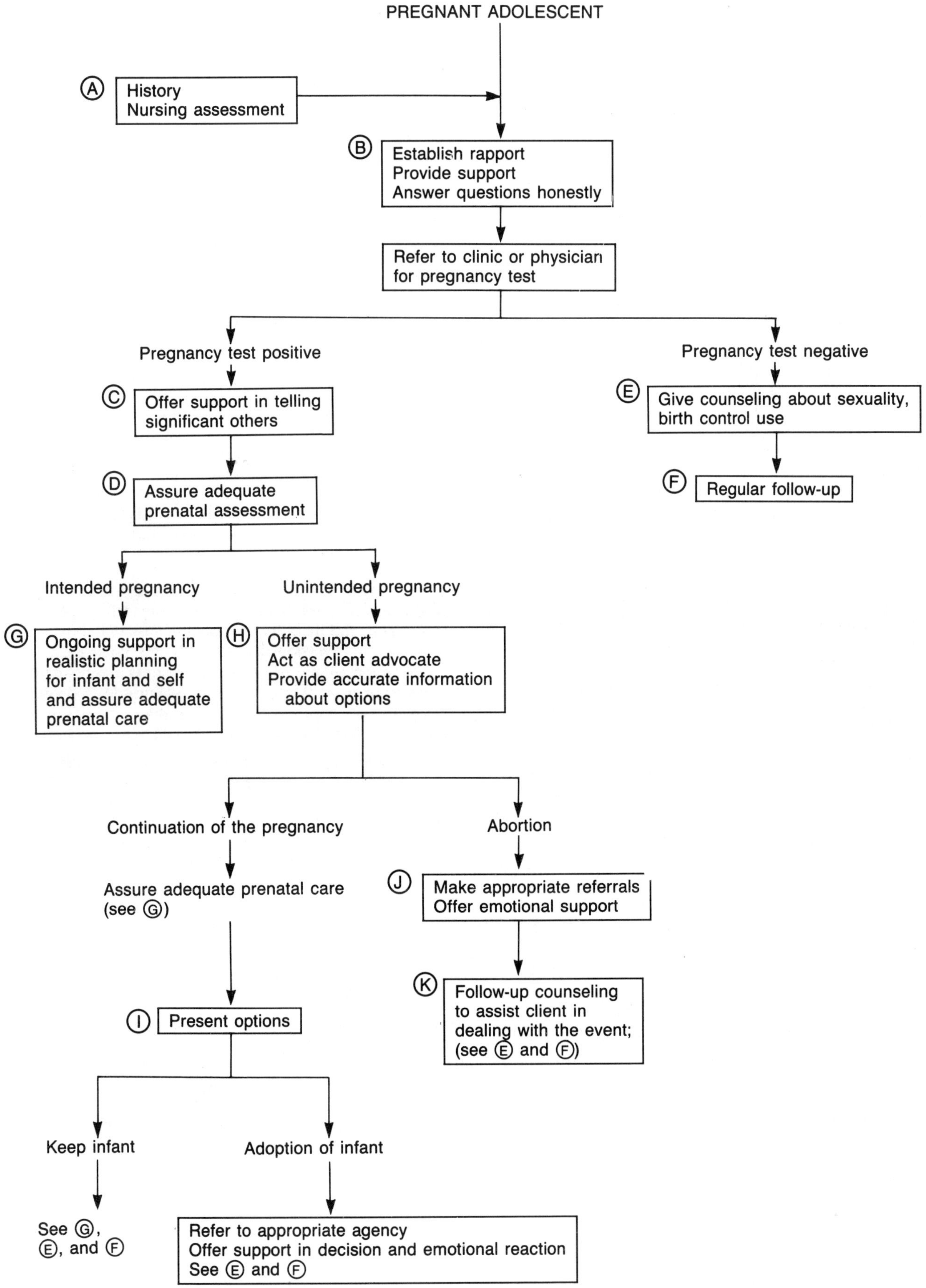

PREGNANT ADOLESCENT
Ⓐ
History
Nursing assessment
Ⓑ
Establish rapport
Provide support
Answer questions honestly
Refer to clinic or physician
for pregnancy test
Pregnancy test positive
Pregnancy test negative
Ⓒ
Offer support in telling
significant others
Ⓔ
Give counseling about sexuality,
birth control use
Ⓓ
Assure adequate
prenatal assessment
Ⓕ
Regular follow-up
Intended pregnancy
Unintended pregnancy
Ⓖ
Ongoing support in
realistic planning
for infant and self
and assure adequate
prenatal care
Ⓗ
Offer support
Act as client advocate
Provide accurate information
about options
Continuation of the pregnancy
Abortion
Assure adequate prenatal care
(see Ⓖ)
Ⓙ
Make appropriate referrals
Offer emotional support
Ⓚ
Follow-up counseling
to assist client in
dealing with the event;
(see Ⓔ and Ⓕ)
Ⓘ
Present options
Keep infant
Adoption of infant
See Ⓖ,
Ⓔ, and Ⓕ
Refer to appropriate agency
Offer support in decision and emotional reaction
See Ⓔ and Ⓕ

SINGLE-PARENT FAMILY

Andrea Baumann
Sheryl L. Boblin

A single-parent family is defined as a family in which one parent is caring for a child or children in a single dwelling home. In 1980, single-parent families represented close to 20 percent of all families in the United States. The large majority of these are parented by females. This family constellation may result from death of a spouse, separation, divorce, or single parenting without marriage. The adjustments to single parenthood by both parent and child may be many, depending upon the circumstances of the family.

A. Death of a spouse is viewed as uncontrollable and generates sympathy. Single parenthood as a result of death of a spouse, although contributing to grief and a sense of loss (see "Widowhood," p 176), is thus likely to result in greater financial security and acceptance by society. Divorce is considered a more controllable situation and implies failure; it is viewed as traumatic to children. Single-parent families of never-married females experience the severest financial difficulties and may be rated lowest in social esteem. Regardless of the reason for single parenthood, the single-parent family is regarded and is tolerated in American society as a temporary state.

B. It is important to recognize that single-parent families cannot be assessed by traditional family standards. The assessment of family strengths and unique communication patterns that develop between parent and children must be recognized. Children may be more independent and decisive and assume some tasks that have been traditionally viewed as parental. The child may take on further responsibilities and share in decision making.

C. There are many immediate adjustments as a result of separation or divorce (p 160). There may be adult social isolation, reduced income, or role change, which require many alterations in life-style for the single parent.

D. With reduced family income or redistribution of income, the parent may have to seek retraining or reeducation in order to secure employment. The parent may require career counseling, assistance with day care, some interim financing such as family service allowance, and assistance with legal services. Another financial burden may be additional help for child care and housekeeping.

E. The loss of role and reformation of a new role may take some time and cause additional stress. The client may have to relocate and develop new social contacts, a stressful situation at the best of times. A woman may move from a prescribed housewife role into a working-mother role. Conversely, a man may have to assume many household duties and family organizational functions.

F. If there is social isolation, the presence of an extended family may neutralize some of the stress encountered. The nurse therapist can assist the single parent by utilizing guidance in order to decrease the amount of stress. For long-term support, joining single parent groups, cooperative day-care organizations, and other help and support groups can be of value; these groups may provide emotional as well as practical assistance. The extended family may serve as a further support system. It is important that the effect of the extended family on family functioning be assessed.

G. Crisis intervention approaches (see "Decision Making During a Crisis State" [p 10] and "Outpatient Crisis Group" [p 142]) are necessary for the interim period. The need for social support will vary over time. Social losses can occur relatively soon after separation or divorce. Child-related problems, however, are likely to continue beyond the crisis period. Once the family is organized, the therapist can play continuing supportive and educational roles. The therapist can help the family develop contingency plans for such things as illness or disputes over custody and access.

H. Continuing therapeutic support is required for feelings of grief and loss, self-blame, and possible feelings of low self-esteem and inability to cope. Because of the extensive changes in responsibilities, activities, finances, and living arrangements, psychological distress may result in depression (see "Major Depressive Episodes," p 46). However, with appropriate tangible support, major social and economic obstacles may be overcome.

I. The nurse therapist can help the family adapt to the initial crisis and the resultant changes in family roles and communication patterns. Vulnerability to the effects of stressors can be reduced by anticipatory guidance and support. These strategies can buffer stressors and can assist in promoting a functional family system.

References

Collinson RC, Futrell J. Family therapy for the single parent system. J Psychiatr Ment Health Serv 1982; 20:16–20.

Leahey M, Wright LM. Families and life threatening illness. Springhouse, PA: Springhouse, 1987.

Gels C, Highley B, Roberts B, Martinson I. Toward a science of family nursing. Menlo Park, CA: Addison Wesley, 1989.

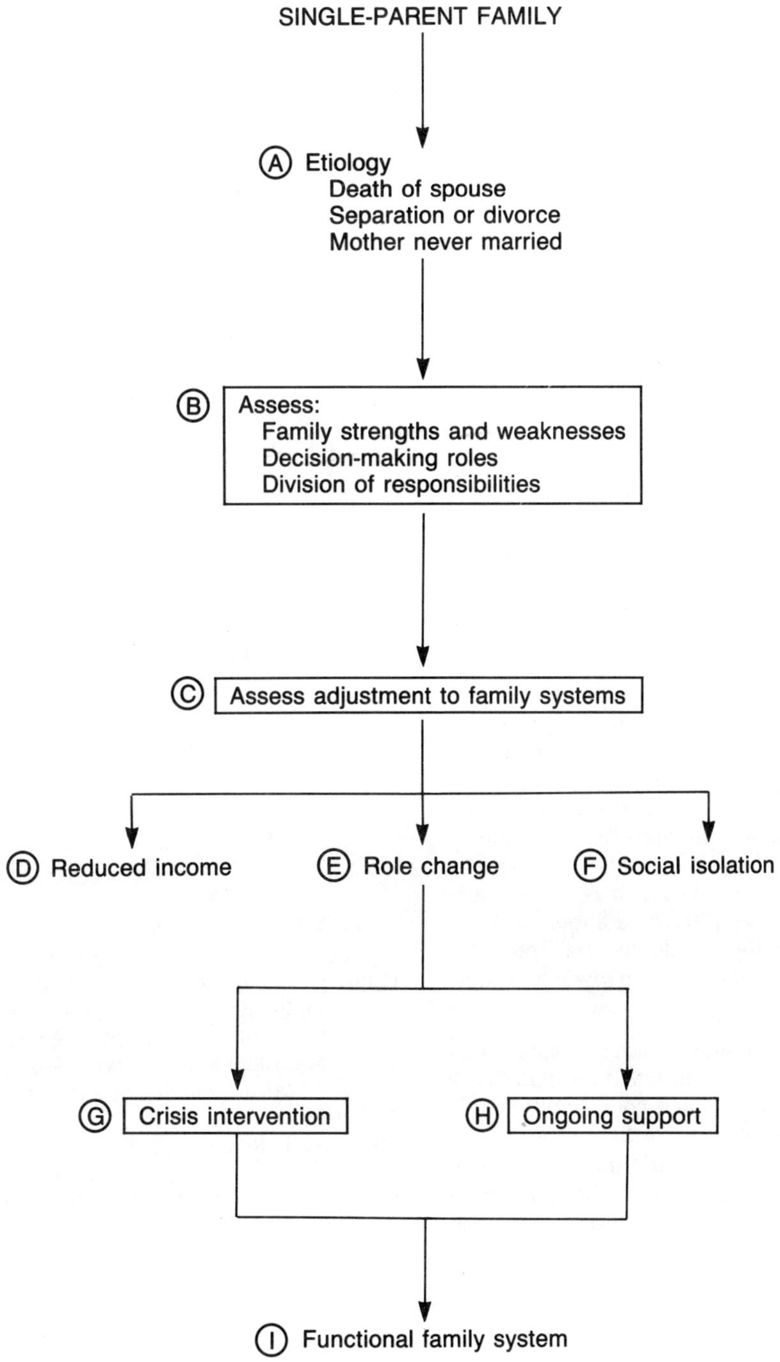
SINGLE-PARENT FAMILY
Ⓐ Etiology
Death of spouse
Separation or divorce
Mother never married
Ⓑ Assess:
Family strengths and weaknesses
Decision-making roles
Division of responsibilities
Ⓒ Assess adjustment to family systems
Ⓓ Reduced income
Ⓔ Role change
Ⓕ Social isolation
Ⓖ Crisis intervention
Ⓗ Ongoing support
Ⓘ Functional family system

DIVORCE AND SEPARATION

Ann C. Beckingham
Andrea Baumann

Pressures on families in modern society are very great. Today's families operate at a high level of emotional intensity, which results in a higher divorce rate. Divorce rates have been on the increase since the early 1970s. Financial and emotional cost may be high. Escaping from destructive relationships may be the most effective way of dealing with unsolvable problems.

A. Higher divorce and/or separation rates are frequently related to teenage pregnancy, lower socioeconomic status, and geographic locations. There are many extended grounds for divorce and separation. Some examples are physical and psychological abuse, alcoholism and other psychopathologies, as well as other mutual incompatibilities.

B. Marriage is considered traditionally in society as a positive state. Consequently, separation and divorce are seen as stressors. Assessment of the characteristics of the loss (see p 198) and stages of the grieving process (see p 192) are necessary. The meaning of the loss to the client is important to ascertain. There is a stigma attached to divorce and dissolution of family that results in overwhelming feelings of failure and guilt. This is reinforced by the lengthy process of service of notice and appeal. If the divorce is contested on issues such as custody, support, and property, this may lead to additional feelings of powerlessness (see p 184) and depression. The client may be seen in hospital with depression (p 46) or anxiety attack.

C. The overall goal of nursing intervention is to support individuals, couples, and groups to retain the stability of the family system through divorce counseling. People need to maintain a balanced view of themselves as well as achieve some psychological closure. Initial crisis intervention techniques (pp 10, 12, 106) may be required in the early stages of the decision to divorce a partner. Interventions may occur at the primary, secondary, and tertiary level of care. Family therapy (p 170), psychotherapy (p 112), and group therapy (pp 136, 138, 142) may be necessary to assist in decreasing anxiety and maintaining positive family functioning during times of crisis. Financial and custodial concerns may be referred to legal aid if necessary. Supportive counseling must continue because ambivalence and internal conflict may exist long after the divorce.

D. An integrative approach to meet long-term needs may be necessary, and includes referral to health-care and other professionals. It is important to assist the client(s) to reach final resolution about their decisions for separation or divorce in order to get on with their new lives. When there are children involved, many decisions have to be made regarding custody, support, and division of finances. Resuming single status may be a temporary or final choice for the client. Ideally, decisions can be made that work out to the mutual advantage of those involved, and mutually defined goals can be met.

References

Beyers B. Dealing with divorce: a group therapy intervention for women. Perspect Psychiatric Care 1987–88; XXIV:91–100.

Gilliss C, Highley B, Roberts B, Martinson I. Toward a science of family nursing. Reading, MA: Addison-Wesley, 1988.

Leavitt M. Families at risk. Primary prevention in nursing practice. Boston: Little, Brown, 1982.

Nett E. Canadian families past and present. Toronto: Butterworths, 1988.

Messinger L. Remarriage: a family affair. St. Paul, MN: Plenum Press, 1984.

Runyon N. Divorce: its impact on children. Perspect Psychiatric Care 1987–88; XXIV:101–105.

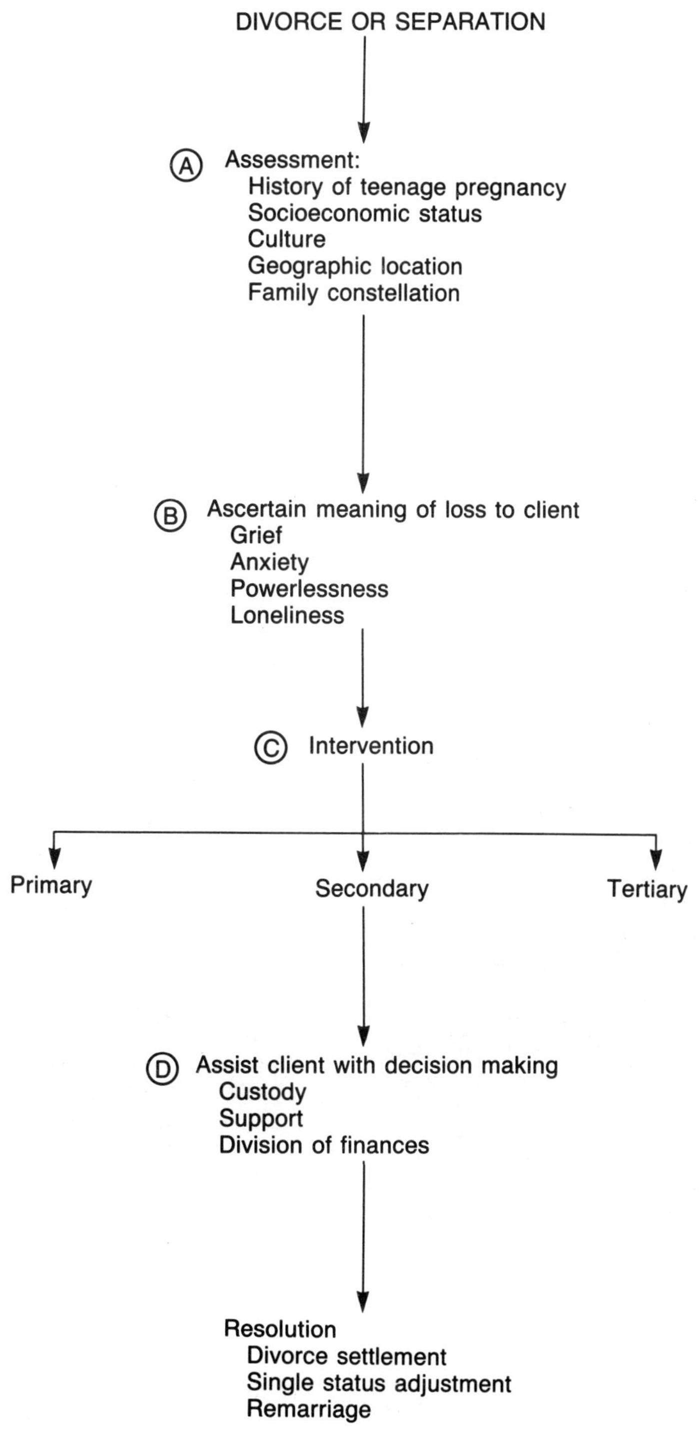
DIVORCE OR SEPARATION
(A) Assessment:
History of teenage pregnancy
Socioeconomic status
Culture
Geographic location
Family constellation
(B) Ascertain meaning of loss to client
Grief
Anxiety
Powerlessness
Loneliness
(C) Intervention
Primary
Secondary
Tertiary
(D) Assist client with decision making
Custody
Support
Division of finances
Resolution
Divorce settlement
Single status adjustment
Remarriage

INCEST

Deborah Antai-Otong

A. When incest is confirmed or suspected, it is essential for nurses to know the legal definition of incest in their state or province. Incest is usually defined as a sexual contact between family members or surrogate family members. Depending on the state, the extent of sexual contact may range from fondling to actual intercourse. Incest is a symptom of a severely dysfunctional family system, often characterized by blurred boundaries and roles, a dysfunctional marital dyad, substance abuse, and poor impulse control. Family members are frequently isolated and have poor self-esteem. The family history often reveals child abuse by one or more of the parents. Nurses obtaining the history from the child and/or family members must not allow personal feelings to interfere with providing a warm, nonjudgmental atmosphere. Incest victims frequently blame themselves for the disclosure and family separations. Sometimes they disclose their family secret to friends or a teacher or counselor. These clients are referred to child protective agencies, and the family and victim enter treatment as a result. Sometimes family members' probation officers make referrals to treatment centers. The nurse may be involved in evaluating the child when incest is suspected.

B. When incest is suspected or confirmed, the nurse must report the incident to a child protective agency. Be aware of institution and state laws about reporting child abuse. Assess the child's feelings about incest victims and their family members. A child's reaction to incest is often determined by the nurse's attitude. Avoid becoming emotional or hysterical about the incident; a warm, nonjudgmental attitude allows the child to ventilate feelings and describe the incident more easily. Recognize that the entire family system is a victim of incest and that efforts to strengthen and support the family system are essential during the course of treatment. The child (victim) must be protected from further injury and assured that he or she is not responsible for what happened. The child needs to understand that it was the parents' job to provide protection and this was not done. This type of intervention minimizes self-blame and guilt in the child. The nurse must be empathetic and nonjudgmental to all family members. During the nursing assessment, interview the child, parents, and other family members separately initially and later as a group. Explore the victim's feelings and reasons for disclosure of the incident. Inform the child as well as other family members of the consequences of the disclosure. If the child and family members were referred by a child protective agency, they have already been informed of the possibility of family separation. Incest throws the family system into disequilibrium. The nurse may be confronted by angry, hostile parents. Protection of the child is essential, and this may require that the parent who perpetrated the act move out of the home. The child frequently feels guilty and anxious about the separation and must be assured often that this is necessary. Elicit information from the family about past psychiatric treatment, substance abuse, history of child abuse, and suicide attempts. During the initial family interview, observe family dynamics, roles, and patterns of communication and interaction. Assess and document the marital dyad in the history. Avoid being overly critical of the parents, but do not condone their lack of protection for the child. Inform the parents that this behavior is unacceptable and must not be allowed to continue. Inform the parents of the harmful consequences to children of blurred parental roles.

C. The physical examination is a critical part of treatment and represents an essential part of the legal process. This procedure is usually done when incest is suspected. The nurse's presence allays anxieties and fears in the child during the examination.

D. Encouraging the parents to deal with their dysfunctional marital dyad is an essential aspect of treatment. Assist them to identify their dysfunction, teach them how to parent, and provide avenues to deal with stress, problem-solve, and communicate effectively. Family therapy teaches members how to identify healthy boundaries, promote effective interaction and communication, facilitate a positive self-image, and deal with stress more effectively.

References

Gottlieb B. Incest: therapeutic intervention in a unique form of sexual abuse. In: Warren CG, ed. Rape and sexual assault. New York: Aspen Corporation, 1980:121–139.

Justice B, Justice R. The broken taboo. New York: Human Sciences Press, 1979.

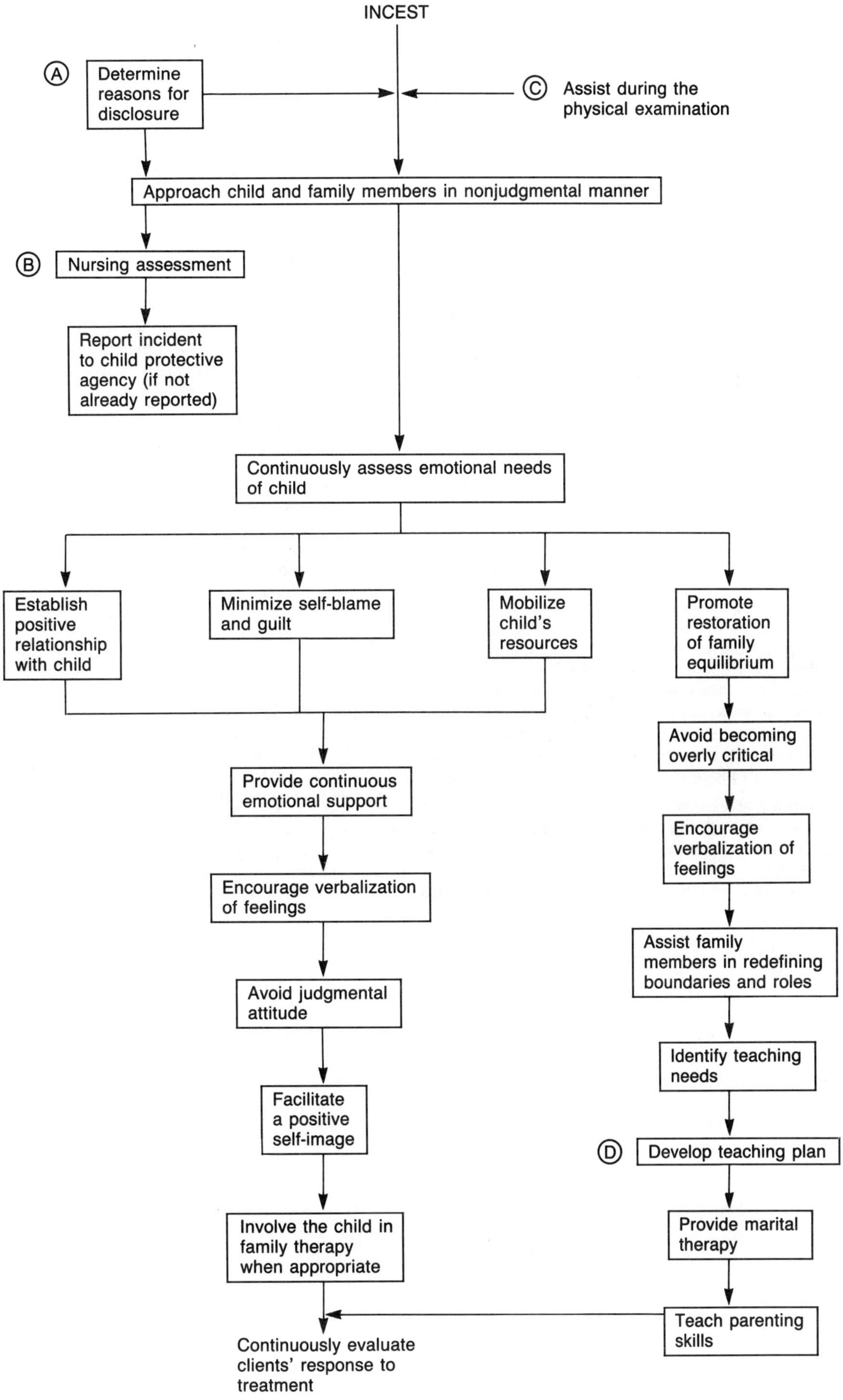
INCEST
Ⓐ Determine reasons for disclosure
Ⓒ Assist during the physical examination
Approach child and family members in nonjudgmental manner
Ⓑ Nursing assessment
Report incident to child protective agency (if not already reported)
Continuously assess emotional needs of child
Establish positive relationship with child
Minimize self-blame and guilt
Mobilize child's resources
Promote restoration of family equilibrium
Provide continuous emotional support
Encourage verbalization of feelings
Avoid judgmental attitude
Facilitate a positive self-image
Involve the child in family therapy when appropriate
Avoid becoming overly critical
Encourage verbalization of feelings
Assist family members in redefining boundaries and roles
Identify teaching needs
Ⓓ Develop teaching plan
Provide marital therapy
Teach parenting skills
Continuously evaluate clients' response to treatment

A COUPLE PRESENTS WITH A PROBLEM

S. Taylor Stephens

A. When a couple initiates contact with the nurse therapist by telephone or in person, the nurse therapist meets with the couple to obtain a history of the problem, determines their individual perceptions of the factors contributing to the problem, and determines previously used coping strategies and their effectiveness. An understanding of the Family Life Cycle (FLC) is useful to the nurse therapist as a developmental context within which to understand all families. The FLC consists of distinctive phases and major tasks: (1) marriage or living together while establishing a relationship of fairness and trustworthiness; (2) birth of first child and integrating the couple's relationship with their child with the relationship already existing between them; (3) individuation of the child(ren) while balancing the child(ren)'s autonomy and maintaining a reasonably fair balance of accountability between parents and child(ren) without expecting too little or too much of the child(ren); (4) individuation of the adolescent and redefining the terms of the parent-child relationship without negating the child(ren)'s trustworthiness, with particular attention paid to autonomy, responsibility, and control; (5) departure of child(ren) and separating without severing family ties plus finding a new focus for the parents' lives; and (6) aging of the parents requiring them to face and accept a variety of losses, including relational losses with family and friends, loss of meaningful work, diminished strength and energy, and financial losses (sometimes), and eventually each parent individually faces his or her death and must come to terms with lifetime accomplishments and failures.

B. The nursing assessment, which may encompass several sessions; first, with the couple together, and then with each partner individually, should provide a profile of the course of the couple's problems: their difficulties, their strengths, the duration of the problems, coping strategies used, problematic family behaviors, and family relationships. Inquiry should be made as to any physical problems of the partners, along with a list of drugs, including alcohol, used by either partner.

C. If the problem is a personal problem of one partner, initiate outpatient individual therapy. If it appears to be a marital problem (see also "Intimacy," p 196), couples therapy is indicated, particularly if there is sexual dysfunction (pp 220, 224). When the problem is that of poor communication between parents and children, outpatient family therapy is indicated (p 170).

D. The nurse therapist's goal is to promote more effective functioning within the couple's interactions with each other. When individuals are able to "own" their own behaviors, choose more effective means of coping, communicate effectively with each other and their children without the active interventions of the nurse, and negotiate more effectively for their needs, then the nurse has provided effective therapy to replace dysfunctional behaviors. The nurse therapist then discharges the individual or couple from therapy with appropriate referrals to community resources.

References

Beavers WR. Successful marriage: a family approach to couples therapy. New York: WW Norton, 1985.

Karpel MA, Strauss ES. Family evaluation. New York: Gardner Press, 1983.

Mirkin M, Koman S, eds. Handbook of adolescents and family therapy. New York: Gardner Press, 1985.

Pasquali E, et al. Mental health nursing: a holistic approach, 2nd ed. St. Louis: CV Mosby, 1985.

Scarf M. Intimate partners: patterns in love and marriage. New York: Random House, 1987.

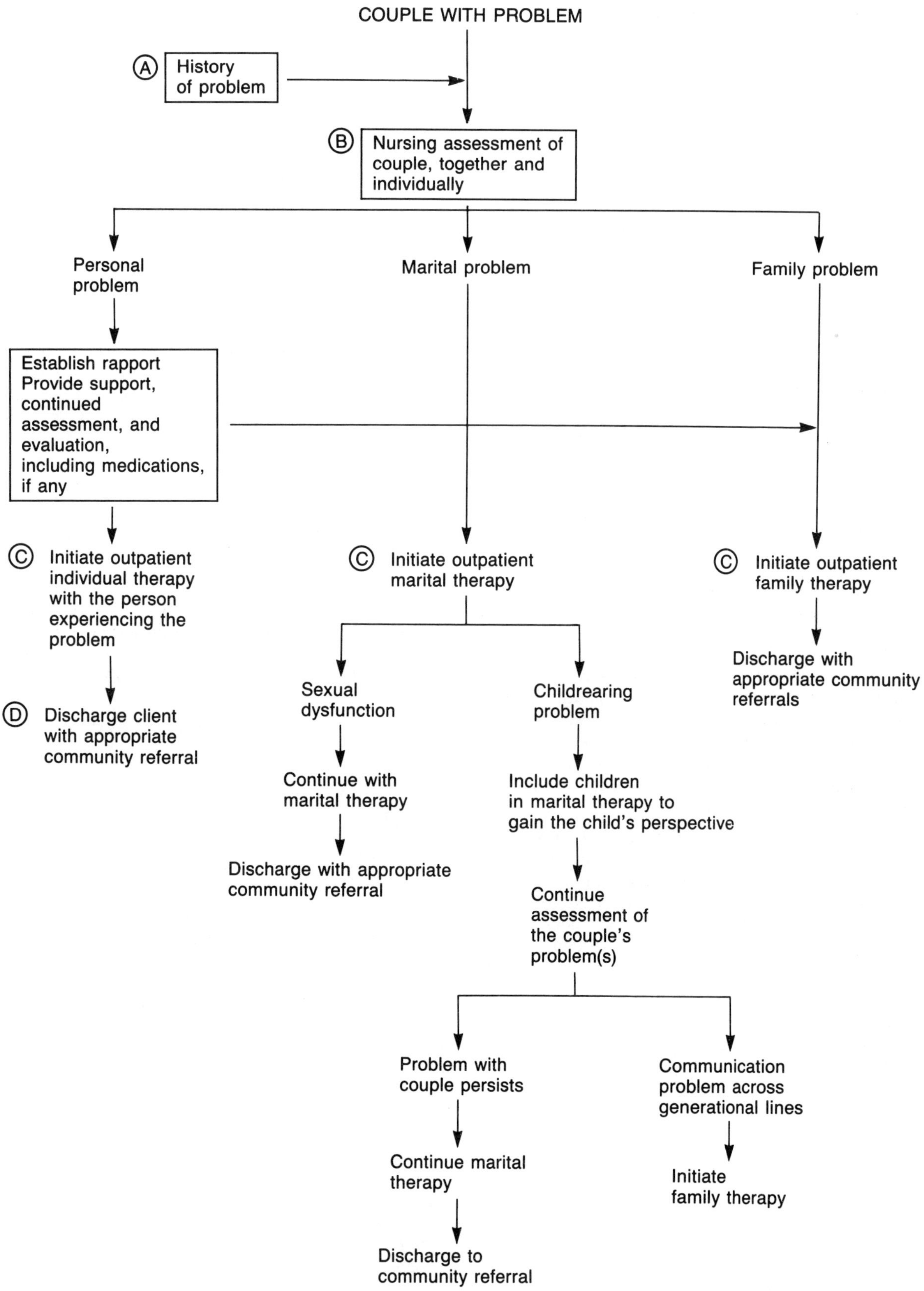
COUPLE WITH PROBLEM
A History of problem
B Nursing assessment of couple, together and individually
Personal problem
Marital problem
Family problem
Establish rapport Provide support, continued assessment, and evaluation, including medications, if any
C Initiate outpatient individual therapy with the person experiencing the problem
C Initiate outpatient marital therapy
C Initiate outpatient family therapy
D Discharge client with appropriate community referral
Sexual dysfunction
Childrearing problem
Discharge with appropriate community referrals
Continue with marital therapy
Include children in marital therapy to gain the child's perspective
Discharge with appropriate community referral
Continue assessment of the couple's problem(s)
Problem with couple persists
Communication problem across generational lines
Continue marital therapy
Initiate family therapy
Discharge to community referral

BLENDED FAMILIES

Andrea Baumann
Ann C. Beckingham

The family is defined as a human group with significant emotional bonds, usually living together. There are many variations of family constellations; thus, there is greater acceptance in society today of alternative family life-styles. A blended family consists of a couple, one or both having been previously married with no children or children from one or both marriages. The previous relationships and/or marriages may have been dissolved through divorce and separation or death of a spouse.

A. Statistics vary depending on geographic location; however, an average of one out of five marriages is a remarriage. Divorced men remarry with more frequency than women. Remarriage occurs, most often, soon after a final separation. Remarriage among widows does not occur as quickly after the loss of a spouse. Women often remarry for financial and security reasons, and men for psychological and emotional reasons. The rate of success of remarriages is 50 percent, and remarriages are reported to be happier.

B. While assessing the existing relationships, it may be found that roles are blurred and that they overlap and conflict with previous relationships and expectations. Since one or both partners were married before, they may enact unconscious roles from previous relationships. This may be without purposeful intention. Unless the effect of role definition is understood and articulated by both partners, eventual conflict may result. Clarity in role definition and expectation assists the couple to work together effectively in a marital dyad.

C. Financial burdens arise from the fact there are more family members to be cared for. The costs of former divorce and remarriage may be high. Communication about the allocation of financial resources has to be open because there are many new factors to consider. In the early stages of the remarriage, financial burden may involve alimony, a second residence, and commitments to an extended family.

D. The effect on the children varies depending on the number of children, their ages, their relationship with previous spouses, and the time since the last marriage or death of a spouse. The children's status must be redefined within the context of the new family structure. There may be interpersonal problems arising from previous situations that need to be dealt with. Role sets are more extended and relationships are more complex. This could be confusing for the children, who already are dealing with loss. It is important to deal with the losses from the previous marriage and present expectations of role function. Family members may have different concepts of role norms and goals. It has been found that parents who have a clearly defined concept of the roles and obligations promote a healthier relationship among stepchildren from previous marriages.

E. One of the most effective therapeutic interventions is anticipatory planning and guidance prior to, and at the beginning of, the new blended relationship. Community support groups or group therapy have proven to be of value in providing a forum for sharing expectations and implementing effective communication skills.

F. The sharing of mutual concerns, anxieties, and subsequent decision-making strategies promote the successful fulfillment of roles and functions within a new family structure, leading to successful family reconstitution.

References

Gilliss C, Highley B, Roberts B, Martinson I. Toward a science of family nursing. Reading, MA: Addison Wesley, 1988.

Leavitt M. Families at risk. Primary prevention in nursing practice. Boston: Little, Brown, 1982.

Nett E. Canadian families past and present. Toronto: Butterworths, 1988.

Messinger L. Remarriage: a family affair. St. Paul, MN: Plenum Press, 1984.

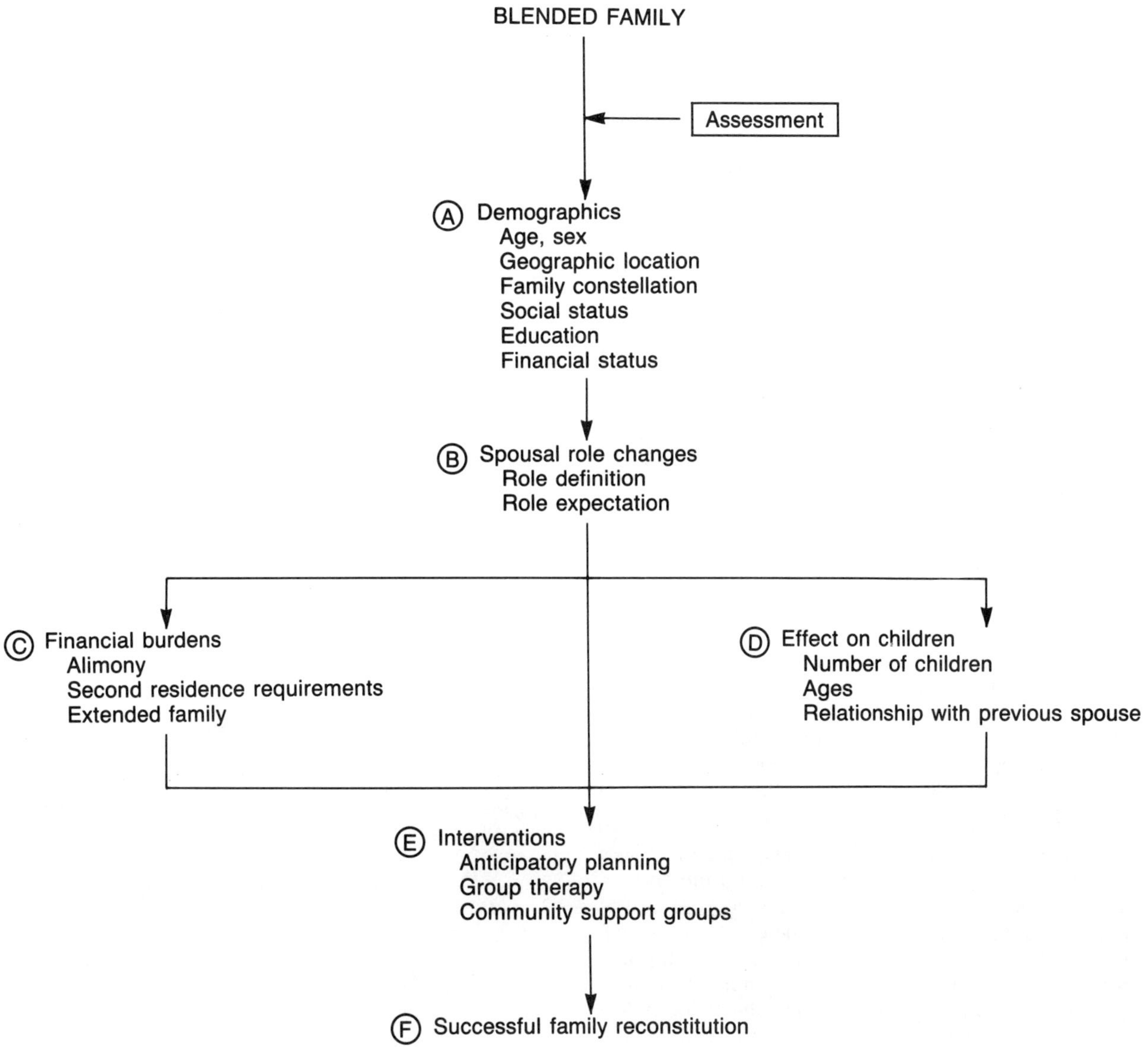
BLENDED FAMILY
Assessment
(A) Demographics
Age, sex
Geographic location
Family constellation
Social status
Education
Financial status
(B) Spousal role changes
Role definition
Role expectation
(C) Financial burdens
Alimony
Second residence requirements
Extended family
(D) Effect on children
Number of children
Ages
Relationship with previous spouse
(E) Interventions
Anticipatory planning
Group therapy
Community support groups
(F) Successful family reconstitution

CHILD ABUSE

B. Helen Thomas

Child abuse is a growing problem in our country. It may be reported by school officials or members of the community, or the child may be brought to the emergency department. Often patients may be admitted for other diagnoses and abuse may be discovered. Although the patient is already hospitalized, the same process should occur. This chapter refers to physical abuse specifically, but a similar decision-making process should occur in cases of neglect.

A. Three factors are important when physical abuse is initially suspected: is the accident age-appropriate, is the explanation consistent with the injury, and have the parents sought treatment as soon as realistically possible? Acts of omission and commission constitute abuse; therefore, injuries resulting from inadequate supervision can be abusive (often considered neglect).

B. Nursing assessment involves assessment of the actual injury as well as parental response to the injury and parent-child interaction during the assessment. In cases of abuse, parents may overreact to a relatively minor injury or not appear to react to a serious one. Abuse should be suspected when the child is overly compliant during the physical examination and does not cry or seek support from his or her parents or when parents do not support the child.

C. Abusive parents are usually frightened of their behavior and of its consequences. They may be hostile and angry. They are very sensitive to negative responses. The nurse needs to be nonjudgmental and give positive feedback to them for bringing the child for treatment. Establishing favorable rapport enables the nurse to collect more information about the family and the incident. Any inconsistencies should be identified and clarification sought.

D. Health teaching regarding home safety and child development may be necessary. Referral to community health nursing to assess home safety and parenting skills may be required.

E. Reporting of cases of nonaccidental injury is governed by state or provincial laws. Know the law in your area and follow it. To minimize parental hostility, explain why you are making the report and that the Child Protective Agency will try to help the family.

F. If this case goes to court, the chart may be subpoenaed. Clearly chart the following: description of actual injury and history of it; parental response; treatment of the injury; time of notification of the Child Protection Agency; intake worker with whom you spoke; and mutually agreed upon plan. Take photographs if possible.

G. Admission to hospital may occur for two reasons: the extent of the injury requires inpatient care, or it separates parents and child for a "cooling-off" period during which additional data can be obtained and long-term plans initiated.

H. Assessments are crucial in the long-term planning for the family. Parent-child interactions, including quotes, should be charted. Absence of parents should also be noted. Child development should be assessed and charted. Any unusual child behavior should be noted as well as the child's reaction to the parents' presence.

I. The nursing care plans should include a clear outline for activities each day. These children need to be able to depend on a routine. Continuity of a single nurse will maximize the impact of care, because both abused children and their parents are very mistrustful. The nurse should be supportive during parental visits and assist the parents to identify parenting problems. Many of these parents have unrealistic expectations of their children, based on a lack of knowledge about normal child development.

References

Anderson CL. Assessing parenting potential for child abuse risk. Pediatr Nurs 1987; 13:323–327.

Kaufman J, Zigler E. Do abused children become abusive parents? Am J Orthopsychiatry 1987; 57:186–192.

Morgan J. What can nurses learn from structured observations of mother-infant interactions? Iss Comprehens Pediatr Nurs 1987; 10:67–73.

Rhodes AM. The nurse's legal obligation for reporting child abuse. Maternal Child Nurs 1987; 12:313–317.

Thomas BH. Nursing strategies: child abuse and maltreatment. In: Foster R, Hunsberger M, Anderson J, eds. Family-centered nursing care of children. Philadelphia: WB Saunders 1989:1077–1107.

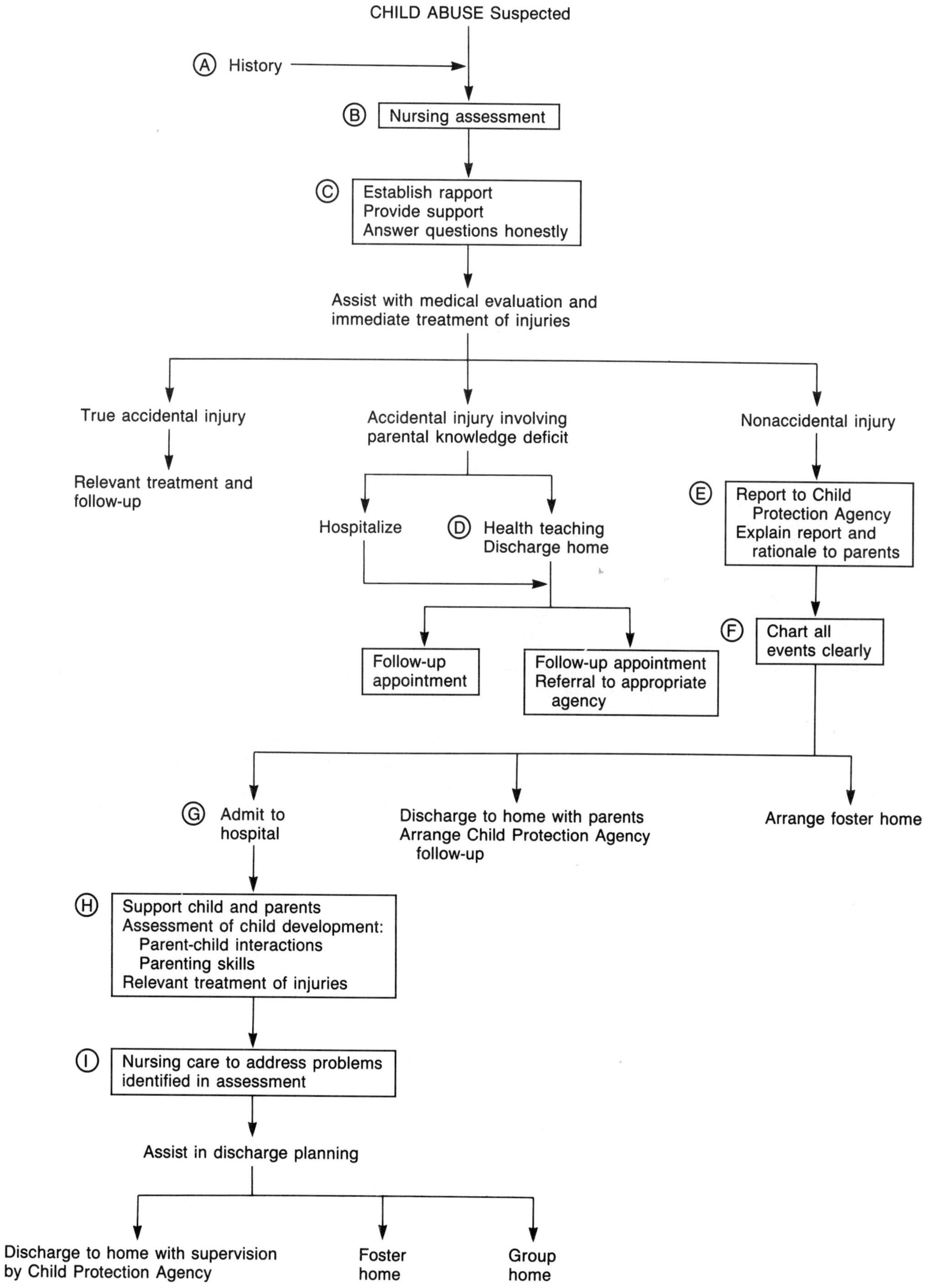
CHILD ABUSE Suspected
Ⓐ History
Ⓑ Nursing assessment
Ⓒ Establish rapport
Provide support
Answer questions honestly
Assist with medical evaluation and immediate treatment of injuries
True accidental injury
Relevant treatment and follow-up
Accidental injury involving parental knowledge deficit
Hospitalize
Ⓓ Health teaching
Discharge home
Follow-up appointment
Follow-up appointment
Referral to appropriate agency
Nonaccidental injury
Ⓔ Report to Child Protection Agency
Explain report and rationale to parents
Ⓕ Chart all events clearly
Ⓖ Admit to hospital
Discharge to home with parents
Arrange Child Protection Agency follow-up
Arrange foster home
Ⓗ Support child and parents
Assessment of child development:
Parent-child interactions
Parenting skills
Relevant treatment of injuries
Ⓘ Nursing care to address problems identified in assessment
Assist in discharge planning
Discharge to home with supervision by Child Protection Agency
Foster home
Group home

FAMILY THERAPY

Deborah Antai-Otong

A. The initial phase of family therapy begins with the nurse psychotherapist gathering and organizing background information from family members. Information may include a genogram to identify past and present psychiatric and medical history, substance abuse, family values, and roles. Information gathered should also include successful and unsuccessful family suicide attempts and threats. Family members often seek treatment when there is a crisis and often present with complaints of one family member's behavior or problem. They are often in an irritable and agitated mood and are seeking immediate resolution of the crisis. The nurse must assess the marital dyad and assume that it is the source of the crisis until proven otherwise. The role of the nurse also involves assisting the family to identify the presenting problem and establish realistic expectations and goals from treatment. The initial assessment determines interactional and communication patterns, boundaries, intimacy, and the family's general affect. As previously mentioned, the marital dyad is the usual source of conflict, which involves issues related to power, conflict resolution, and ineffective problem-solving patterns. Through the course of family therapy the nurse must offer marital therapy to the couple to deal with these issues.

B. Numerous reasons for seeking family or marital therapy may be identified during the initial assessment phase and may include ineffective conflict resolution, which precipitates a family crisis, and dysfunction in the family system, which may result in ineffective parenting roles and family violence.

C. The nurse must identify intimacy patterns in the marital dyad and recognize their effects on the resolution of family conflicts. Encourage activities that enhance and strengthen this dyad, and provide activities that challenge dysfunctional patterns. Offer adaptive options and coping patterns to assist development of effective problem-solving patterns.

D. Family sculpting and role playing allow the nurse and family members opportunities to identify ineffective coping patterns and blurred or enmeshed boundary issues. These techniques allow family members to "play out" these patterns and learn new, more effective patterns of communication and conflict resolution.

E. Family violence often results from substance abuse (see pp 30 to 40) and/or past generational family violence patterns. These behaviors must be suspected in families that exhibit high stress and strong affects such as anger.

References

Duvall E. Family development. 4th ed. Philadelphia: JB Lippincott, 1970.

Hogarth CR. Families and family therapy. In: Johnson BS, ed. Psychiatric mental health nursing: adaptation and growth. Philadelphia: JB Lippincott, 1986:207–208.

Minuchin S. Families and family therapy. Cambridge, MA: Harvard University Press, 1974.

Papp P. Family choreography. In: Guerin PJ, ed. Family therapy. New York: Gardner Press, 1976.

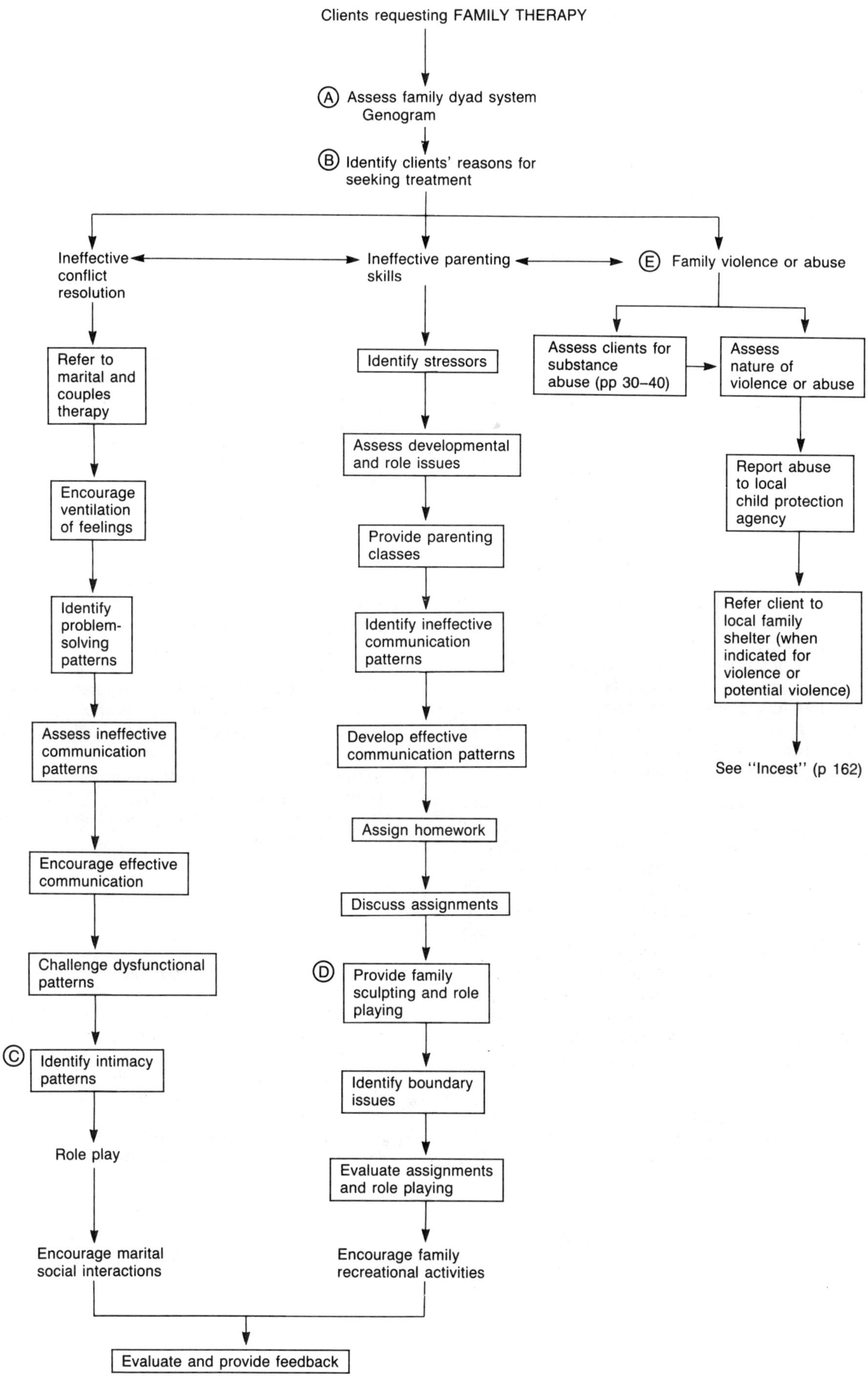
Clients requesting FAMILY THERAPY
Ⓐ Assess family dyad system Genogram
Ⓑ Identify clients' reasons for seeking treatment
Ineffective conflict resolution
Ineffective parenting skills
Ⓔ Family violence or abuse
Refer to marital and couples therapy
Encourage ventilation of feelings
Identify problem-solving patterns
Assess ineffective communication patterns
Encourage effective communication
Challenge dysfunctional patterns
Ⓒ Identify intimacy patterns
Role play
Encourage marital social interactions
Identify stressors
Assess developmental and role issues
Provide parenting classes
Identify ineffective communication patterns
Develop effective communication patterns
Assign homework
Discuss assignments
Ⓓ Provide family sculpting and role playing
Identify boundary issues
Evaluate assignments and role playing
Encourage family recreational activities
Assess clients for substance abuse (pp 30–40)
Assess nature of violence or abuse
Report abuse to local child protection agency
Refer client to local family shelter (when indicated for violence or potential violence)
See "Incest" (p 162)
Evaluate and provide feedback

THE AGING FAMILY AS CLIENTS

Ann C. Beckingham

In 1984, Christie-Seely defined *family* as "a group of people—often but not necessarily related by blood or marriage—with a commitment to live with and care for one another over time." Family health is frequently described in terms of the family's or family members' interprofessional relationships, developmental tasks, family processes, behaviors, functioning, organization, and family integration. The term *familial health*, which connotes the family as a system within a structural framework and as the social agent in the promotion of health and well-being, has also been proposed. The elderly person is defined as being 65 years of age or over. Therefore, the aging family is one in which any member is 65 years of age or more.

A. One can say that the family is a system composed of parts that interact in a given environment. Understanding systems theory is basic to both the family-oriented approach and the approach using the family as a decision-making unit. The family is the basic system in one's life. This system in turn is interrelated with and part of the larger environment or the suprasystem. In an extensive review of the literature on systems theory and its application in working with families, Wright and Leahey (1984) found no clear agreement on the primary concepts of systems theory. They described the family using the analogy of a mobile. Family analyses must take into account not only the interrelationships of the parts, but also the parts in relation to the whole. According to Levitt (1982) the family is an emotional buffer between the individual and the impersonal, stressful society we live in.

B. Some families manage well on their own. Other families may experience a great sense of need or crises, but hesitate to ask for help for fear of losing their independence or self-esteem. The assessment process is not simple because many variables operate simultaneously in the family system. Assessment includes structural, functional, and developmental concepts simultaneously along with sociocultural, developmental, physiologic, belief, and psychological variables. A meaningful assessment approach must be viewed in terms of a continuum of family and individual needs, and includes observation of the individual and the environment. For a discussion on intergenerational relations, refer to Connides (1989).

C. Intervention for the aging family is dependent on the needs of the elderly for a certain level of care. Also, consideration of the degree of support they are receiving from the family or other domestic care-giver should be evaluated. If nursing intervention is required after assessment, an accurate picture of the degree of functional deterioration in an individual family member is also needed. Information on the likely speed and extent of further change could be of great value to the family and to health professionals seeking a more appropriate care plan for that family. For example, families could be helped by improved knowledge of the likely outcome of chronic illnesses, and of support that could be made available to them as an illness progresses. With the focus on keeping the elderly family at home in the community as long as possible, essential criteria include those of acceptability, affordability, and accessibility of services. Proactive strategies that support autonomy and independence should be developed.

D. Each step in caring for the aging family as clients involves decision-making skills. An elderly family in a crisis situation may have neither the time nor the experience to use a rational decision-making approach (see "Decision Making During a Crisis State," p 10). Lack of familiarity with the complex health-care system in itself can stress the family members. Family-centered nursing emphasizes the continuity of services and comprehensive, collaborative team work. The nurse's role in family assessment and management in the community is of utmost importance. Nursing considers the family as the main focus of health care; therefore, the main emphasis is on health promotion, disease prevention, disability postponement, and primary, secondary, and tertiary care. The family's importance as a social institution has been the ideal focus for policy initiatives.

References

Christie-Seely I, ed. Working with the family in primary care: a systems approach to health and illness. New York: Praeger, 1984.

Connides IA. Family ties and aging. Toronto: Butterworths, 1989.

Leavitt MB. Families at risk: primary prevention in nursing practice. Boston: Little, Brown, 1982.

Wright LM, Leahey M. Nurses and families: a guide to family assessment and intervention. Philadelphia: FA Davis, 1984.

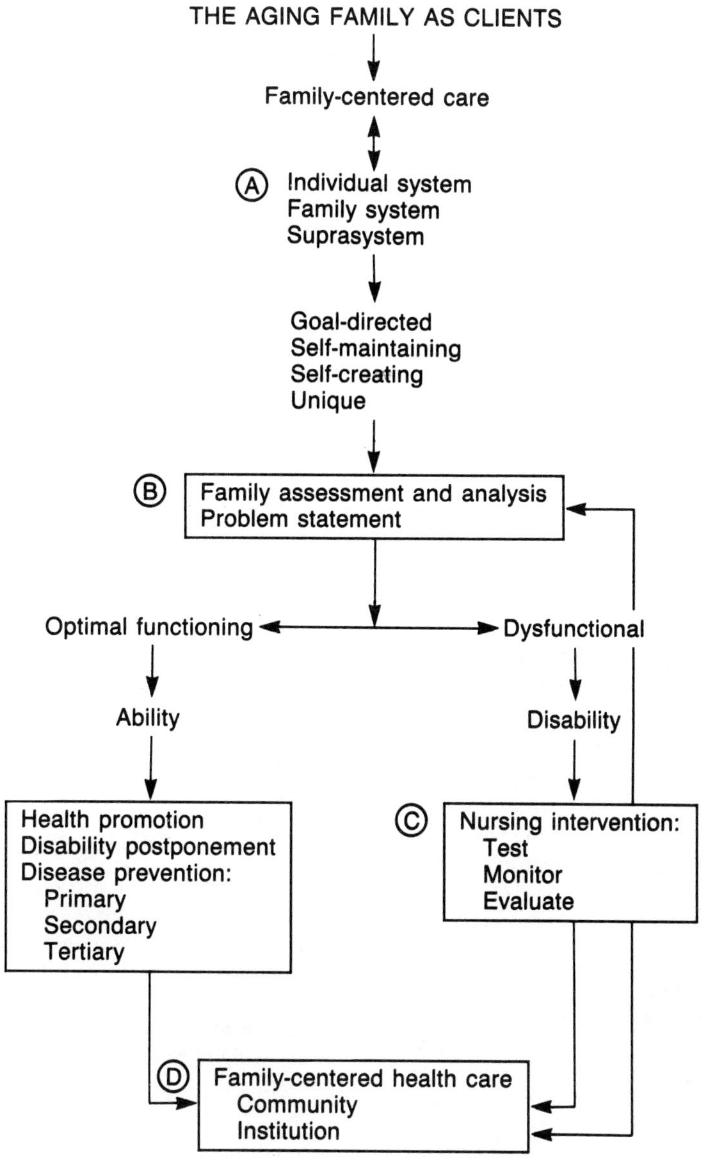
THE AGING FAMILY AS CLIENTS
Family-centered care
A
Individual system
Family system
Suprasystem
Goal-directed
Self-maintaining
Self-creating
Unique
B
Family assessment and analysis
Problem statement
Optimal functioning
Dysfunctional
Ability
Disability
Health promotion
Disability postponement
Disease prevention:
Primary
Secondary
Tertiary
C
Nursing intervention:
Test
Monitor
Evaluate
D
Family-centered health care
Community
Institution

ELDER ABUSE AND NEGLECT

Elizabeth Podnieks

Physical and emotional impairments increase with age, and older persons may develop dependent relationships that can place them at risk for maltreatment. Elder abuse is mistreatment of older people by those in a position of trust, power, or responsibility for their care. Neglect is the deprivation of basic needs and may be intentional or unintentional. Elder abuse takes place in the home, in institutions, and in the community. It is not restricted to any single economic, social, or cultural group.

High-risk clients include women, elders living with their abuser, the old-old (over 75 years of age), those dependent on someone else for their care needs, isolated elders, and those who demonstrate problematic behavior (incontinence, night wandering, or aggression). Potential perpetrators may suffer from alcoholism, drug addiction, medical problems, or psychopathology.

Communication skills and empathy are needed to establish a trusting relationship with the client.

A. The history obtains background information from the client and the primary caregiver. It should be examined for any inconsistencies, e.g., frequent falls, injuries, "accidents," or examples of the client's explanation not matching the results of the physical examination. A history of seeking medical attention from a variety of doctors or health-care facilities is characteristic of a family in an abusive cycle.

B. Determine if the client is in immediate danger, whether hospitalization is required, whether it is safe for the client to remain with the caregiver, how long the maltreatment has been going on, whether the client is able to function alone, and whether there is an available support system (family, friends). Evaluate whether the perpetrator is willing to accept help and admit to the abusive behavior. Establish the competence of the client. Competent clients have the right to make their own choices. If clients are incompetent, a substitute decision-maker is appointed.

C. The physical assessment may reveal bruises, injuries related to sexual abuse, fractures, burns, or rope marks. Indicators of neglect are dehydration, malnutrition, inadequate personal hygiene, over- or undermedication, untreated medical problems, and inappropriate clothing. Cognitive or affective functioning indicates the client's mental status. Depression or passive behavior may suggest powerlessness and resignation to a longstanding abusive situation. Be alert for signs of chemical restraints (tranquilizers or hypnotics) in the client presenting with confusion, disorientation, or lethargy.

D. The psychosocial assessment usually reveals low self-esteem, isolation, feelings of humiliation, and inadequacy. Observe the interaction between the client and caregiver to determine their relationship. Assess culture and values. Is the abusive behavior an acceptable norm for the client? Indicators of financial or material exploitation are based on the client's appearance and the physical environment.

E. Causes of elder abuse and neglect are explained by a variety of theories. Recent research suggests that elder abuse is related to the psychopathologic state of the perpetrator and to substance abuse. Family dysfunction is also associated with abusive behavior patterns. There is a growing awareness that much of the abuse of older persons is, in fact, spouse abuse grown old.

F. The nursing diagnosis should be formulated only after all multidisciplinary assessments are completed. Signs and symptoms of elder abuse may actually be due to the aging process. Accurate and comprehensive documentation must be maintained on an ongoing basis.

G. Intervention strategies are directed toward the client, the care provider, and the family. Primary prevention increases the awareness of elder abuse and neglect through professional and public education. Secondary prevention includes a wide range of services that are required to provide adequate care to the client and family: health and medical services, nutrition services, homemaker services, alternative housing, financial counseling, legal assistance, and social and supportive services. Tertiary prevention maximizes self-care capabilities of the client and ensures ongoing counseling of the perpetrator.

H. Case management is directed toward recognition of the client's right to self-determination, provision of safety, availability of a continuum of community-based services, maintenance of the family unit, and use of the least restrictive alternative in practice and treatment. Institutionalization is a last resort. Nurses must support clients in pressing criminal charges in cases of assault, forgery, and theft.

I. To guarantee client safety, reassessment of care through ongoing monitoring by geriatric and geropsychiatric teams is necessary. Revisions are made with the changing health and service needs of the client, perpetrator, and family. Abuse and neglect may be alleviated through case management (see p 128) and the provision of services. In long-term abusive patterns, the only resolution may be the separation of the client from the perpetrator. The client must be involved in relocation strategies. The client's autonomy and dignity always take precedence over the desire to provide "rescue." Should the client choose not to accept services, maintain contact and reassure the client that help is always available.

References

Fulmer T, O'Malley T. Inadequate care of the elderly—a health care perspective on abuse and neglect. New York: Springer, 1987.

Pillemer K, Wolf R, eds. Elder abuse: conflict in the family. Dover, MA: Auburn House, 1986.

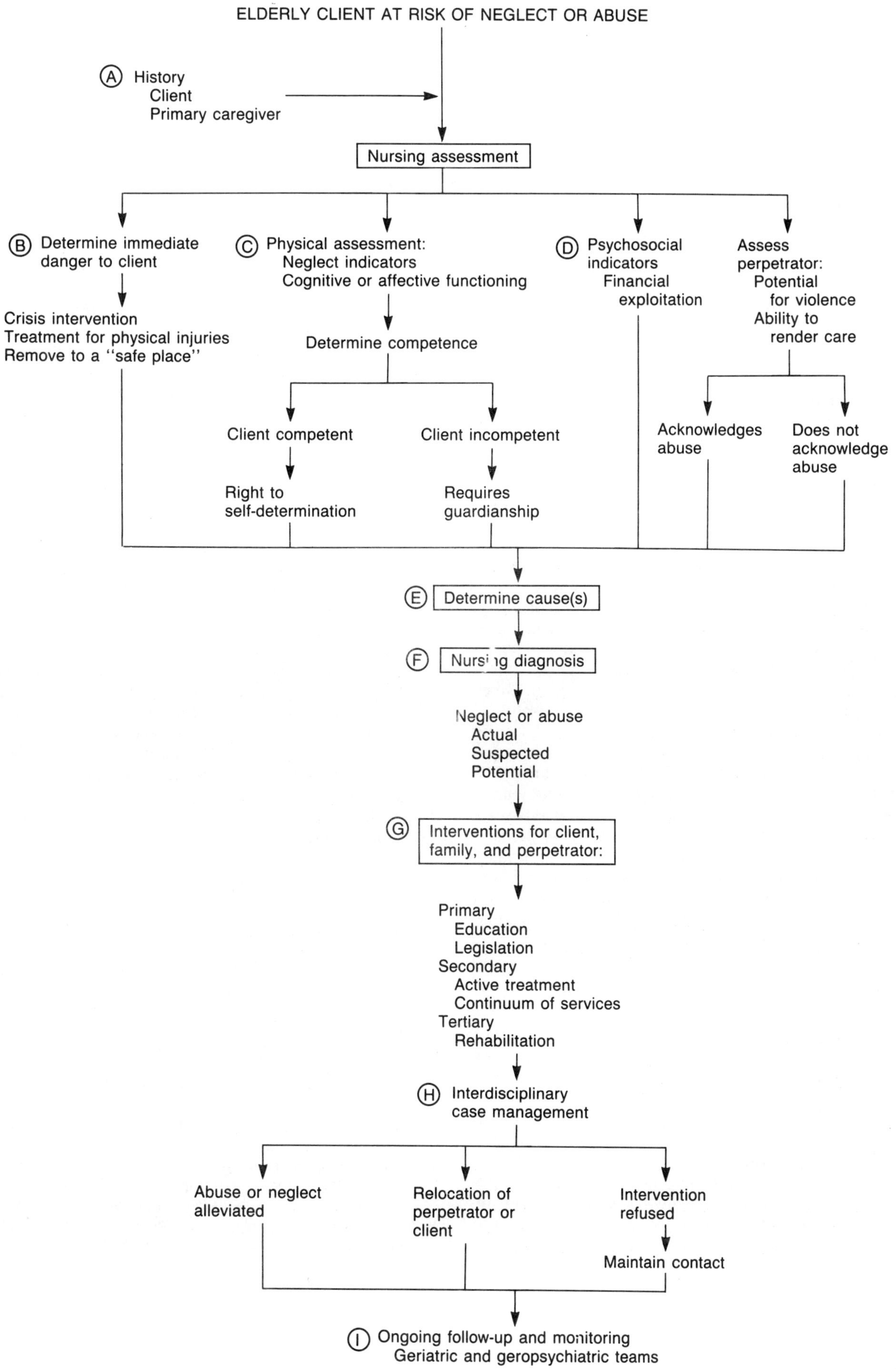
ELDERLY CLIENT AT RISK OF NEGLECT OR ABUSE
(A) History
Client
Primary caregiver
Nursing assessment
(B) Determine immediate danger to client
Crisis intervention
Treatment for physical injuries
Remove to a "safe place"
(C) Physical assessment:
Neglect indicators
Cognitive or affective functioning
Determine competence
Client competent
Right to self-determination
Client incompetent
Requires guardianship
(D) Psychosocial indicators
Financial exploitation
Assess perpetrator:
Potential for violence
Ability to render care
Acknowledges abuse
Does not acknowledge abuse
(E) Determine cause(s)
(F) Nursing diagnosis
Neglect or abuse
Actual
Suspected
Potential
(G) Interventions for client, family, and perpetrator:
Primary
Education
Legislation
Secondary
Active treatment
Continuum of services
Tertiary
Rehabilitation
(H) Interdisciplinary case management
Abuse or neglect alleviated
Relocation of perpetrator or client
Intervention refused
Maintain contact
(I) Ongoing follow-up and monitoring
Geriatric and geropsychiatric teams

WIDOWHOOD

Barbara Brown

Three out of four married women are likely to be widowed during their lifetime. The death of a spouse results in deep feelings of anguish, profound life disruptions, and a complex readjustment. Grieving is a normal adaptive response that enables a widow to resolve the death, regain a sense of well-being, and reinvest in new relationships. However, grieving can take its toll and is often at the root of many emotional and physical problems. Evidence suggests that early interventions can be successful in reducing the damaging effects of grieving (i.e., morbid and pathologic grief reactions).

A. A thorough multidimensional model for bereavement assessment that encompasses social, psychological, situational, spiritual, and physical factors is essential. This assessment assists in creating a profile of the widow, determining the phase of the grief process, and identifying the risk potential for morbid grief reactions. The one consistent predictor of adjustment to widowhood is social support. Tasks of grief work require encouragement, empathy, and sustenance gained from positive relationships. Social roles change as a wife becomes a widow, and she is often ostracized in her new role, finding herself isolated and lonely. The repertoire of coping strategies resulting from previous experience with losses and separation should be explored. The widow who has dealt successfully with other crises may be better equipped to deal with the loss of her husband. Death never occurs at a right time, but the time of death can affect the grieving process. Sudden or accidental death may result in difficulties, yet the widow whose husband dies after a prolonged illness is also viewed at risk. The younger widow with children at home is more vulnerable to poor bereavement outcomes. Many widows live in poverty; at best, their income drops by 44 percent. There may be some initial anger directed at their faith; however, this should subside in time, leaving no bitterness. Gass found that many widows feel closer to God and use prayer to deal with their grief (see "Spiritual Distress," p 204). Numerous physical and emotional symptoms are linked to the normal grieving process, yet grieving is often masked by depression, anxiety, and psychosomatic conditions.

B. The assessment guides the nurse to develop nursing diagnoses related to anticipatory, normal, unresolved, or complicated grieving. In turn, appropriate and individualized nursing interventions can be planned and implemented. Monitor the grief process and facilitate grief work. Grieving has been conceptualized as a process of flexible phases. In his work with widows, Bowlby offered the following phases of the grieving process: numbing, yearning and searching, disorganization and despair, reorganization and resolution. The course of grief for widows can be as prolonged as 4 or more years after the death. The nurse-client relationship serves as the vehicle to facilitate grief work and integrates the counseling principles of grieving as outlined by Worden. Helping the widow to actualize the loss and interpreting normal behavior are prominent interventions. Listening to the widow's experiences over and over again in a patient, accepting and nonjudgmental manner is paramount. This takes on added importance when family and friends are uncomfortable or simply unable to listen any more, not understanding the underlying premise. "I thought I was going crazy" is a common statement and interpreting behavior as a component of normal grieving brings considerable relief. Coordinating complementary resources such as a referral to a widow-to-widow support group is often required. The more complex and complicated grief reactions may require a referral to a mental health agency or psychiatrist.

C. Evaluation focuses on the content and the goals of the grieving process as facilitated through grief work. The accomplishment of the grieving goals often gives rise to issues of self-esteem, problem solving, and personal control for widows. Exploring new aspirations and goals, as well as other support systems, may rest on the widow's ability to deal with these issues. Shifting from "we" to "I" indicates a redefinition of identity and the ability to stand alone. When terminating the relationship with a widow, follow-up past the anniversary date of the death is crucial because a resurgence of emotional and physical reactions may occur. The more complicated grief patterns, including unresolved, delayed, chronic, masked grief, and/or depression, suicidal behaviors, and physical health deterioration, may warrant referral and possible hospitalization.

References

Bowlby J. Attachment and loss. Vol 3. Sadness and depression. New York: Basic Books, 1980.

Dimond MJ. Bereavement for widows. J Psychosoc Nurs Ment Health Serv 1983; 21(9):27–30.

Forchuk C, Brown B. Establishing a nurse-client relationship. J Psychosoc Nurs Ment Health Serv 1989; 27(2):30–34.

Gass KG. Coping strategies of widows. J Gerontol Nurs 1987; 13(6):29–33.

Peplau HE. Interpersonal relations in nursing. New York: GP Putnam, 1952.

Rando TA. Grief, dying and death: clinical interventions for caregivers. Champaign, IL: Research Press, 1984.

Windholz MJ, Marmar CR, Horowitz MJ. Review of the research on conjugal bereavement: impact on health and efficacy of intervention. Comprehens Psychiatry 1985; 26(5):433–447.

Worden JW. Grief counselling and grief therapy: a handbook for the mental health practitioner. New York: Springer, 1982.

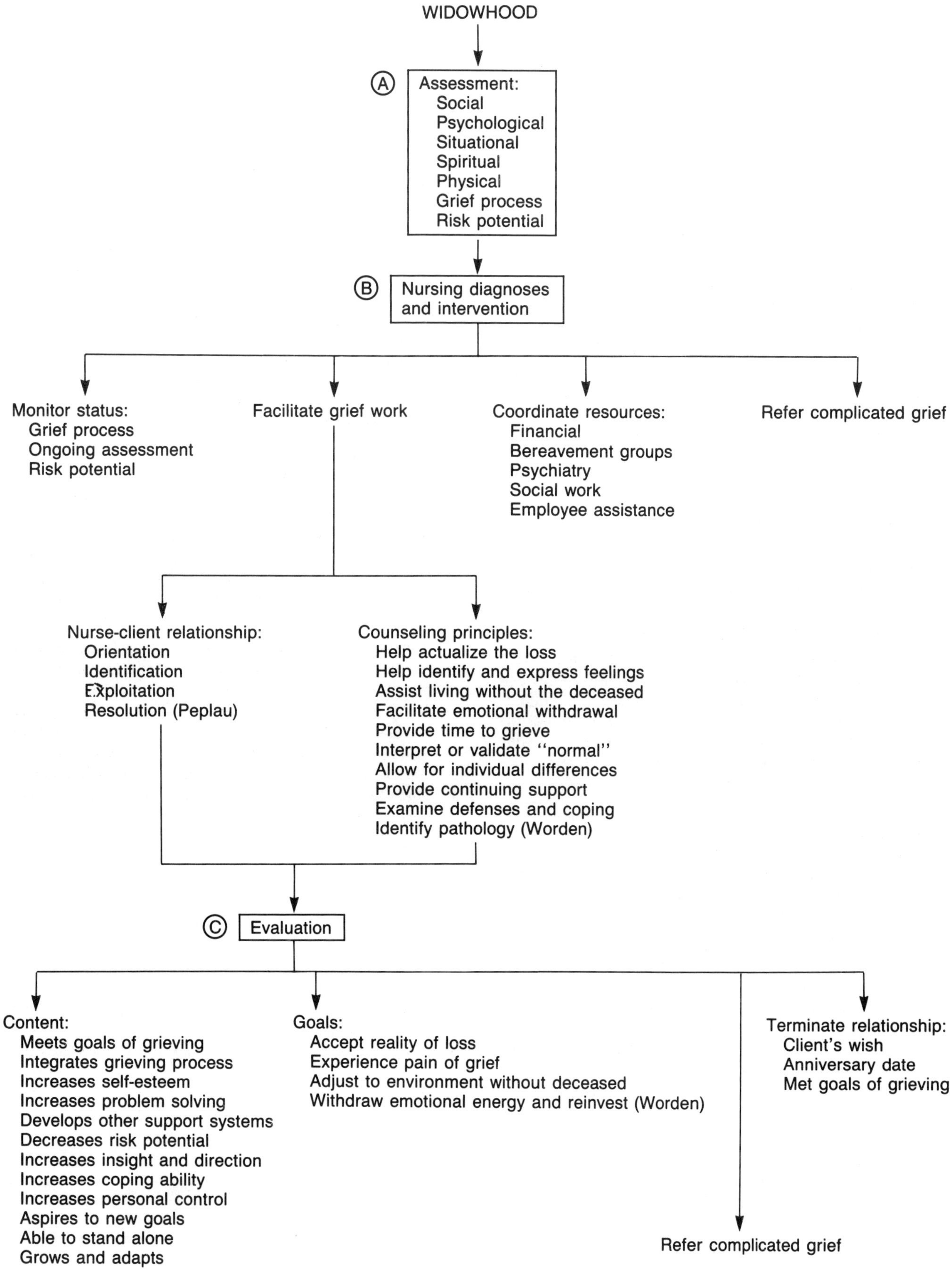
WIDOWHOOD
Ⓐ Assessment:
Social
Psychological
Situational
Spiritual
Physical
Grief process
Risk potential
Ⓑ Nursing diagnoses and intervention
Monitor status:
Grief process
Ongoing assessment
Risk potential
Facilitate grief work
Coordinate resources:
Financial
Bereavement groups
Psychiatry
Social work
Employee assistance
Refer complicated grief
Nurse-client relationship:
Orientation
Identification
Exploitation
Resolution (Peplau)
Counseling principles:
Help actualize the loss
Help identify and express feelings
Assist living without the deceased
Facilitate emotional withdrawal
Provide time to grieve
Interpret or validate "normal"
Allow for individual differences
Provide continuing support
Examine defenses and coping
Identify pathology (Worden)
Ⓒ Evaluation
Content:
Meets goals of grieving
Integrates grieving process
Increases self-esteem
Increases problem solving
Develops other support systems
Decreases risk potential
Increases insight and direction
Increases coping ability
Increases personal control
Aspires to new goals
Able to stand alone
Grows and adapts
Goals:
Accept reality of loss
Experience pain of grief
Adjust to environment without deceased
Withdraw emotional energy and reinvest (Worden)
Terminate relationship:
Client's wish
Anniversary date
Met goals of grieving
Refer complicated grief

CO-DEPENDENCE

Karen Perkins

A. The concept of co-dependence has developed since the 1970s when it was used to describe the often similar behavioral clusters exhibited by the spouses of alcoholics. In fact, the concept was often referred to as "co-alcoholism," whether the spouse was an alcoholic or not. Since then, the concept has been greatly expanded and, along with the term "adult children of alcoholics" (ACoA), has become a buzz word of the late eighties. There is no generally accepted definition of the term co-dependence. Most writers active in the field of behavioral science define co-dependence as a pathologic condition in which an individual's preoccupation with a relationship or other individual results in an exaggerated pattern of learned maladaptive behaviors, beliefs, and feelings that result in leading a life of chronic suffering and ineffectiveness.

B. Co-dependence is thought to develop when significant others, especially parents, invalidate one's observations, feelings, and reactions. Self-doubt develops, and family rules and secrets are internalized. Feelings, especially painful ones, are pushed aside, and healthy grieving over a variety of losses is seldom accomplished. All of these conditions contribute to the blocking of many developmental aspects of the emotional self.

C. There are approximately six major parental or primary caregiver conditions that foster co-dependence. These include alcoholism and/or chemical abuse, parental co-dependent interactional behaviors, chronic mental illness, dysfunctional physical illness, a behavioral cluster of extreme rigidity, punitiveness, judgmentalism, perfectionism, and child abuse.

D. Children raised in households in which a parent or primary caregiver is chronically ill and emotionally and/or physically unavailable often adopt a caretaker's role. Such children may overidentify with the ill parent to the point of fusion. Often a vague sense of being the cause of the family's problems may evolve.

E. A growing body of literature reports an increase in the number of patients who grew up in families that appear "normal" but were really dysfunctional. There was no evidence of substance abuse in these families; however, common qualities included extreme rigidity, punitiveness, judgmentalism, a demand for perfection, and a cold and distant family atmosphere.

F. Child abuse is not confined to the dramatic accounts of severe physical or sexual abuse that make the daily news. Psychological and emotional abuse as well as subtle forms of sexual abuse are often not recognized as such by the victim, perpetrator, or mental health provider. These less obvious forms of abuse become the basis upon which a deep-seated sense of shame and low self-esteem inevitably develop.

G. As one begins to feel more and more out of control, the need to control intensifies. Compulsive behaviors may develop as a way to decrease temporarily the level of chronic tension related to the need to be always in control. Psychosomatic illnesses (p 70) may develop as a result of chronic tension and stress.

H. As many as 14 potential "core issues" have been identified as having direct relevance to the recovery process of the co-dependent patient. The eight most commonly identified issues are trust, control, feelings, all-or-none thinking and behaving, low self-esteem, high tolerance for inappropriate behavior, neglect of one's own needs, and being overly responsible. Difficulty in handling and appropriately resolving conflict and the fear of abandonment are two other major areas of concern.

I. Because of extensive media coverage, a large segment of the general public has been exposed to the concept of psychologically oriented self-help groups such as ACoA and Survivors of Incest. Such groups have begun to demystify the psychological jargon associated with basic psychodynamic theory. As client advocates, mental health nurses have a responsibility to help their clients differentiate between those groups and individuals which may be helpful and those which may be harmful.

References

Beattie M. Co-dependent no more. New York: Harper & Row, 1987.

Schaef AW. When society becomes an addict. San Francisco: Harper & Row, 1987:1–150.

Whitfield CL. Healing the child within. Deerfield Beach, FL: Health Communications, 1987.

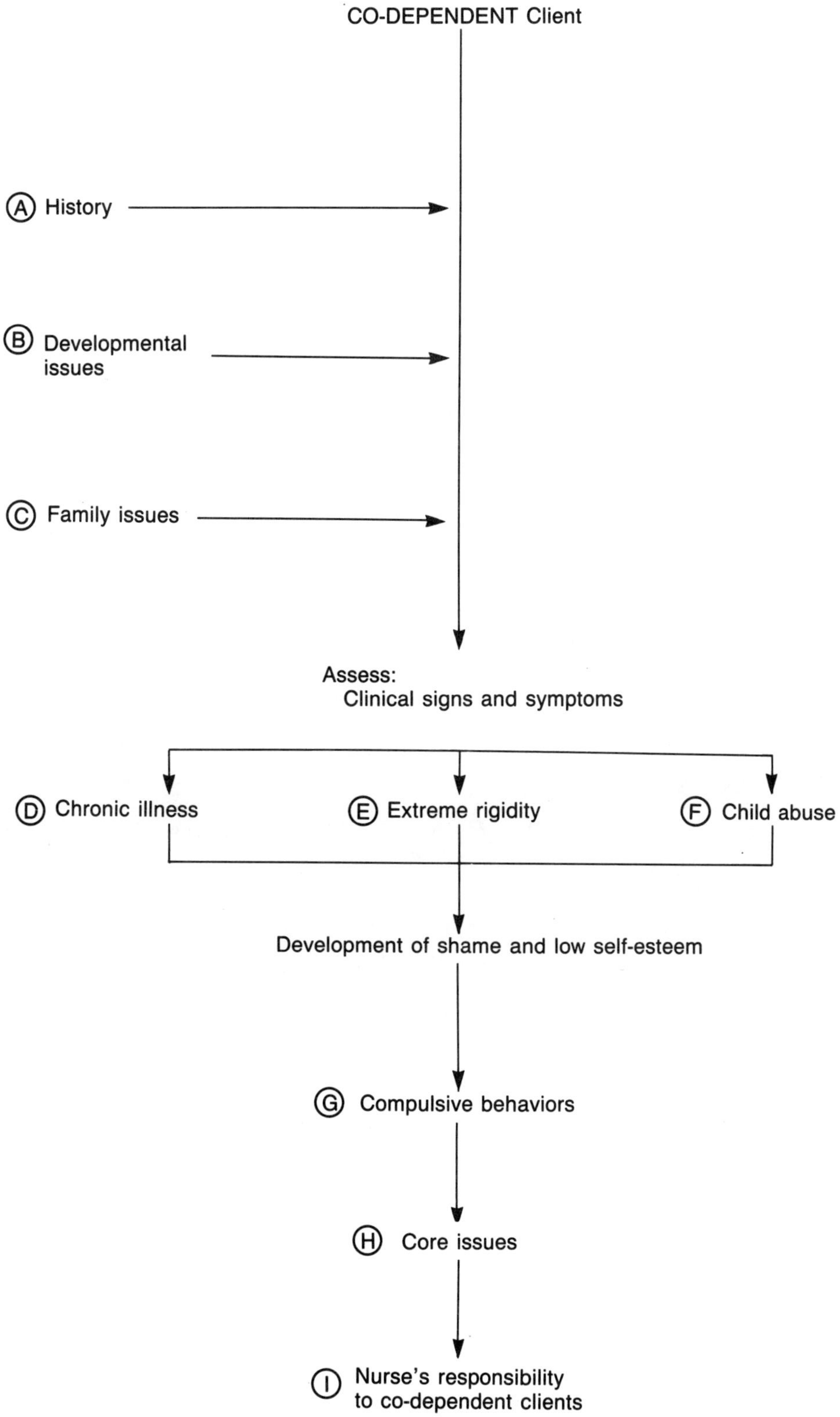
CO-DEPENDENT Client
(A) History
(B) Developmental issues
(C) Family issues
Assess:
Clinical signs and symptoms
(D) Chronic illness
(E) Extreme rigidity
(F) Child abuse
Development of shame and low self-esteem
(G) Compulsive behaviors
(H) Core issues
(I) Nurse's responsibility to co-dependent clients

V PSYCHOSOCIAL CONCEPTS AND ISSUES

PERCEIVED UNCERTAINTY

Roberta Ronayne

Uncertainty is a cognitive state that occurs when the client is unable to structure or categorize an event because sufficient cues are lacking. Uncertainty arises in situations when the client is unable to assign definite value to an event or situation and/or is unable to accurately predict outcomes.

A. A brief history should include information about illness, the symptoms at onset, pattern (including remissions and exacerbations), treatment (including compliance with prescribed regimens), and underlying stress.

B. The nursing assessment should identify the client's perception of the illness situation. Factors influencing perception include the client's subjective appraisal of personal experiences and information from others related to diagnosis, symptoms, treatment, seriousness of illness and prognosis, and personal variables such as age, level of education, and knowledge of illness.

C. Uncertainty should be assessed initially during the early phase of illness and reassessed at frequent intervals throughout the course of illness because the focus, intensity, and duration of uncertainty may vary over time.

D. Clients experience uncertainty related to diagnosis, symptoms, treatment, and prognosis. Four factors contribute to uncertainty: ambiguity concerning the state of illness, complexity regarding treatment and system of care, lack of information about diagnosis and seriousness of illness, and unpredictability about the course of illness and prognosis.

E. Although clients experiencing uncertainty use a variety of coping modes to deal with their situation, the strategies utilized are neither inherently adaptive nor maladaptive. Techniques that are effective in one situation may not be in the next, and those that may be effective for one person may not be for another. When coping modes fail to lessen the threat associated with uncertainty, clients experience and exhibit increased levels of stress. Intrapsychic modes are used more frequently than direct action or information seeking modes. Intrapsychic modes such as avoidance, denial, and vigilance help regulate emotion by making the client feel better. Action-oriented strategies such as biofeedback, exercise, and compliance, help regulate emotion and facilitate behavior change. Seeking information provides data necessary to make decisions about management of stressful situations. Clients may seek out only information that is congruent with their desire, thereby avoiding dissonant information, or they may search for information which will help them to understand their present status, to reinterpret past events, and to anticipate the future.

F. Providing clients with information about illness, its cause, symptoms, treatment, and system of care, enhances congruency between experienced and expected events. It also reduces the unfamiliar and frightening nature of the illness situation, thereby enabling a more accurate interpretation of current health status and more realistic expectations about the future. Providing immediate and relevant feedback about progress and the small gains that have been made enables clients to determine their position on the illness trajectory and to develop realistic expectations for the future. Interaction with others through social support networks enables clients to clarify their perceptions of illness and to examine and test out new resources for coping with uncertainty.

G. The goal of intervention is to reduce the client's level of uncertainty so that other aspects of illness can be considered. Continued monitoring and evaluation are necessary to detect changes in level of uncertainty.

References

Folkman S, Schaefer C, Lazarus RS. Cognitive processes as mediators of stress and coping. In: Hamilton V, Warburton DM, eds. Human stress and cognition: an information processing approach. Chichester, England: John Wiley, 1979.

Mishel MH. The measurement of uncertainty in illness. Nurs Res 1981; 30:258–263.

Mishel MH, Braden CJ. Uncertainty: a mediator between support and adjustment. West J Nurs Res 1987; 9(1):43–57.

Mishel MH, Braden CJ. Finding uncertainty: antecedents of uncertainty in illness. Nurs Res 1988; 37:98–103.

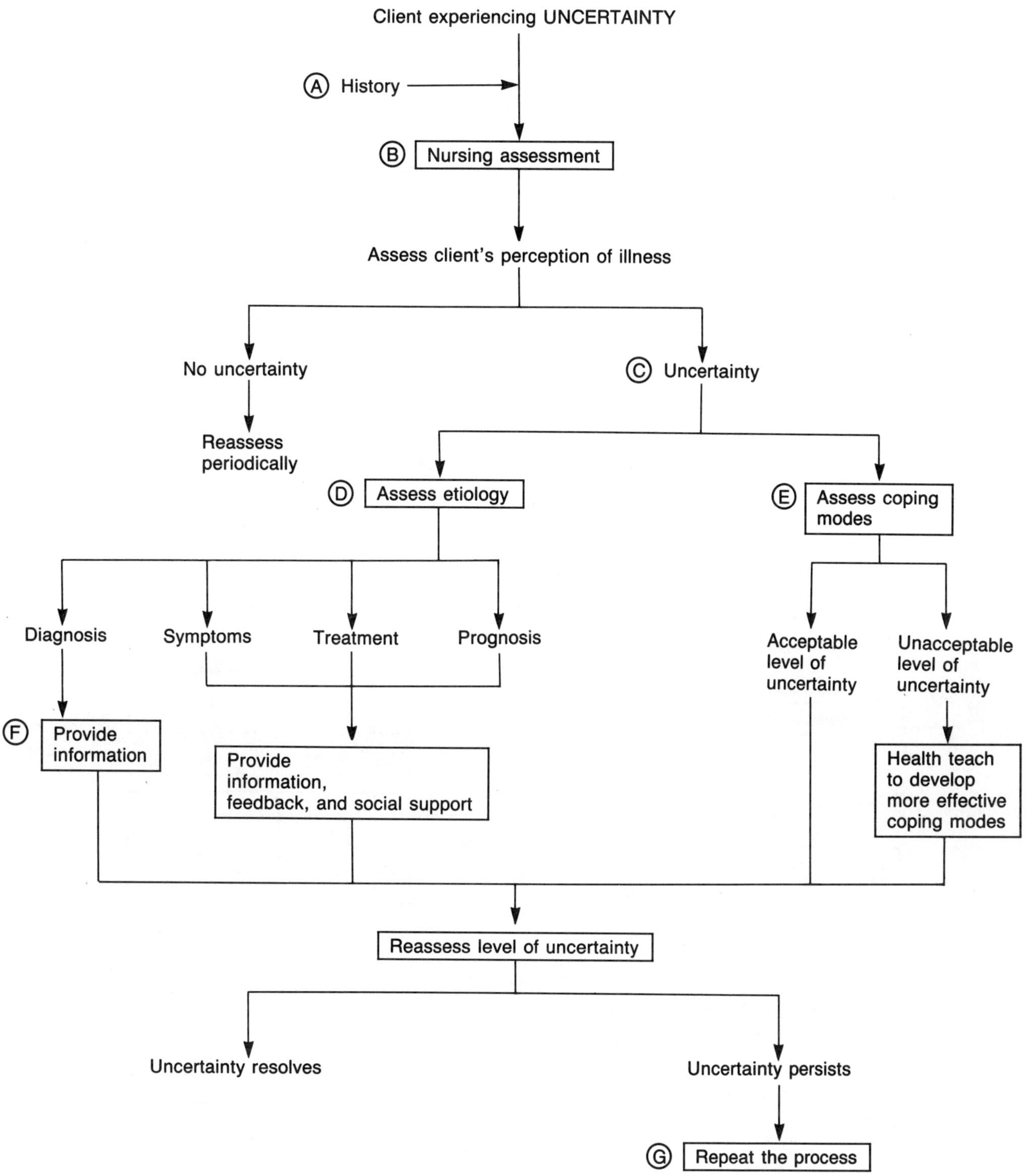
Client experiencing UNCERTAINTY
(A) History
(B) Nursing assessment
Assess client's perception of illness
No uncertainty
Reassess periodically
(C) Uncertainty
(D) Assess etiology
(E) Assess coping modes
Diagnosis
Symptoms
Treatment
Prognosis
Acceptable level of uncertainty
Unacceptable level of uncertainty
(F) Provide information
Provide information, feedback, and social support
Health teach to develop more effective coping modes
Reassess level of uncertainty
Uncertainty resolves
Uncertainty persists
(G) Repeat the process

POWERLESSNESS

Andrea Baumann

Powerlessness is defined as the perception of a loss of personal control over events or situations in one's life. This state was observed as early as 1963 by Melvin Seeman in his work with institutionalized persons. The phenomenon is a result of a complex interaction between past experience and adjustment to a present situation. It may follow from a series of life events over which a person has been perceived to have little control.

A. Severity of illness, previous adjustment pattern, present coping mechanisms, and support systems in the environment are all important data to elicit from the client and family. A history of chronic illness and frequent hospitalization can result in a perception of loss of control over both one's body and the surrounding environment. The client enters hospital relatively unaware of the dynamics of organizational systems. There is a system of rules, regulations, and communication patterns that may be overwhelming and may enhance preexisting feelings of powerlessness. A client may become resigned to having little control over outcome if hospitalization is coupled with potential loss of community ties and isolation from significant others.

B. Assessment should include the use of Miller and Oertel's (1986) powerlessness behavioral assessment tool (Fig. 1). This four-point rating scale examines the following areas: verbal and emotional responses, interest in activities of daily living, and motivation for learning. Feelings of worthlessness, feeling alone, and lack of interest are not uncommon symptoms when a person becomes resigned to having no control over outcome.

C. The first goal of therapy is to mobilize the client's physical and psychic energy. Initial treatment of depression (see p 46) may be necessary. Through positive encourage-

	Patient Behaviors	Nurse Rating of Behaviors: 1 Never	2 Occasionally	3 Frequently	4 Always
VERBAL RESPONSE	Verbal expressions of lack of control over what is happening				
	Verbal expressions of doubt that self-care measures can affect outcome				
	Verbal expressions of giving up				
	Verbal expressions of fatalism				
EMOTIONAL RESPONSE	Withdrawal				
	Pessimism				
	Undifferentiated anger				
	Diminished patient-initiated interaction				
	Submissiveness				
PARTICIPATION IN ACTIVITIES OF DAILY LIVING	Nonparticipation in daily personal hygiene				
	Noninterest in treatments				
	Refusal to take food or fluids				
	Inability to set goals				
	Lack of decision making when opportunities are provided				
	Dependency on others for activities of daily living				
INVOLVEMENT IN LEARNING ABOUT CARE RESPONSIBILITIES	Lack of questioning concerning illness				
	Low level of knowledge of illness after being given information				
	Lack of knowledge related to treatment				
	Lack of motivation to learn				

Figure 1 Powerlessness behavioral assessment tool. (From Miller JF, Oertel CB. Powerlessness in the elderly: preventing hopelessness. In: Miller JF, ed. Coping with chronic illness: overcoming powerlessness. Philadelphia: FA Davis, 1985:127.)

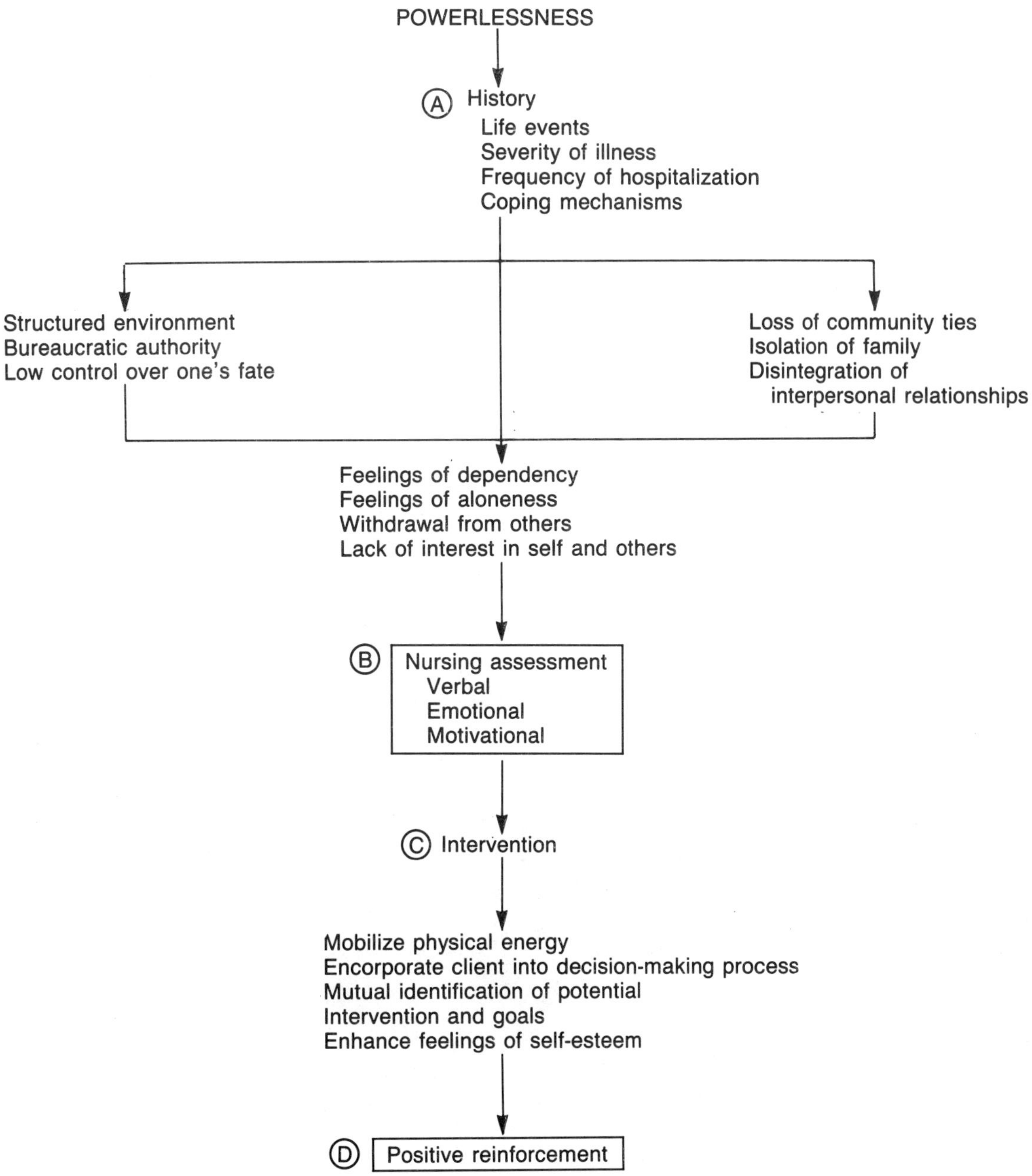

ment and support, the client can become an integral participant in the decision-making process. The sharing of information about treatment is essential. The client should be allowed control over those treatment decisions that are possible. Mutual identification of potential interventions encourages conscious activity on the part of the client to plan the care.

D. The overall goal is to help the client set realistic goals and to feel more in control of outcomes. It is important to set goals that can be achieved; then the client can see progress in decision-making capabilities. Short-term goals that are readily attainable are most suitable for initial treatment. Recognition of progress is necessary to allow the client to build up the confidence to be able to take control over the environment. Positive reinforcement encourages ongoing progress in the client's ability to make decisions and thus reduces the feelings of powerlessness.

References

Carpenito L. Nursing diagnosis application to clinical practice. 2nd ed. Philadelphia: JB Lippincott, 1987.

Miller JF, Oertel C. Powerlessness in the elderly: preventing hopelessness. In: Miller JF, ed. Coping with chronic illness: overcoming powerlessness. Philadelphia: FA Davis, 1985.

Seeman M. Alienation and social learning in a reformatory. Am J Sociol 1963; 69:270–273.

Townsend M. Nursing diagnosis in psychiatric nursing. Philadelphia: FA Davis, 1988:128–130.

HOPELESSNESS

Deborah Antai-Otong

Hopelessness is frequently described as a feeling of "giving up." Frequently hopelessness accompanies depression and presents a worrisome picture to the nurse. These clients are often apathetic, detached from others, have a poor self-concept, and are self-deprecating.

A. Encourage clients who complain of feeling hopeless to identify recent stressors or major life-style changes. Include family members to clarify and verify this information. Approach the client and family members in a warm, caring, and respectful manner.

B. The nurse must assess the client for symptoms of major depression and suicide potential (see "Major Depressive Episodes" [p 46] and "Suicide Attempt" [p 42]). Assess the client's current support system, coping capacities, problem-solving skills, and mental and physical status.

C. Clients feeling hopeless sometimes isolate themselves or feel alienated. The nurse must mobilize the client's resources and support system. Improving the client's self-respect and integrity are key issues in dealing with hopelessness.

References

Beck AT, Rush AJ, Shaw BF, Emery G. Cognitive therapy of depression. New York: The Guilford Press, 1979.

Miller JF. Coping with chronic illness. Philadelphia: FA Davis, 1983.

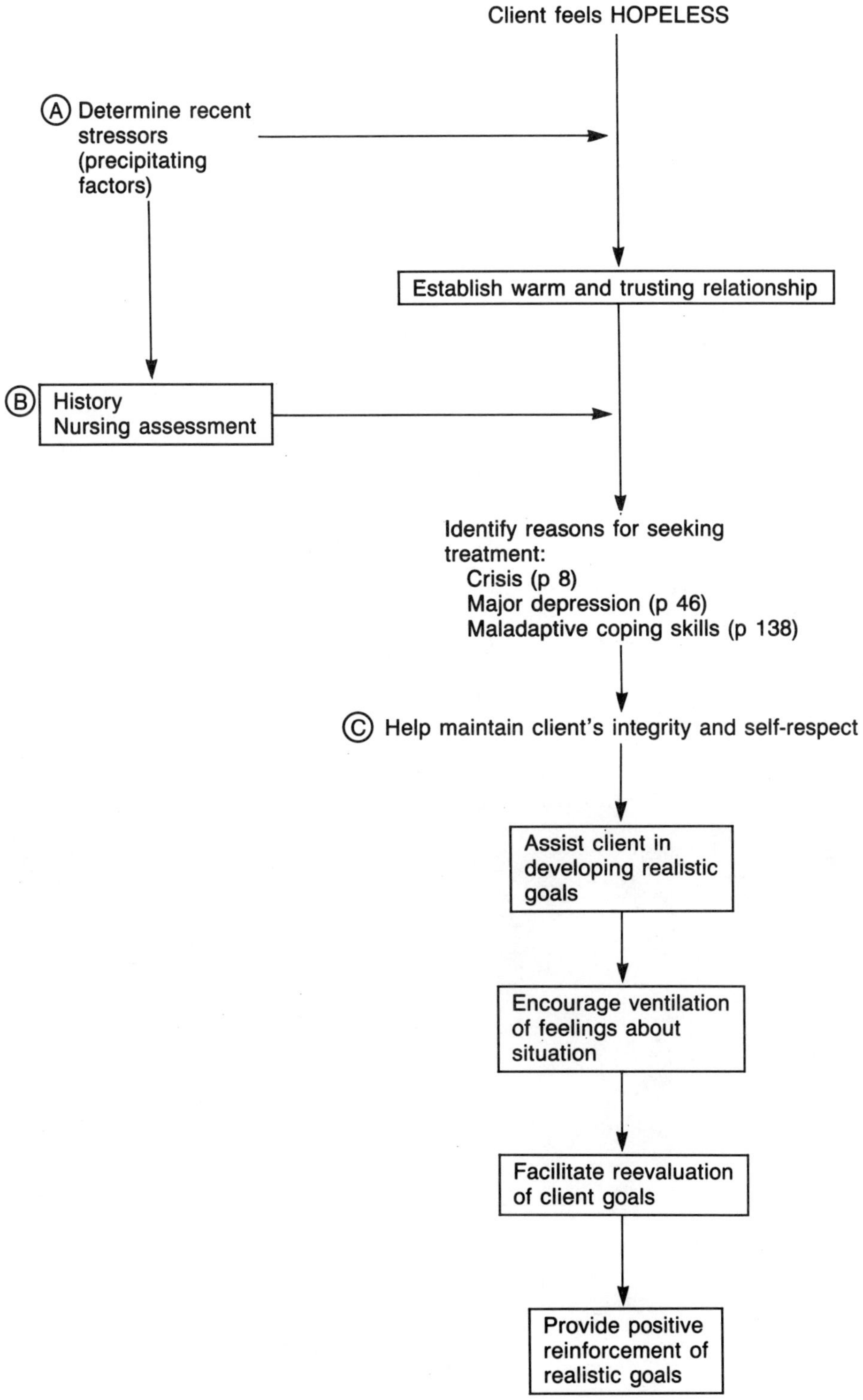

Client feels HOPELESS
Ⓐ Determine recent stressors (precipitating factors)
Establish warm and trusting relationship
Ⓑ History
Nursing assessment
Identify reasons for seeking treatment:
Crisis (p 8)
Major depression (p 46)
Maladaptive coping skills (p 138)
Ⓒ Help maintain client's integrity and self-respect
Assist client in developing realistic goals
Encourage ventilation of feelings about situation
Facilitate reevaluation of client goals
Provide positive reinforcement of realistic goals

LONELINESS

Deborah Antai-Otong

A. Loneliness is a subjective experience that sometimes results from dissatisfaction in current social relationships and not having expectations met. Loneliness is frequently experienced by depressed clients. These individuals must be assessed for symptoms of major depression and suicide potential (see "Major Depressive Episodes" [p 46] and "Suicide Attempt" [p 42].) Loneliness may also result from stressful situations or major life-style changes. Clients suffering from loneliness frequently complain of feelings of inadequacy and alienation. Other factors that may contribute to loneliness include personality traits such as shyness, poor self-esteem, and poor social skills. These traits can interfere with development of social and interpersonal skills.

B. In addition to the parameters discussed in "Major Depressive Episodes" (p 46), the history must include recent stressors, and significant life-style changes, and past and present coping patterns. Determine the duration of current feelings of loneliness, past experiences, and problem-solving skills. Include also the client's level of function over the past year.

C. For further discussion of assessment, see page 46.

D. Pathologic loneliness may be manifested by chronic social isolation and impaired social skills. Certain psychiatric illnesses may interfere with developing interpersonal relationships and must be identified and treated appropriately, i.e., schizophrenias, schizoid personality. For a discussion of appropriate interventions see pages 72, 74, and 128.

Reference

Peplau LA, Perlman D. Loneliness: a source book of current theory, research, therapy. New York: John Wiley, 1982.

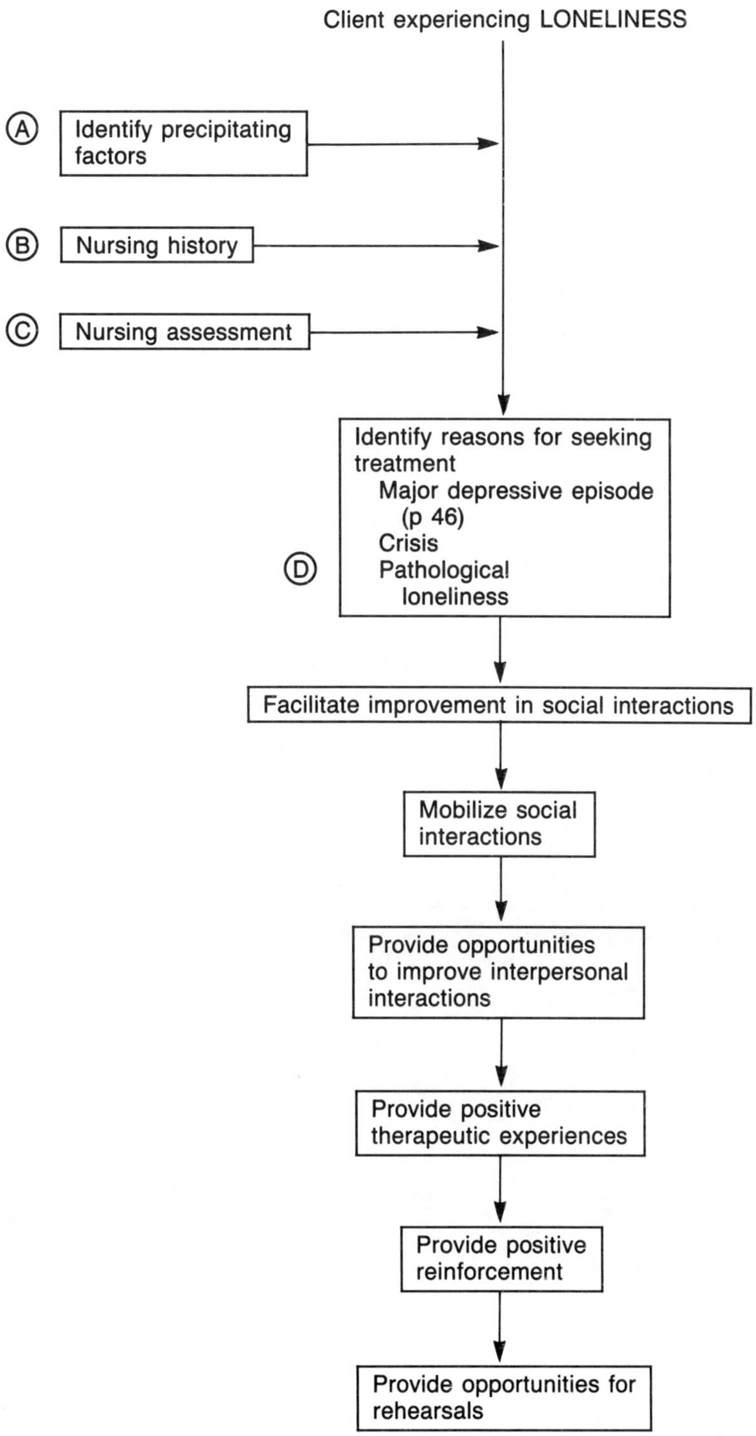
Client experiencing LONELINESS
Ⓐ Identify precipitating factors
Ⓑ Nursing history
Ⓒ Nursing assessment
Ⓓ Identify reasons for seeking treatment
Major depressive episode (p 46)
Crisis
Pathological loneliness
Facilitate improvement in social interactions
Mobilize social interactions
Provide opportunities to improve interpersonal interactions
Provide positive therapeutic experiences
Provide positive reinforcement
Provide opportunities for rehearsals

ANGER

Nona Flye

A. Angry behavior may accompany a number of psychiatric disorders. The client exhibiting angry behavior should undergo a thorough psychiatric and medical assessment. The medical examination includes a neurologic work-up to rule out disorders such as brain tumor, temporal lobe epilepsy, and trauma that may have resulted in brain damage. Assess the client's feelings of powerlessness (p 184) and loss of control, issues which increase the likelihood of anger.

B. A client exhibiting disruptive behavior may shout, threaten, destroy property, become physically abusive to others, make unrealistic demands, and demonstrate inability to reason. These individuals often have a low tolerance to frustration and poor impulse control. Persistent agitation and restlessness may require restraint and/or seclusion.

C. Anxiolytic agents such as lorazepam (Ativan) produce rapid sedation within minutes after parenteral injection. Assess and document the client's response to this medication. The initial dose may be larger than the maintenance regimen. The client usually becomes more cooperative and less agitated within a short time and more amenable to treatment after several hours or days. When clients exhibit psychotic behavior, neuroleptics are prescribed which may produce a wide range of side effects including dystonia (p 78), extrapyramidal symptoms, (p 80), and akathisia. These symptoms are very frightening to the client.

D. Clients with lengthy histories of inappropriate expression of anger are often unaware of the destructive nature of this behavior. Encourage clients to discuss these feelings and the precipitating events that trigger anger. Assess how anger has been handled in the past and how people reacted to it. Approaching clients in a calm, concerned manner encourages them to talk about reasons for current angry feelings. These measures minimize and de-escalate hostility and aggressive behaviors. They also allow the client to gain control over his thoughts and behavior.

E. The nurse is in an opportune position to teach clients how to relax and gain control over current angry feelings and learn more appropriate coping patterns. The client must understand that anger is normal and appropriate under certain conditions, but certain behaviors and expressions of anger are not acceptable. The nurse can point out strategies and focuses that help the client stay in control and express anger in a more appropriate manner. For a description of some appropriate interventions see pages 118, 120, 122, and 124.

References

Rubin TI. The angry book. New York: Collier MacMiilan, 1978.
Taylor CM. Mereness' essentials of psychiatric nursing. 12th ed. St. Louis: CV Mosby, 1986.

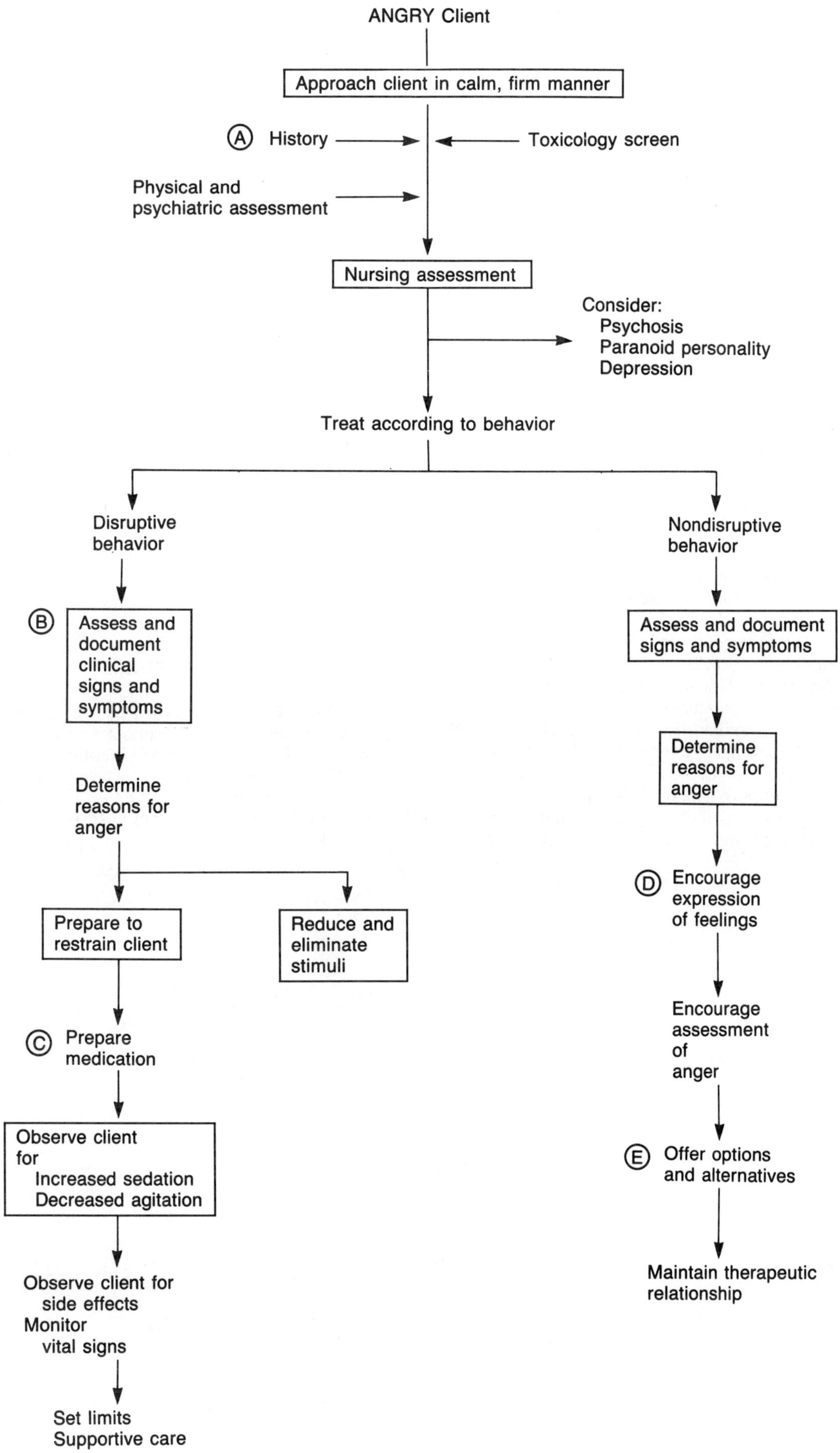
ANGRY Client
Approach client in calm, firm manner
(A) History
Toxicology screen
Physical and psychiatric assessment
Nursing assessment
Consider:
Psychosis
Paranoid personality
Depression
Treat according to behavior
Disruptive behavior
Nondisruptive behavior
(B) Assess and document clinical signs and symptoms
Assess and document signs and symptoms
Determine reasons for anger
Determine reasons for anger
Prepare to restrain client
Reduce and eliminate stimuli
(D) Encourage expression of feelings
(C) Prepare medication
Encourage assessment of anger
Observe client for
Increased sedation
Decreased agitation
(E) Offer options and alternatives
Observe client for side effects
Monitor vital signs
Maintain therapeutic relationship
Set limits
Supportive care

GRIEF AND BEREAVEMENT

Deborah Antai-Otong

A. Most people have experienced grief at some time. Grief often results from significant or anticipated losses of significant others. It is usually experienced as a normal reaction and seldom requires intervention. Some clients fail to grieve because of social or psychological reasons. These individuals require support and empathy from nurses. The nurse's responsibilities include determining the significance of the loss and available resources. Assess the cause of the loss (i.e., illness), current support systems, past and present coping patterns, and familial and cultural influences that may possibly influence the grief reaction (see "Loss," p 198). Often these clients present requesting medication for sleep or depression. Medications should be avoided or used cautiously in clients suffering from grief.

B. Clients experiencing normal grief reactions typically present in psychiatric settings with symptoms of depression. They may have somatic complaints of decreased appetite, sleeplessness, fatigue, and difficulty concentrating. Often they complain of sadness, despair, anger, and guilt; they may be preoccupied with the deceased person and report frequent dreams. Four stages of grief have been described by Bowlby and Parkes (1970): (1) numbness and disbelief, (2) anger and preoccupation with the deceased, (3) disorganization, and (4) reorganization. The scope of these symptoms may range from several months to years. The nurse needs to determine the stage of grief, recognizing the need to mobilize psychosocial support and facilitate adaptive coping skills to promote reorganization and prevent a pathologic grief reaction. A differential diagnosis of normal grief reaction versus major depression must be established during the initial assessment. In both instances the client may experience sadness, decreased appetite, sleeplessness, and social isolation, but with a normal grief reaction the duration is shorter. Clients with this reaction eventually find enjoyment and reorganization in their life-style and recognize that their sadness is related to a loss. Depressed clients complain of not knowing why they are feeling sad and are more likely to threaten suicide than those experiencing a normal grief reaction.

C. A pathologic grief reaction often results when the client denies or inhibits the normal grief process. The client fails to deal with the reality of the loss, which may be demonstrated by experiencing the physical symptoms of the deceased or presenting with false euphoria. These clients often complain of extreme guilt and self reproach. If this course is allowed to continue, psychosis and/or symptoms of major depression will ensue.

References

Bowlby J, Parkes CM. Separation and loss. In: Anthony EJ, Koupernick C, eds. International yearbook for child psychiatry and allied disciplines. New York: Wiley-Interscience, 1970.

Burgess AW. Psychiatric nursing in the hospital and community. 4th ed. Englewood Cliffs, NJ: Prentice-Hall, 1985.

Lindemann E. Beyond grief: studies in crisis intervention. New York: Jason Aronson, 1979.

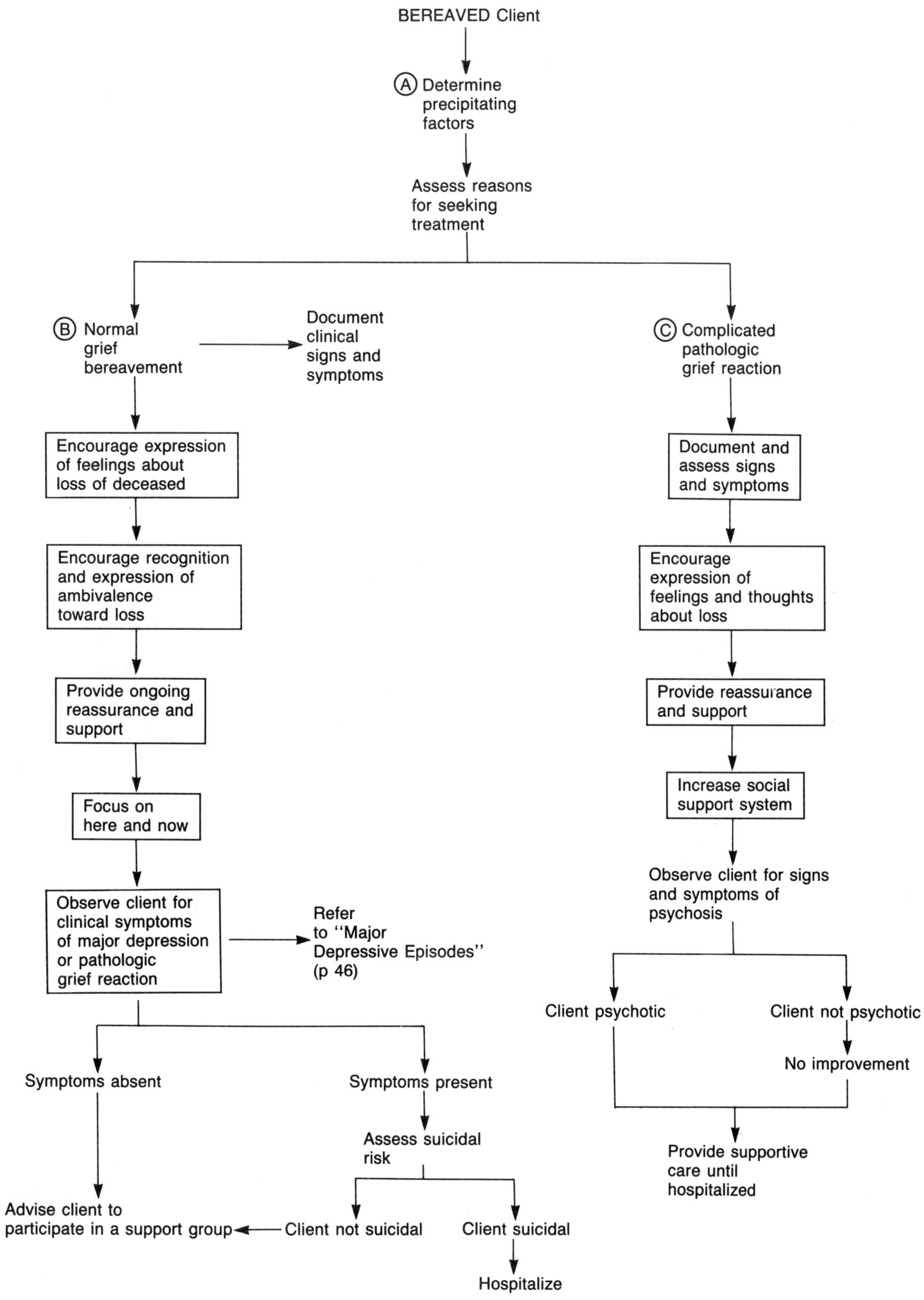
BEREAVED Client
(A) Determine precipitating factors
Assess reasons for seeking treatment
(B) Normal grief bereavement
Document clinical signs and symptoms
Encourage expression of feelings about loss of deceased
Encourage recognition and expression of ambivalence toward loss
Provide ongoing reassurance and support
Focus on here and now
Observe client for clinical symptoms of major depression or pathologic grief reaction
Refer to "Major Depressive Episodes" (p 46)
Symptoms absent
Symptoms present
Assess suicidal risk
Advise client to participate in a support group
Client not suicidal
Client suicidal
Hospitalize
(C) Complicated pathologic grief reaction
Document and assess signs and symptoms
Encourage expression of feelings and thoughts about loss
Provide reassurance and support
Increase social support system
Observe client for signs and symptoms of psychosis
Client psychotic
Client not psychotic
No improvement
Provide supportive care until hospitalized

DENIAL

Cheryl Forchuk
Jan Westwell

A. Denial is a process in which the individual disowns unpleasant or painful reality. It is an internal and unconscious process. The nurse can only observe behavior and speculate as to what is happening. When the nurse is confronted with a situation in which an individual does not acknowledge the apparent "obvious," denial may or may not be involved. Differences in perceptions, values, or available information may explain the apparent denial. Another possibility is that the individual, at a conscious level, may choose to not discuss the issue.

B. Denial assists the individual to avoid painful feelings created by conflicting thoughts and/or emotions. Nurses need to accept the protective function of denial. This includes self-awareness of feelings and actions in situations where someone may be using denial.

C. Speculate what specific thoughts and/or feelings are creating conflict or pain within the individual. Discuss with the individual, in a nonconfronting manner, a related but less anxiety-provoking part of the conflict. Careful listening is a starting point that allows both the nurse and the individual to become aware of the issues.

D. Assessment includes the nurse's judgment of whether or not denial is creating a problem for the individual. Although denial cannot be directly confirmed, the effect or influence of denial may be observed.

E. If, in the nurse's assessment, the individual's use of denial is not causing the individual any problems, no further intervention may be required at this time.

F. Discussion may allow alternate views of the conflict, or alternate ways of dealing with the pain, to become apparent. This seldom happens within one interview, but usually is a process that unfolds over time. The individual may persist in the use of denial if the pain of accepting reality is unconsciously too difficult to bear.

References

Dorpat TL. The cognitive arrest hypothesis of denial. Int J Psychoanal 1983; 64:47–58.

Forchuk C, Westwell J. Denial. J Psychosoc Nurs 1987; 25(6):9–13.

Lazarus RS. The costs and benefits of denial. In: Dohrenwend BS, Dohrenwend BP, eds. Stressful life events and their contexts. New York: Prodist Publications, 1981.

Westwell J, Forchuk C. Denial: buffer and barrier. Can Nurse (in press).

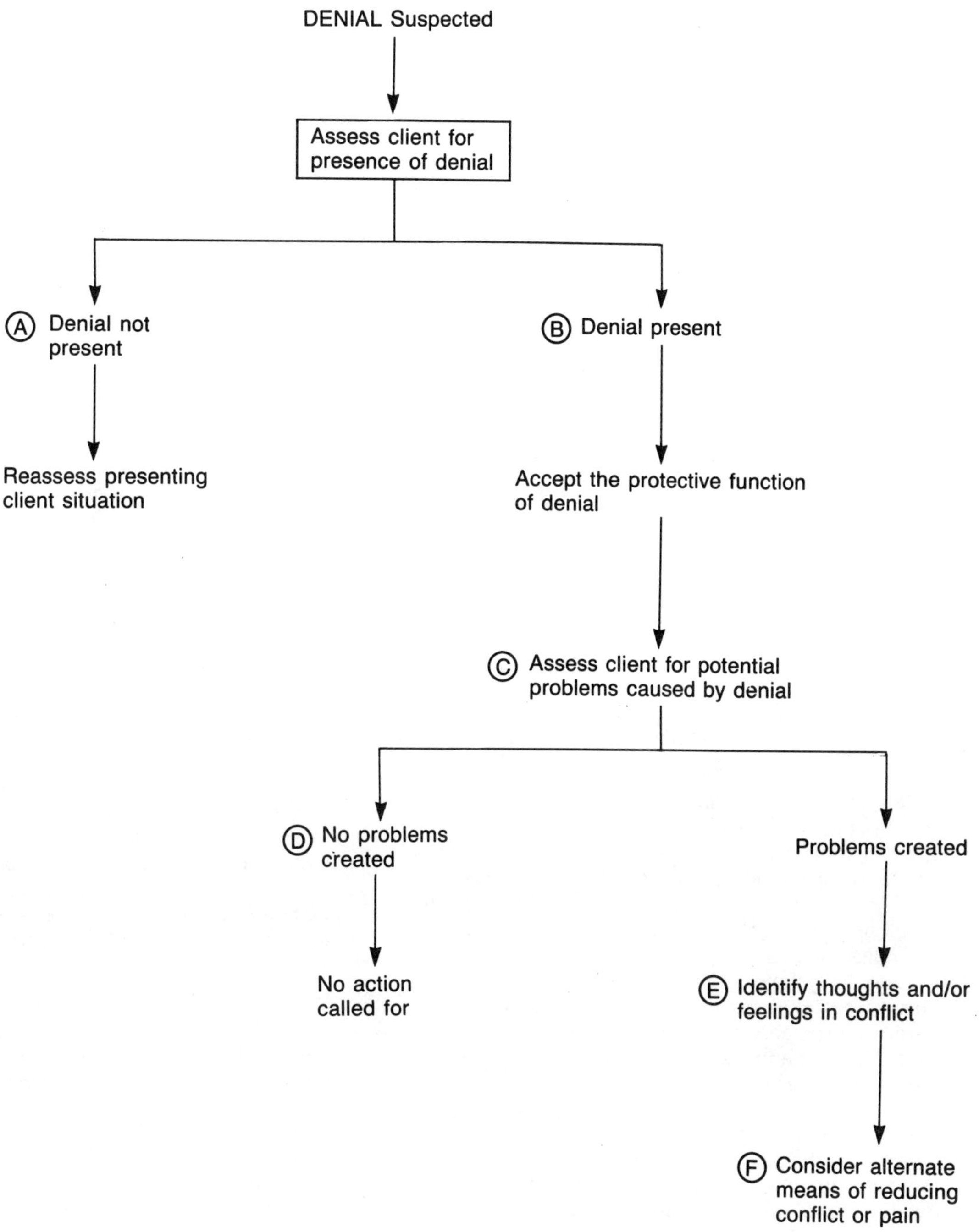

Adapted with permission from: Forchuk C, Westwell J. Denial. J Psychosoc Nurs 1987; 25(6):12.

INTIMACY

Nancy E. Johnston

A. Intimacy is an essential ingredient of a satisfying marital relationship. It may be assessed by evaluating four major interrelated dimensions. One important dimension to assess is conflict resolution. Couples seeking greater intimacy may frequently require assistance in identifying sources of conflict. The nurse-therapist, operating from a neutral position, assists the couple to explore and relinquish rigid positions in favor of more viable and flexible compromises.

B. Assess effective communication and the expression of affection, which have been correlated significantly to marital adjustment. Explore each partner's history and style of communicating and encourage greater self-disclosure. The goal of therapy is to access, express, and reprocess the emotional responses underlying each partner's interactional positions and thereby facilitate a shift in these interactional positions toward greater accessibility and responsiveness. Identify problematic patterns of interaction and encourage reenactment of these scenarios in therapy. Explore emotional responses as they occur and reframe interactions by accessing underlying feelings.

C. Cohesion and compatibility are closely related concepts that describe the feelings of commitment the couple has to the marriage and the degree to which the couple is able to work and play together comfortably. Assess the levels of diversity and complementarity with a view to developing and reinforcing mutuality. Effecting a shift in individual values and attitudes is often necessary in order to create a psychological climate that is conducive to the development of realistic goals and expectations. Once tension and defensiveness have been reduced, it is possible to promote the development and sharing of common interests, activities, and friends. Dyadic closeness is strongly related to the ability of young married couples to relinquish strong emotional ties with significant others, including the family of origin. Assess the degree to which strong bonds with others beyond the marital dyad jeopardize the ability of the couple to access each other's capacity for giving and receiving emotional nurturance.

D. Identity and sexuality are vital aspects of intimacy. Identity is the couple's level of self-confidence and self-esteem. The capacity of the individuals within the dyad to develop a strong marital identity is predicated on the ego strength of the individuals and the previous accomplishment of normative developmental tasks. Individuals who have strong personal identities are able to negotiate effectively with their partners to obtain the nurturance and support required to develop deeper levels of trust and intimacy. In some marriages individuals with incomplete identity development may find within the marriage the resources needed to compensate for previous deficiencies. In these cases the nurse-therapist acts to support the accessibility of available resources while ensuring that the potential for unhealthy dependency states is avoided. In other cases it may become apparent that individual deficits are too great and resources too meager to bring about the desired enhancement of the marital relationship. Sexuality refers to the degree to which sexual needs are communicated and fulfilled by the marriage. Frequently sexual dysfunction develops as a symptom of ineffective functioning in the dimensions described above. To the extent that these dimensions of marital function can be improved, sexual satisfaction may also be enhanced. However, since all dimensions of marital function are interrelated, it may be most effective to treat sexual dysfunction at the same time that other dimensions are being addressed. Nurses with advanced training in human sexuality are competent to intervene effectively in this area. Those without advanced training are more comfortable assessing the problem and referring the couple. It is frequently desirable for therapists with different areas of speciality to collaborate in the treatment of the couple.

E. Since marital happiness has been found to be strongly related to the absence of neuroticism in the spouses, it is appropriate to investigate the possibility of psychopathology in either or both of the individuals if, despite careful assessment and appropriate therapeutic intervention, no appreciable changes in intimacy occur. If the psychopathology is mild, short-term psychotherapy may prove to be efficacious. When there is evidence of psychosis or severe depression, a referral for psychiatric evaluation and possible chemotherapeutic support is appropriate.

F. When desirable changes to the dyadic relationship cannot occur for a variety of reasons, reassess the commitment to the relationship. In some cases separation and divorce may prove to be acceptable options. In other cases religious or ethical prohibitions may prevent spouses from parting. Then it becomes necessary to support the spouses to continue to offer what they can to each other while building alternative supports that will supply the recognition and satisfaction necessary to maintain self-esteem.

References

Frey J III, Holley J, L'Abate L. Intimacy is sharing hurt feelings: a comparison of three conflict resolution models. J Marr Fam Ther 1979; 5(2):35.

Johnson SM, Greenberg LS. Emotionally focused marital therapy: an overview. Psychotherapy: Theory, Research, Practice 1987; 24:552–560.

Shaeffer MT, Olson DH. Assessing intimacy: the PAIR inventory. J Marr Fam Ther 1981; 7(1):47–60

Waring EM, McElrath D, Lefcoe D, Weisz G. Dimensions of intimacy in marriage. Psychiatry 1981; 44:169–175.

Waring E, Patton D, Neron C, Linker W. Types of marital intimacy and prevalence of emotional illness. Can J Psychiatry 1986; 31:720–725.

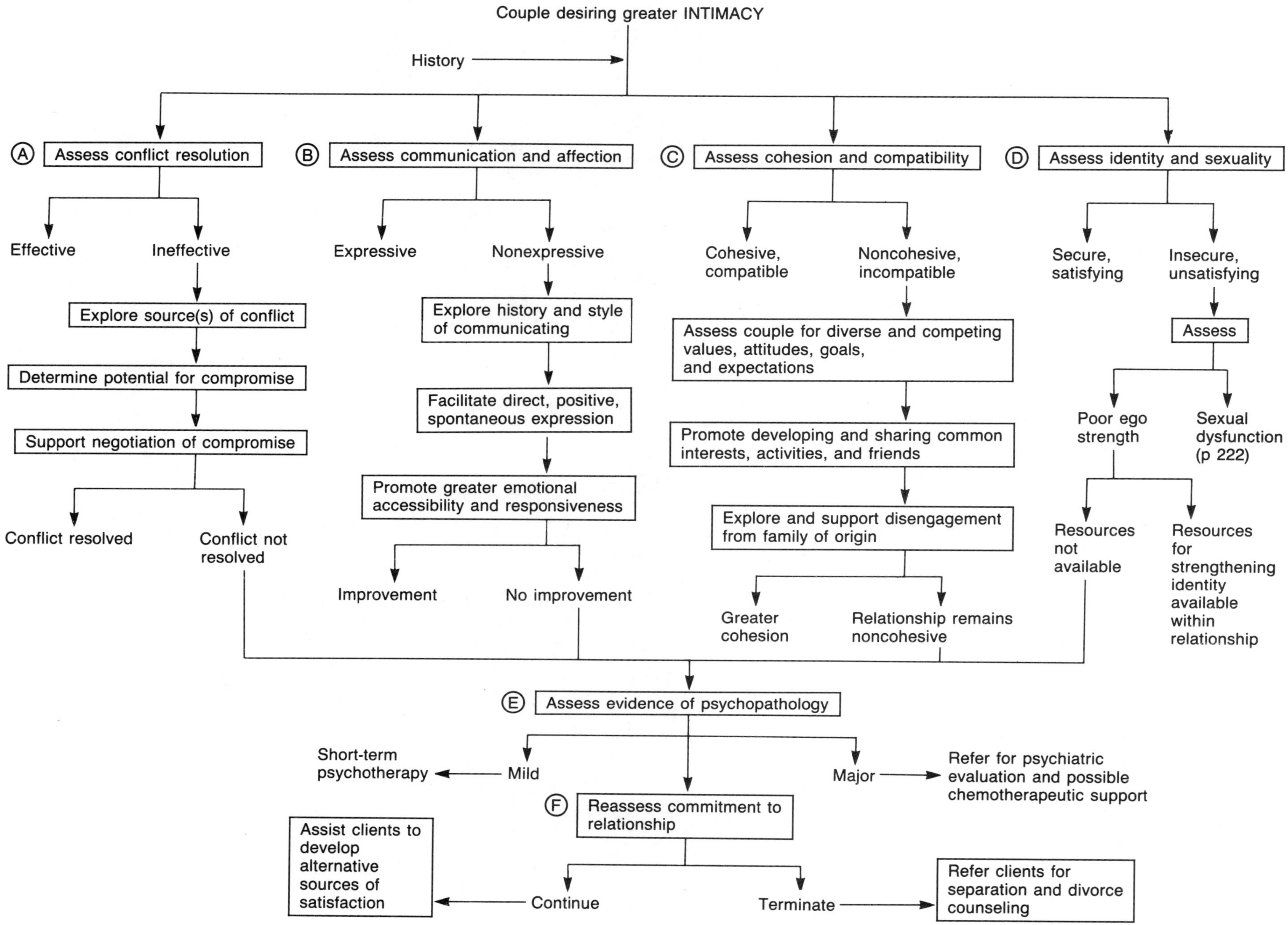
Couple desiring greater INTIMACY
History
A Assess conflict resolution
Effective
Ineffective
Explore source(s) of conflict
Determine potential for compromise
Support negotiation of compromise
Conflict resolved
Conflict not resolved
B Assess communication and affection
Expressive
Nonexpressive
Explore history and style of communicating
Facilitate direct, positive, spontaneous expression
Promote greater emotional accessibility and responsiveness
Improvement
No improvement
C Assess cohesion and compatibility
Cohesive, compatible
Noncohesive, incompatible
Assess couple for diverse and competing values, attitudes, goals, and expectations
Promote developing and sharing common interests, activities, and friends
Explore and support disengagement from family of origin
Greater cohesion
Relationship remains noncohesive
D Assess identity and sexuality
Secure, satisfying
Insecure, unsatisfying
Assess
Poor ego strength
Sexual dysfunction (p 222)
Resources not available
Resources for strengthening identity available within relationship
E Assess evidence of psychopathology
Short-term psychotherapy
Mild
Major
Refer for psychiatric evaluation and possible chemotherapeutic support
F Reassess commitment to relationship
Assist clients to develop alternative sources of satisfaction
Continue
Terminate
Refer clients for separation and divorce counseling

LOSS

M. Anne Wyness

Loss is an integral part of human experience. It may be defined as a state of being without something that has or could have had meaning for an individual or family. Loss has many meanings because each individual has a distinct life history of contact with loss and beliefs about loss that reflect that life experience.

A. Loss may occur because of maturational events or unpredictable events. Major loss frequently results from chance events such as traumatic injury or acute or chronic illness. The loss associated with growth and development is expected. Experiences with separation and loss are essential for the development of personal autonomy and a sense of mastery. These experiences influence responses to loss arising because of unpredictable events.

B. Unpredictable events can lead to several types of loss. Probably the most profound is loss of a loved or valued person, usually through death. Loss of a body part or function results in loss of some aspect of the physical self and frequently leads to other losses. Social role or status loss occurs when membership in a group that provides interpersonal satisfaction and consensual validation of beliefs and values is altered (e.g., loss of a job). Loss of possessions includes loss of valued external objects such as money or home.

C. Characteristics of loss are linked to the source and type of loss. Certain characteristics are common to all losses. Each individual processes loss in his own idiosyncratic way. Self-concept, the mental picture of one's identity, abilities, and worth that develops through and functions in relation with others, is threatened when loss occurs. This threat to self-concept helps determine the meaning the loss has for the individual. Every loss involves change, and one loss may cause additional or future losses. The loss may be sudden or insidious, temporary or permanent.

D. Grieving is the total response (thoughts, feelings, behaviors) to the emotional suffering caused by loss. Reactions to loss are exceedingly complex and are based on a number of internal and external factors. During the grieving process, basic patterns of response blend into and replace each other. It is important not to impose a particular model of grieving. Experiences should be explored with the individual and family to arrive at a common definition of the situation as it really exists. Loss through death has some unique aspects—the finality and inability to control death. Loss associated with chronic disease may result in a loss situation with no foreseeable closure or resolution.

E. Assessment of individual and family responses to loss is the basis for facilitating grief work. Because of the temporal dimensions of grieving, assessment should be an ongoing process. Each individual's response to loss and influencing factors such as age, sex, and personality should be assessed. Risk assessment to determine individuals and families who may have particular problems with grief work is important as is consideration of social and cultural factors.

F. Health professionals who work with individuals and families experiencing loss are vulnerable to their own feelings of loss and grief. These feelings must be recognized and positive coping enhanced through supportive collegial relationships.

G. Based on analysis of assessment data, nursing diagnoses are established and interventions are designed. The main objective is to help the individual and the family as a group to cope in productive ways with the losses and changes they are experiencing. Examples of approaches that may facilitate grief work, when used in the context of a therapeutic relationship, are provided.

H. Evaluation focuses on the outcomes of the grief work. The goals set by the individual and family and their success in achieving them should be considered. Ideally, grieving leads to growth through resolution of the loss or adaptation to it.

I. Complicated grief reactions such as chronic grief, delayed grief, and exaggerated grief require care by health professionals with particular expertise. Referral to the appropriate professional is the nurse's responsibility.

References

Benoliel JQ. Loss and adaptation: circumstances, contingencies and consequences. Death Stud 1985; 9:217–233.

Benoliel JQ. Loss and terminal illness. Nurs Clin North Am 1985; 20:439–449.

Bowlby J. Attachment and loss. Vol 3: Loss, sadness and depression. New York: Basic Books, 1980.

Martocchio BC. Grief and bereavement, healing through hurt. Nurs Clin North Am 1985; 20:327–341.

Werner-Beland JA. Grief responses to long-term illness and disability. Reston, VA: Reston Publishing, 1980.

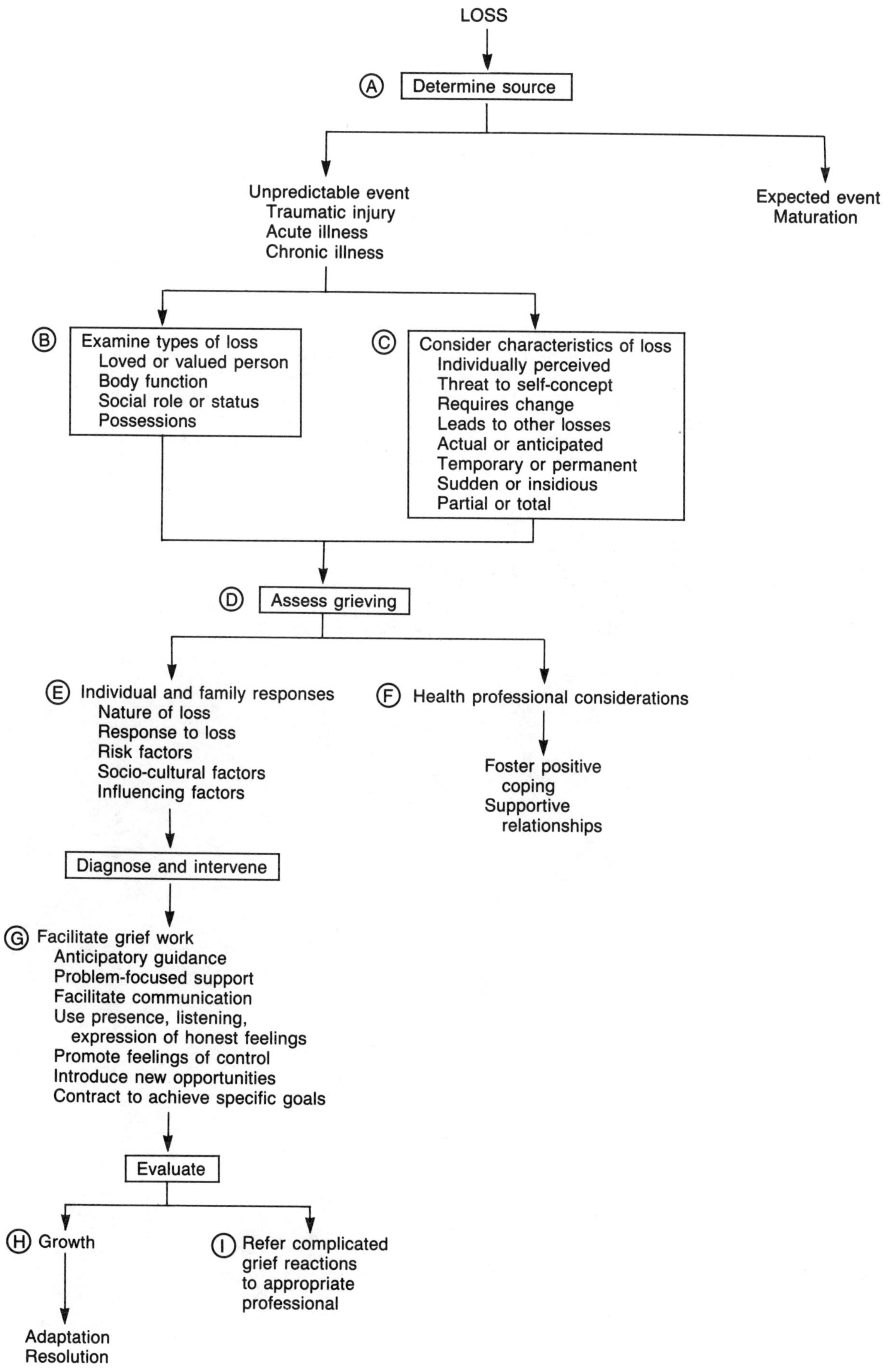
LOSS
(A) Determine source
Unpredictable event
Traumatic injury
Acute illness
Chronic illness
Expected event
Maturation
(B) Examine types of loss
Loved or valued person
Body function
Social role or status
Possessions
(C) Consider characteristics of loss
Individually perceived
Threat to self-concept
Requires change
Leads to other losses
Actual or anticipated
Temporary or permanent
Sudden or insidious
Partial or total
(D) Assess grieving
(E) Individual and family responses
Nature of loss
Response to loss
Risk factors
Socio-cultural factors
Influencing factors
(F) Health professional considerations
Foster positive coping
Supportive relationships
Diagnose and intervene
(G) Facilitate grief work
Anticipatory guidance
Problem-focused support
Facilitate communication
Use presence, listening, expression of honest feelings
Promote feelings of control
Introduce new opportunities
Contract to achieve specific goals
Evaluate
(H) Growth
Adaptation
Resolution
(I) Refer complicated grief reactions to appropriate professional

ALTERED BODY IMAGE

Deborah Antai-Otong

A. Clients experiencing significant physical losses or changes in body function exhibit some degree of altered body image. The nurse plays a key role in assisting clients through this difficult period. Provide an accepting and caring atmosphere that allows the client to express feelings and assist them to understand their meaning. Ventilation allows the client and family members to deal with these changes and develop coping skills. Reassure the client and family members that their feelings are normal. Frequently clients and family members gauge their reactions to their physical changes by those of the nurse. During the initial history taking interview, be aware of facial expressions and body language that might be interpreted by the client as a negative reaction. Clients and family members are sensitive to negative reactions in the nursing staff. These negative reactions can in turn reinforce the client's already altered body image. The history must include past and present medical treatment, psychiatric history, and current medications. Determine whether there have been recent physical changes and/or losses and explore the client's perception of them. Identify the client's support systems, coping patterns, and problem-solving skills. Assess current mental status and observe the client for signs and symptoms of major depression (p 46) and suicide risk (p 42). During the assessment, reinforce adaptive behaviors and mobilize the client's resources and support system.

B. Sometimes in spite of support from nurses and family members, clients may develop maladaptive coping patterns and behavior. Manifestations of maladaptive reactions include social isolation and exaggerated negative self-image. Continue to assess the client for symptoms of major depression and suicide risk periodically.

C. Increasing the client's support system and resources is essential when clients choose to isolate themselves. Family members and significant others must be actively involved in treatment. The nurse and other community resources must be used to facilitate a supportive environment. For further discussion on support groups, see "Support and Life Skills Groups" (p 138).

References

Beck AT, Rush AJ, Shaw BF, et al. Cognitive therapy of depression. New York: Guilford Press, 1979.

Harris M. Helping the person with an altered self-image. Geriatr Nurs 1986; 7:90–92.

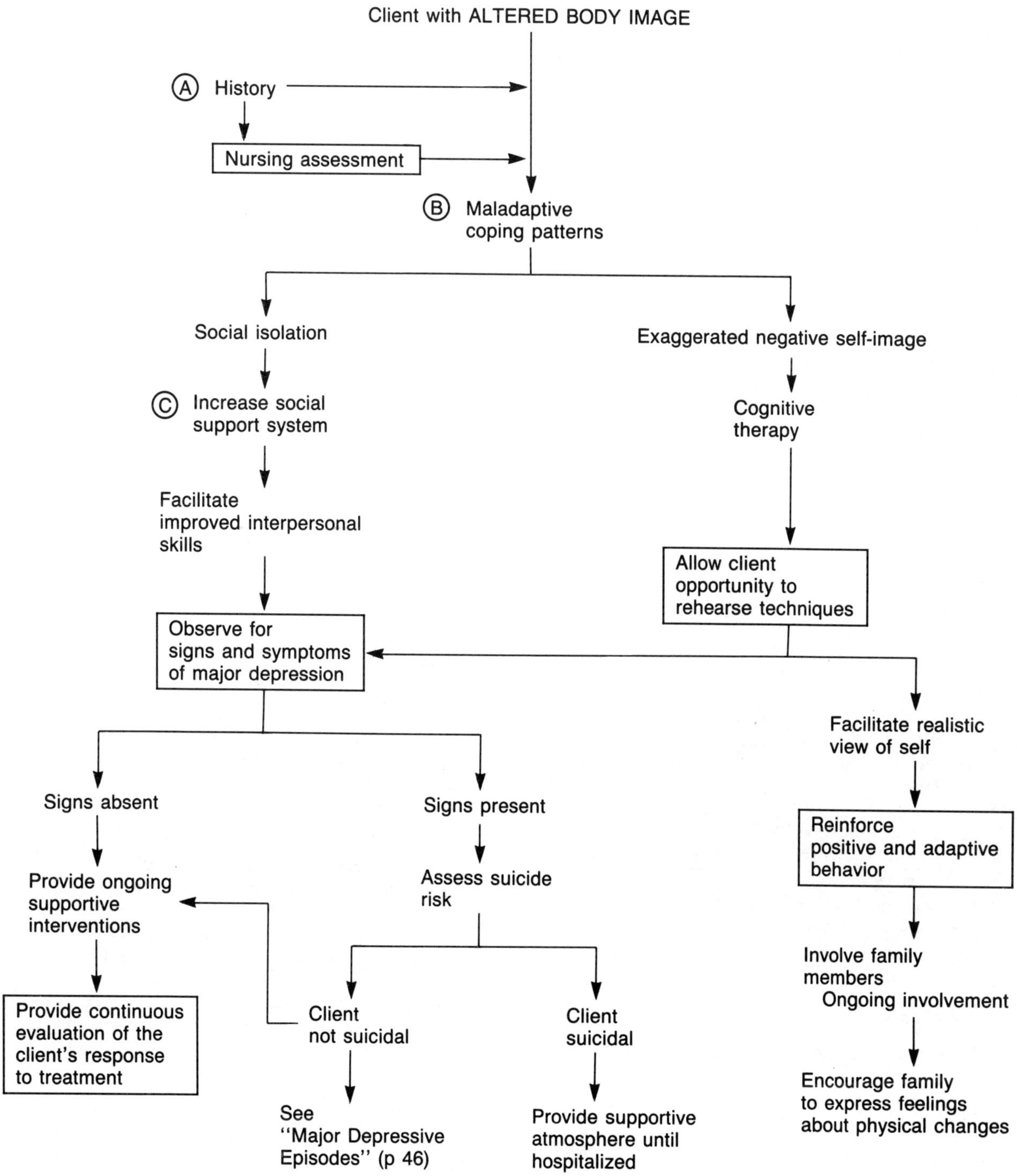
Client with ALTERED BODY IMAGE
Ⓐ History
Nursing assessment
Ⓑ Maladaptive coping patterns
Social isolation
Exaggerated negative self-image
Ⓒ Increase social support system
Cognitive therapy
Facilitate improved interpersonal skills
Allow client opportunity to rehearse techniques
Observe for signs and symptoms of major depression
Facilitate realistic view of self
Signs absent
Signs present
Reinforce positive and adaptive behavior
Provide ongoing supportive interventions
Assess suicide risk
Involve family members
Ongoing involvement
Provide continuous evaluation of the client's response to treatment
Client not suicidal
Client suicidal
Encourage family to express feelings about physical changes
See "Major Depressive Episodes" (p 46)
Provide supportive atmosphere until hospitalized

STRESS

Guirosebegum N. Jiwani

Stress is a hypothetical abstraction that possesses no independent existence and can be identified only when changes in the individual are manifested. Stress results from a demand to change or adapt, a perceived threat, a challenge to one's ability to cope or perform, or unmet needs or lack of available resources. If persistent and intense, stress has the potential for reducing the person's level of health, including causing sudden death. Factors influencing the stress response include: (1) nature of stressor—type, intensity, scope, and meaning of the stressor for the individual; (2) duration of exposure to stressor—longer duration requires greater energy expenditures; (3) number of stressors—timing and clustering of events simultaneously make it more difficult to deal favorably with the events; and (4) limitations of the system—genetic uniqueness including previous experience with comparable stressors affect the stress response.

A. Certain balancing factors that affect the return to equilibrium are perception of the event, available coping mechanisms, and situational supports.

B. If the event is not perceived as a threat and no subjective discomfort results, the goal must be health promotion and prevention of stress-related illnesses. Prevention strategies are aimed at (1) identifying high-risk individuals, (2) creating and increasing availability of support systems and community resources that enhance individual independence and autonomy, (3) hot lines for people under acute stress (e.g., suicide, child abuse prevention), and (4) public education and steps to reduce risks of abuse and violence. Health promotion strategies include health education and counseling, stress appraisal and management programs that are multidimensional in nature, allowing for individual choice, anticipatory planning, and wellness programs. Successful participation in any health promotion or prevention program requires rapport with the client, client receptivity and motivation, and the client's expectation of perceived benefits.

C. The intensity of the stress experience is determined by the degree of perceived threat in terms of controllability, responsibility, uniqueness, and how well the person feels he or she can deal with the identified danger. Frain and Valiga defined four levels of stress to assist nurses in their assessment of clients experiencing stress.

D. As anxiety increases, the person becomes more immobilized, and a sense of disequilibrium or crisis results. The client may not connect the stressful event to the actual crisis situation. Crisis intervention as a short-term modality focuses on the healthy resolution of the immediate issue through the mobilization of social, environmental, and intrapersonal resources, with the return to at least precrisis functioning. It is important to establish structure and develop a client contract that facilitates crisis resolution (see "Crisis State," p 8, and "Decision Making During a Crisis State," p 10). The nurse communicates sensitivity and uses sound therapeutic communication skills. The client's sense of self-worth and personal strength is affirmed. The nurse assists the client in gaining understanding of the relationship between the crisis and the event(s) in his or her life and fosters realistic perception of the event(s). The nurse needs to be aware of his or her personal strengths and limitations and assist the client in mobilizing support systems and community resources appropriately.

E. Inadequate resolution of crisis results in chronic stress for the individual. Continued or chronic stress imposes great demands on the person's physiologic and psychological integrity. Assessing the severity of impact of the stress on the client is critical. Prompt assessment of the symptom level including appropriate treatment may reduce the level of decompensation resulting from stress.

F. Inpatient care is indicated when the symptom level is high. The decision to seek hospitalization for the client comes when his or her personal resources are exhausted and he or she is deemed incapable of self-care. Hospitalization also occurs if there is need for security and protection of the client (e.g., client with suicidal or homicidal tendencies). Psychiatric disorders such as anxiety disorders, mood disorders, somatoform disorders, psychosis, substance abuse, including delayed grief reactions and severe character pathology and/or decompensation, require multifaceted treatment and specific nursing interventions. Individual therapy may be long and intensive; in addition, self-help or professionally led support groups, including family therapy, may be necessitated.

G. If the high symptom level persists, long-term inpatient care and further referral may be warranted. If symptoms are relieved considerably, careful discharge planning to facilitate community readjustment is done. Linkages to outpatient services for follow-up care and other community supports are established to help the client maintain optimal health.

References

Aguilera DC, Messick J. Crisis intervention: theory and methodology. 4th ed. St. Louis: CV Mosby, 1982.

Caplan G. Principles of preventive psychiatry. New York: Basic Books, 1964.

Cook JS, Fontaine KL. Essentials of mental health nursing. Redwood City, CA: Addison-Wesley, 1987.

Frain M, Valiga TM. The multiple dimensions of stress. Top Clin Nurs 1979; 1(1):43–52.

Pasquali EA, Arnold HM, DeBasio N, Alesi EG. Mental health nursing: a holistic approach. 2nd ed. St. Louis: CV Mosby, 1985.

Sutterley DC. Stress and health: a survey of self-regulation modalities. Top Clin Nurs 1979; 1(1):1–21.

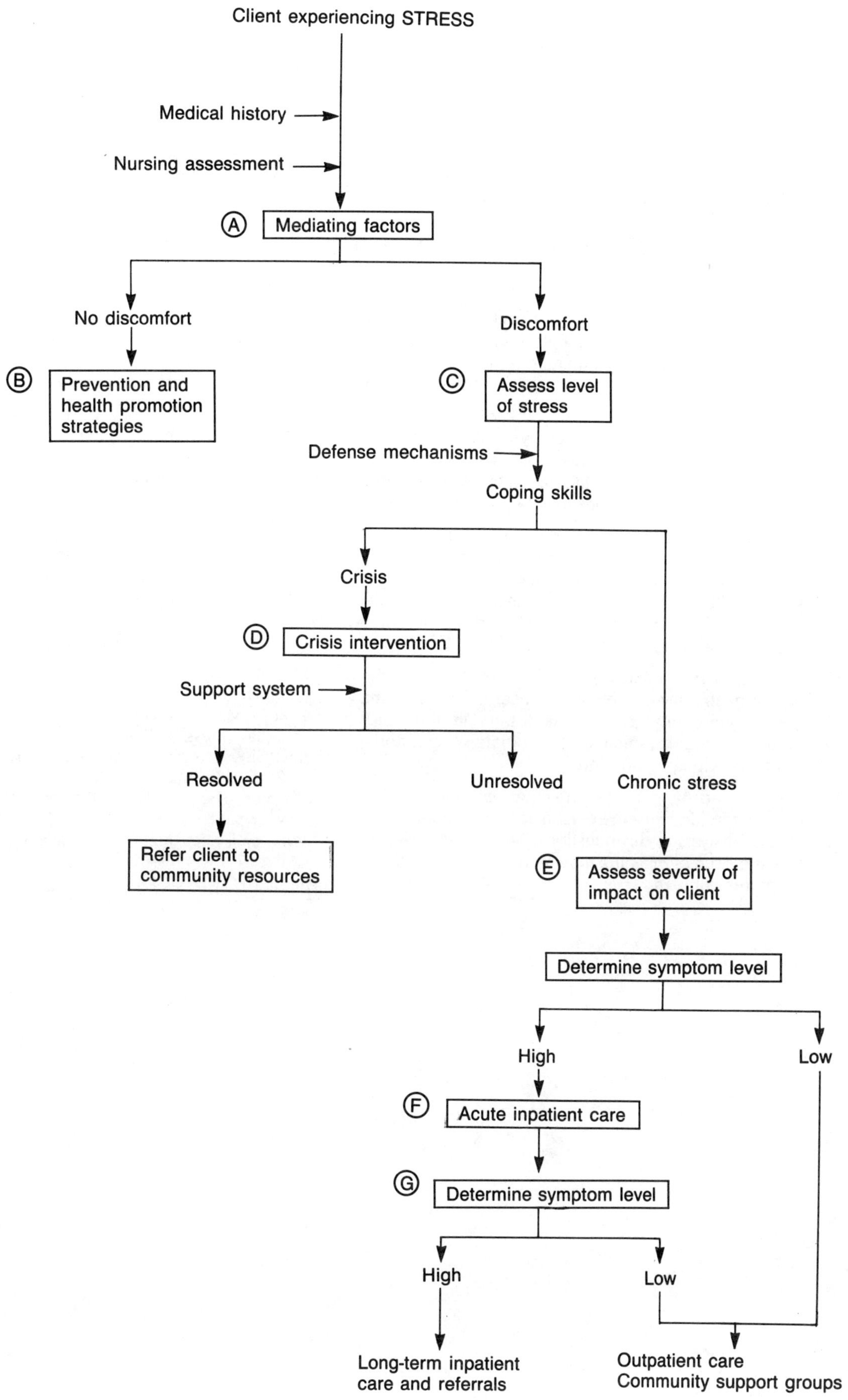
Client experiencing STRESS
Medical history
Nursing assessment
(A) Mediating factors
No discomfort
Discomfort
(B) Prevention and health promotion strategies
(C) Assess level of stress
Defense mechanisms
Coping skills
Crisis
(D) Crisis intervention
Support system
Resolved
Unresolved
Chronic stress
Refer client to community resources
(E) Assess severity of impact on client
Determine symptom level
High
Low
(F) Acute inpatient care
(G) Determine symptom level
High
Low
Long-term inpatient care and referrals
Outpatient care
Community support groups

SPIRITUAL DISTRESS

Viola Duff

Spiritual distress is the state in which the individual experiences or is at risk of experiencing a disturbance in the belief or value system that provides strength, hope, and meaning to life. It pervades a person's entire being and integrates and transcends the biological and psychosocial nature.

A. The assessment of spiritual distress must include both subjective and objective aspects. The client may express anxiety, guilt, doubt, or meaninglessness. Objective data may include refusal of treatment, questioning regarding beliefs or values, or excessive seeking of advice or support for decisions.

B. The nurse must assess his or her own abilities and comfort level to assist with spiritual distress. If this is not his or her area of expertise, collaboration or referral to other nurses or a religious leader may be necessary.

C. Spiritual distress may be related to the inability to practice spiritual rituals. The nurse can assist in eliminating or reducing the contributing factors and encourage spiritual rituals not detrimental to health. For example, a bed may be moved or an area cleared for the client to face ritual directions for prayer.

D. Spiritual distress related to the crises of illness, suffering, or death may create major concerns for the client. Three main components of this distress are the needs for the sense of meaning, a sense of forgiveness, and a sense of belonging and love.

E. "Why is this happening to me?" An existing sense of meaning in life helps the person answer or tolerate the lack of answers to this question. Denial and refusal to face the issue of meaning may require assistance to address this concern.

F. "What did I do to deserve this?" The means of forgiveness is essential in dealing with one's shortcomings. No one lives up to all moral principles. Acceptance of imperfections allows forgiveness from self and others. Expressions of guilt may begin reflection and exploration of avenues of forgiveness.

G. "Why do I feel so alone?" A source of love and relatedness is the resource to be used when this inevitable question arises. The nurse must listen for existing sources and promote recollections of reliance on these.

H. Spiritual distress may be related to conflict between religious or spiritual beliefs and the prescribed health regimen. Resolution may occur with adequate information. If true conflict arises and a compromise cannot be found, informed decision will need to be made by the client.

I. Whether religious philosophy is clearly articulated or is being sought during illness, spiritual help must be based on the client's search for meaning.

References

Carpenito L. Nursing diagnosis: application to clinical practice. Philadelphia: JB Lippincott, 1987:580–592.

Frankl V. Man's search for meaning. New York: Washington Square Press, 1971.

Hubert Sister M. Spiritual care for every patient. J Nurs Educ 1963; 2:115–118.

Peterson E. The physical . . . the spiritual . . . can you meet all your patient's needs? J Gerontol Nurs 1985; 11(1):23–27.

Pumphrey J. Recognizing your patients' spiritual needs. Nursing 77 1977; 64–69.

Ryan J. The neglected crisis. Am J Nurs 1984; 1257–1258.

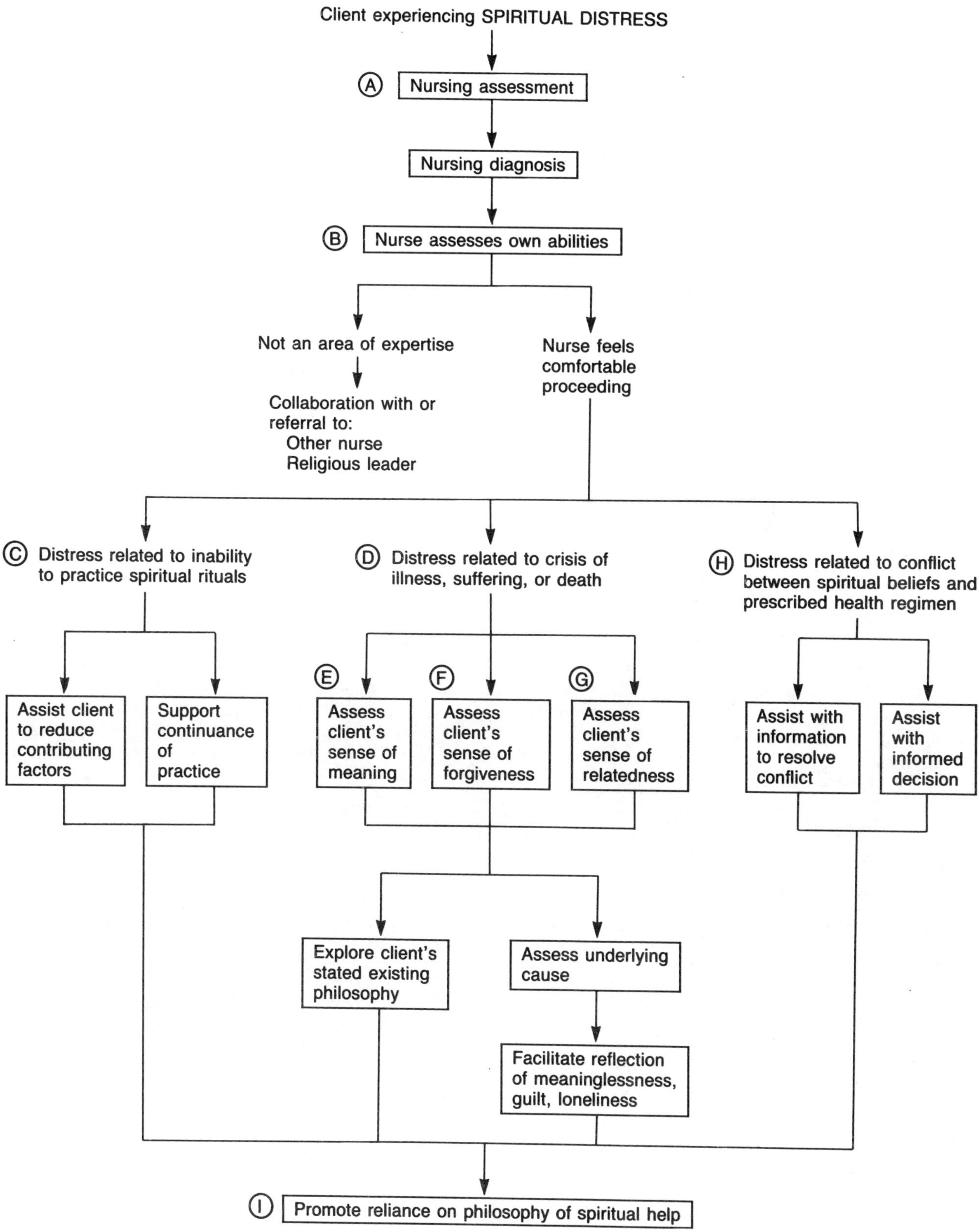

Client experiencing SPIRITUAL DISTRESS
(A) Nursing assessment
Nursing diagnosis
(B) Nurse assesses own abilities
Not an area of expertise
Collaboration with or referral to: Other nurse Religious leader
Nurse feels comfortable proceeding
(C) Distress related to inability to practice spiritual rituals
(D) Distress related to crisis of illness, suffering, or death
(H) Distress related to conflict between spiritual beliefs and prescribed health regimen
Assist client to reduce contributing factors
Support continuance of practice
(E) Assess client's sense of meaning
(F) Assess client's sense of forgiveness
(G) Assess client's sense of relatedness
Assist with information to resolve conflict
Assist with informed decision
Explore client's stated existing philosophy
Assess underlying cause
Facilitate reflection of meaninglessness, guilt, loneliness
(I) Promote reliance on philosophy of spiritual help

NORMALIZATION

Marilyn E. Dewis

Normalization can be defined as all behavioral attempts to live as normally as possible despite the signs and symptoms of chronic illness or disability (see "Chronic Illness," p 212). When normalizing, the individual suppresses the "physiologic imperative" and proceeds with the "activity imperative" as normal. The person with long-term illness strives to reaffirm the personal self, to be as capable as his or her peers, to reduce feelings of being different, and to achieve maximal integration into society.

A. Many disabilities and chronic illnesses render a person stigmatized. The presence of visible symptoms or treatment modalities can result in reactions of avoidance or excessive solicitation. When the symptoms of illness or disability are intrusive, the individual can experience "identity spread," i.e., the assumption by others that he or she is totally incapable of working, acting, or being like other people. This stigma tends to dominate social interactions unless the affected person uses tactics to normalize the situation.

B. The principal strategies employed in normalization are covering up, keeping up, and pacing. Covering up means concealing or minimizing disability and/or symptoms such as pain or fatigue and is an important part of the behavioral repertoire. A deformity may be covered with clothes, or a trembling hand may be held under the table during conversation. It is not a denial of the disease, but rather a rejection by the individual of the handicap as his total identity and as a determinant of social interaction. Keeping up refers to the deliberate and successful carrying out of a planned activity, while covering up, expending increased energy, and perhaps causing exacerbation of symptoms. Pacing refers to balancing the activities of covering up and keeping up with rest so as to avoid periods of immobilization that would be needed to restore energy used in covering up and keeping up. Pacing results from the individual's understanding limitations and abilities and appropriately engaging in activities over a time span that satisfies normative needs without causing undue exhaustion.

C. If effective normalizing does not occur or strategies fail, the individual encounters difficulty in keeping control of interactions. This occurs most frequently when visible symptoms are frightening or repulsive to others, as in movement disorders or facial disfigurement. The result is almost total withdrawal from ordinary interaction, living in the company of others like oneself, or limiting interaction to close family or friends.

D. Normalization implies that through "normal" or valued interaction and positive interpretation, both structures of the individual's environment, the devalued individual becomes more valued in terms of cultural norms. Addressing and referring to individuals in a valued manner (rather than with labels) creates a positive interpretation and a culturally normative image. Successful normalizing strategies can be fostered and encouraged. When covering up is temporarily impossible because of exacerbation of symptoms, the individual can be assisted to justify inaction. Social skills training programs can promote normalization by developing social competence through modeling, role playing (p 126), and social reinforcement, and peer feedback.

E. Strategies aimed at promoting normalization include fostering the individual's attempts to maintain an attractive and socially appropriate appearance. Clothing and grooming can help to divert attention from the disability. Rehabilitative aids such as wheelchairs and braces attract attention to the disability and may increase feelings of stigma. These devices can often be individualized and made less obtrusive. Disabled peers can share inventive strategies for covering up. Family members and friends can be taught to provide appropriate assistance in maintaining a pleasing appearance.

References

Dewis ME. Spinal cord injured adolescents and young adults. The meaning of body changes. J Adv Nurs 1989 (in press).

Miller JS. Chronic illness: overcoming powerlessness. Philadelphia: FA Davis, 1983.

Nelson AL. Normalization: the key to integrating the SCI patient into the community. SCI Nurs 1987; 4(1):3–6.

Strauss AL. Chronic illness and the quality of life. St. Louis: CV Mosby, 1984.

Weiner CL. The burden of rheumatoid arthritis: tolerating the uncertainty. Soc Sci Med 1975; 9:97–104.

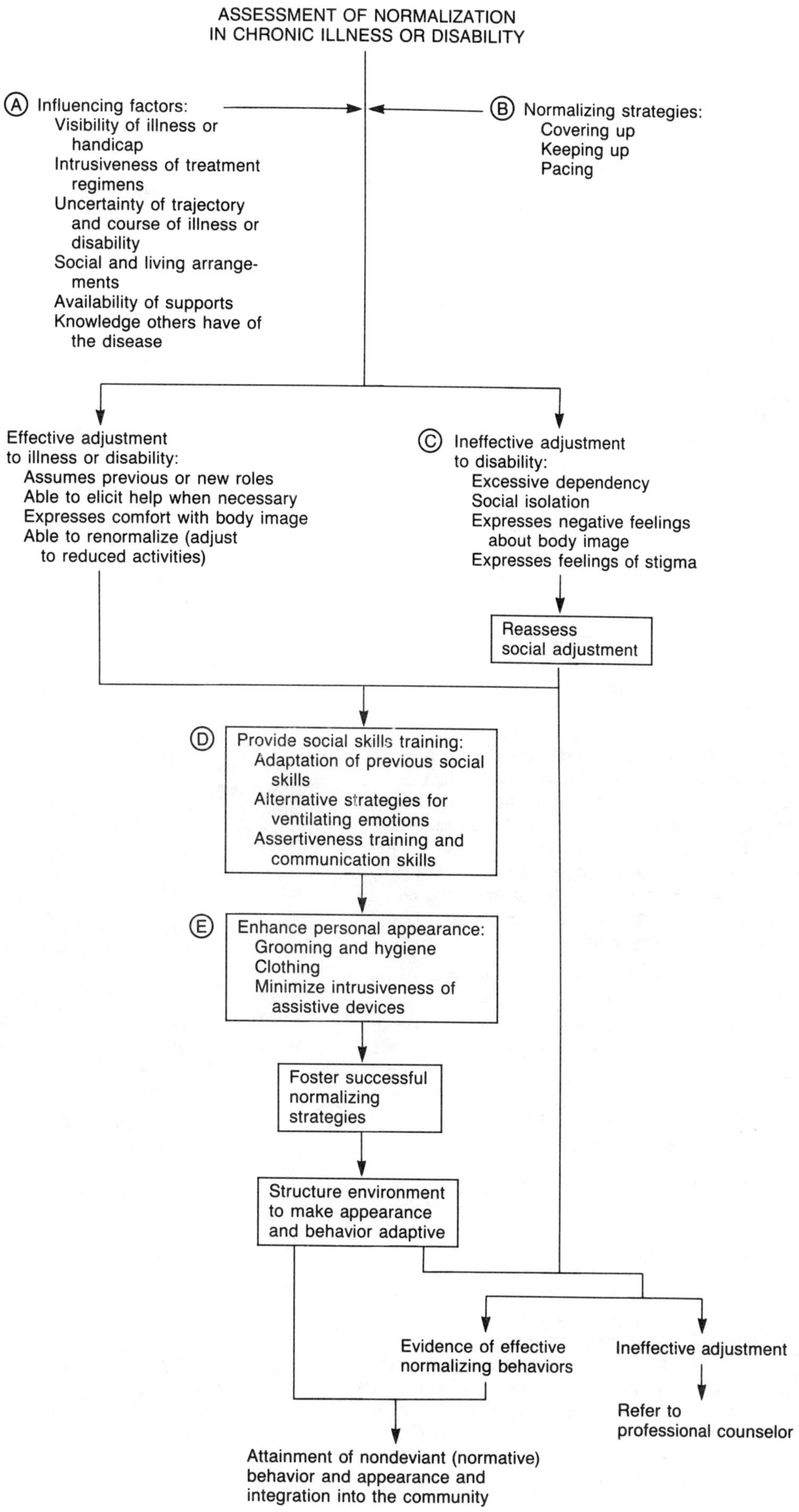
ASSESSMENT OF NORMALIZATION IN CHRONIC ILLNESS OR DISABILITY
(A) Influencing factors: Visibility of illness or handicap; Intrusiveness of treatment regimens; Uncertainty of trajectory and course of illness or disability; Social and living arrangements; Availability of supports; Knowledge others have of the disease
(B) Normalizing strategies: Covering up; Keeping up; Pacing
Effective adjustment to illness or disability: Assumes previous or new roles; Able to elicit help when necessary; Expresses comfort with body image; Able to renormalize (adjust to reduced activities)
(C) Ineffective adjustment to disability: Excessive dependency; Social isolation; Expresses negative feelings about body image; Expresses feelings of stigma
Reassess social adjustment
(D) Provide social skills training: Adaptation of previous social skills; Alternative strategies for ventilating emotions; Assertiveness training and communication skills
(E) Enhance personal appearance: Grooming and hygiene; Clothing; Minimize intrusiveness of assistive devices
Foster successful normalizing strategies
Structure environment to make appearance and behavior adaptive
Evidence of effective normalizing behaviors
Ineffective adjustment
Refer to professional counselor
Attainment of nondeviant (normative) behavior and appearance and integration into the community

NONCOMPLIANCE

Nancy E. Johnston

It has been estimated that of all clients visiting health professionals, 97 percent will receive a diagnosis and related advice pertaining to the eradication or amelioration of the reported symptoms. Despite normative expectations that clients will follow medical advice, the majority fail to follow the recommendations that have been offered. Enabling well people to utilize appropriate mental health measures and encouraging people with addictions, mental illnesses, or other conditions to accept and follow health advice is a significant nursing challenge.

A. Facilitating compliance involves the assessment of contributing factors and the implementation of interventions to promote: awareness of potential and actual disease processes and the health recommendations pertaining thereto (level I); acceptance of the medical regimen or acceptance of the need to effect life-style changes in order to prevent illness and promote recovery (level II); and adjustment to the arduous process of developing new health habits and appropriate health-seeking behaviors (level III).

B. The client's perceived vulnerability to stress and/or mental illness can be related to the willingness to accept health advice. Vulnerability can be conceptualized to include three constituent dimensions: (1) susceptibility, the individual's estimated probability of encountering a specific health threat; (2) severity, the client's perception of the pain and suffering involved; and (3) seriousness, the degree of disablement, life-threat, or stigma likely to result from the disease process. Under ideal conditions of compliance facilitation, the nurse enables the client to be sufficiently anxious yet not overwhelmed by the disease threat. By achieving this balance, the client is encouraged to develop an attitude of cautious hopefulness rather than paralyzing futility.

C. A subsequent step in motivating the client to take recommended action requires that the nurse thoroughly investigate the client's awareness of specific health risks or disease processes. If knowledge is deficient, evaluate the client's readiness to learn. Deploy strategies to overcome anxiety and denial and engender hope if resistance to learning is encountered. Tailor teaching to fit with the client's cognitive abilities and cultural expectations.

D. Although individuals may be well aware of disease risks and medical protocols, compliance is unlikely to occur unless the recommended regimens are acceptable to the client. The nurse gently explores the extent to which the proposed protocol poses a threat to the individual's body image, life-style or autonomy. Enabling the client to maintain a sense of dignity and personal worth while acknowledging the need for limitations and restrictions requires the nurse to convey a deep level of sensitivity, warmth, and faith in the client's ability to successfully confront these issues. Frequently the acceptability of medical regimens is diminished by the disinclination of clients to continue with medications or treatments that cause disagreeable side-effects. Early discontinuance of antipsychotic medication is the major cause of recidivism in the mental health care field. Nurses play a major role in educating clients regarding strategies and options for controlling side-effects, thus rendering the treatment process more acceptable.

E. Research has demonstrated that when clients consider the payoff of compliance to be worthwhile, compliance improves. Frequently clients have difficulty retaining a vision of the long-term gains, especially when daily adherence is so difficult. Structure the therapy to provide opportunity for frequent reflection on the long-term benefits of compliance. This may be accomplished in one-to-one sessions, but is frequently more effective in group self-help sessions. Here clients themselves can provide reinforcement in the form of encouragement and testimonials.

F. Accessibility and ongoing adherence to prescribed protocols may be facilitated by reducing waiting times, providing transportation, or taking the treatment to the client (home-visits). Strategies such as the use of written and verbal instructions, appointment cards, telephone reminders, and special pill containers divided into slots corresponding to the day of the week and equipped with signal alarms have shown some promising results. The use of prompts such as instructions and pictures on refrigerator doors and mirrors have also been shown to be beneficial.

G. Maintaining high compliance with long-term treatments is difficult and unlikely to be achieved without the active involvement of health professionals in providing opportunity for reinforcement of desired behaviors. Since nurses are frequently limited in their ability to support compliant behavior in its natural setting, soliciting additional support from the family is desirable. Group discussions that focus on self-help monitoring and even self-selection of medications from a standardized protocol are other ways of developing social support while minimizing unhealthy dependence. The nurse cultivates a climate that supports the client's self-view as active participant. The use of Swain and Steckel's contingency contracting as well as relapse road-maps are additional techniques that enable the client to exercise personal control in the treatment or therapy process.

References

Becker H, ed. The health belief model and personal health behavior. Thorofare, NJ: Charles B Slack, 1974.

Carpenito L. Nursing diagnosis: application to clinical practice. New York: JB Lippincott, 1983:278–286.

Haynes R, Taylor D, Sackett D. Compliance in health care. Baltimore: Johns Hopkins Press, 1979.

Kluger M, Karras A. Strategies for reducing missed initial appointments in a community mental health center. Commun Ment Health J 1983; 19:137–143.

Rees DW. Changing patient's health beliefs to improve compliance with alcoholism treatment, controlled trial. J Stud Alcohol 1986; 47:436–439.

Steckel S, Swain M. Contracting with patients to improve compliance. Hospitals 1977; 51:81.

Stuart RB, ed. Adherence compliance and generalization in behavioral medicine. New York: Brunner/Mazel, 1982.

Withersty DF, ed. Communication and compliance in a hospital setting. Springfield, IL: Charles C Thomas, 1980.

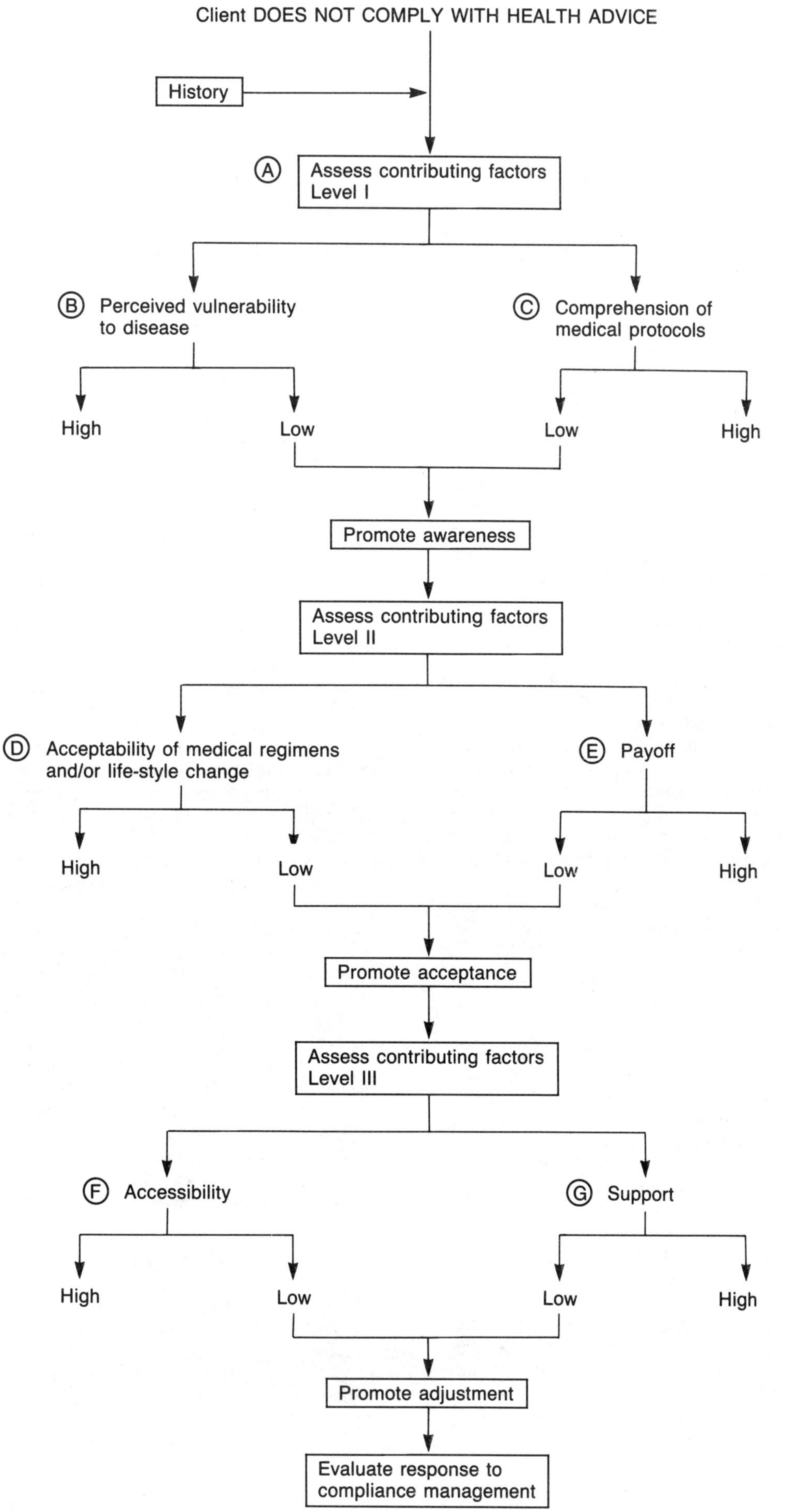
Client DOES NOT COMPLY WITH HEALTH ADVICE
History
Ⓐ Assess contributing factors Level I
Ⓑ Perceived vulnerability to disease
Ⓒ Comprehension of medical protocols
High
Low
Low
High
Promote awareness
Assess contributing factors Level II
Ⓓ Acceptability of medical regimens and/or life-style change
Ⓔ Payoff
High
Low
Low
High
Promote acceptance
Assess contributing factors Level III
Ⓕ Accessibility
Ⓖ Support
High
Low
Low
High
Promote adjustment
Evaluate response to compliance management

CHRONIC PAIN

Frances Fothergill-Bourbonnais

A. Many clients in psychiatric settings complain of pain. The assessment of any client's complaint of pain should include precipitating factors, time factors, and the factors that help and do not help to decrease the pain. The location of the pain is crucial information as well as the client's description of the intensity and severity of the pain. The tendency to presume that the client's initial complaint of pain or pain on admission has not changed can result in missed or delayed medical treatment of acute situations such as chest pain. Acute pain is self-limiting (<6 months) and tends to disappear once the cause of the pain has been removed. Chronic pain is pain that has lasted more than 6 months, occurs frequently and in some cases continuously, and has not responded to appropriate medical treatment. The most common problems clients seek help for are low back pain, neck or shoulder pain, and headaches. For some clients with chronic pain there is a clearly diagnosable cause such as arthritis or nerve damage due to injury. In other situations the origin of the pain cannot be found. Both situations can present a pain problem for which a satisfactory or lasting treatment does not exist.

B. If through assessment the nurse discovers that the pain is different from pain the client has previously experienced, further investigation is warranted to discover the cause. The client needs much reassurance from the nurse as he or she may believe some other problem is developing. Further investigations may be necessary in order to determine the source of this new pain. The nurse must explain specific tests and treatments to the patient and provide support at this time. Respect for the client's expression of pain is crucial. Different cultures, experiences, and values between patient and nurse can result in misconceptions and prejudices, which can interfere with accurate and adequate treatment.

C. Continuous pain with or without pathologic findings can consume the person and affect all aspects of his or her life. The client views the pain as endless, purposeless, and unavoidable. The pain and illness become the focus of the client's life. There are real losses associated with chronic pain such as loss of income or job, loss of physical abilities if there are physical limitations, loss of role in the family, marital discord, and loss of friends and other social contacts. These losses frequently result in depression. The patient feels alone—that no one understands what is happening to him or her. These patients have tried one unsuccessful treatment after another and have frequently taken multiple medications. When no definable physiologic causes can be found or it has been determined that emotional factors are contributing to and aggravating the pain experience, patients may get referred to psychiatric treatment setting or a pain clinic. Referral to a psychiatric treatment setting may be seen by the client as others telling him his pain is not real. The nurse must always remember that no pain is purely physical or purely emotional. All pain has the influence of past experience, anxiety, culture, and meaning of the illness. Acute pain has physiologic indicators resulting from sympathetic nervous system activation: increased pulse, sweating, and nausea. Patients with chronic pain do not demonstrate these physiologic signs, which is why they often do not "appear" to be in pain. However, chronic pain results in sleep disturbances, fatigue, and decreased appetite. Pain tools such as numerical rating scales whereby the client rates his pain from 0 to 10 are useful for acute pain. Chronic pain requires tools such as the McGill Pain Questionnaire that provide more detail of the pain and its impact on the person's life. It is questionable whether the continual use of charts is of value in persons with unresolved or intractable pain because they serve to remind the client of the problem. Pain may become a means of coping with intolerable problems (i.e., severe stress). For example, occasionally there is a relationship between work stress and pain. Factors the nurse could explore in this situation would be the patient's sense of powerlessness at work, inability to cope with work-related stress, and general job dissatisfaction. Therefore, it is important to listen to the emotions expressed while the client is talking about pain.

D. Because clients with chronic pain can present with complicated emotional and social problems, an holistic approach is required. The patient and health care team must work at goals that are realistic as to the degree of pain relief that is achievable and acceptable. Total pain relief may not be possible. Working with family members can facilitate their contribution to the client's recovery. Clients can be taught to block pain sensations by cognitive strategies including distraction, relaxation, guided imagery, biofeedback. Transcutaneous electrical nerve stimulation (TENS) has been used with some success in patients with headaches and low back pain. The nurse must convey confidence to the client that these strategies will help. Chronic pain without definable physiologic cause often responds to antidepressants and phenothiazines, which assist in decreasing the depression associated with chronic pain. The continual use of analgesics is much less effective, and clients can develop analgesic tolerance and dependence sometimes in conjunction with alcohol misuse. Referral to a pain clinic with its multidisciplinary staff and approach can be most beneficial for the client experiencing chronic pain.

References

Beck CK, Rawlins RP, Williams S. Mental health psychiatric nursing: a holistic life-cycle approach. St. Louis: CV Mosby, 1988.

Peck C. Controlling chronic pain. London: Fontana/Collins, 1985.

Walker VA, Dicks B, Webb P. Pain assessment charts in the management of chronic cancer pain. Palliative Med 1987; 1:111–116.

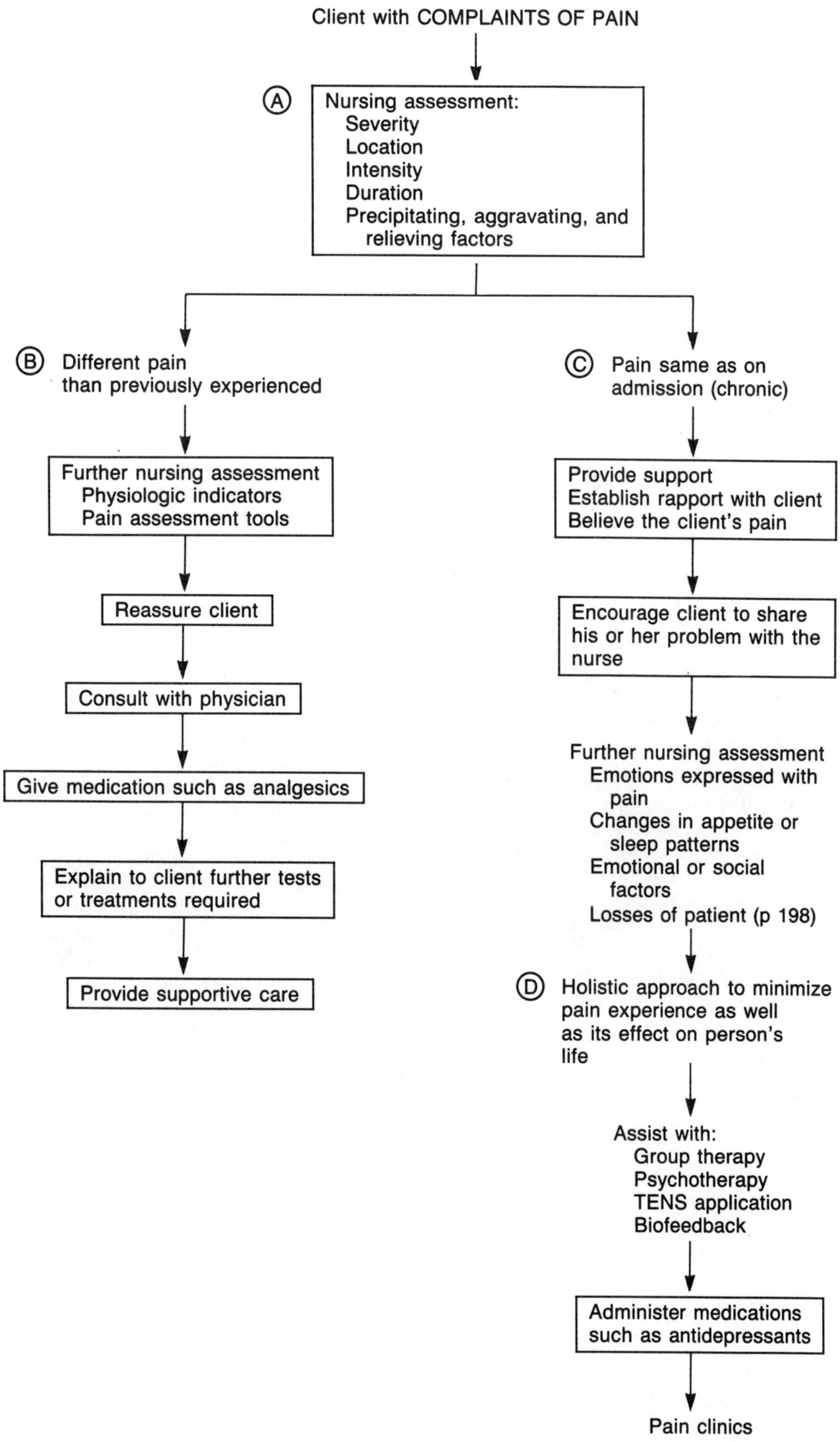
Client with COMPLAINTS OF PAIN
(A) Nursing assessment:
Severity
Location
Intensity
Duration
Precipitating, aggravating, and relieving factors
(B) Different pain than previously experienced
Further nursing assessment
Physiologic indicators
Pain assessment tools
Reassure client
Consult with physician
Give medication such as analgesics
Explain to client further tests or treatments required
Provide supportive care
(C) Pain same as on admission (chronic)
Provide support
Establish rapport with client
Believe the client's pain
Encourage client to share his or her problem with the nurse
Further nursing assessment
Emotions expressed with pain
Changes in appetite or sleep patterns
Emotional or social factors
Losses of patient (p 198)
(D) Holistic approach to minimize pain experience as well as its effect on person's life
Assist with:
Group therapy
Psychotherapy
TENS application
Biofeedback
Administer medications such as antidepressants
Pain clinics

CHRONIC ILLNESS

Roberta Ronayne

A. The onset or exacerbation of a chronic illness, whether mental or physical, almost always results in profound changes in personal identity and established patterns of living. A history of the illness provides information about the etiology of symptoms and facilitates planning immediate and long-term care. Information about symptoms, related to physical health, disturbances in thought, emotion and/or behavior, as well as the precipitating factors, illness pattern (exacerbation, remission), type of onset (insidious, sudden), treatment regimen, and compliance with therapies such as psychotherapy, pharmacotherapy, and group therapy are particularly important.

B. Nursing assessment should focus on identifying the client's perceptions of the illness situation. Perceptions may be influenced by (1) demographic and personal factors such as age, personality, values, beliefs, developmental phase, ego strength, and functional ability; (2) illness characteristics including type of illness, its meaning and stigma, level of knowledge about illness as well as complexity and effectiveness of treatment regimens; and (3) environmental variables such as social identity, socio-occupational status, availability and accessibility of support systems including health professionals, social networks, and financial assistance.

C. Chronically ill persons continuously assess their illness situation in order to control symptoms effectively. Control helps maintain one's personal identity. Loss of control results in loss of identity, increased tension, anxiety and uncertainty about illness, its duration, outcome and treatment. It also interferes with activities of daily living and ability to maintain social relationships. Clients experiencing loss of control tend to respond by either voluntarily or involuntarily relinquishing responsibility for self-care to others such as family and health professionals.

D. Adaptive tasks refer to complex challenges or issues that chronically ill clients must deal with daily in order to achieve and maintain control over the illness situation. Biologic adaptive tasks involve dealing with discomfort, incapacitation, and other symptoms associated with a specific illness. Psychological adaptive tasks involve preserving a reasonable emotional balance and a sense of control over decision making about one's life, preparing for an uncertain future, attaining a satisfactory self-image, and dealing with the hospital environment, treatment procedures, and diagnostic tests. Sociocultural tasks involve sustaining relationships with family and friends, developing and maintaining relationships with health-care professionals, adjusting to role change, and practicing preventive health care. The relative importance of a specific task may vary depending on the individual's appraisal of the illness situation.

E. The coping skills commonly used in chronic illness may be used individually or in various combinations. Skills that are effective in one situation may not be so in another, and those which are effective for a short period may be harmful if used excessively. Effective strategies enable clients to perceive a sense of control and to maintain personal integrity; ineffective strategies result in increased tension and loss of control. Appraisal-focused or cognitive strategies, such as anticipatory planning, avoidance, denial, and minimizing the seriousness of illness, enable clients to understand and find a pattern in illness. Problem-focused or behavior-oriented strategies, such as seeking information and support, learning specific self-care procedures, contracting, and compliance, enable clients to confront the reality of illness by dealing with its identifiable consequences and trying to develop a satisfying life-style. Emotion-focused strategies, such as anger, acting out, and maintaining a sense of hope, help clients to manage the emotions associated with illness and to maintain a sense of equilibrium.

F. Nursing interventions should maximize the client's strengths, potentials, and ability to manage illness effectively on a day-to-day basis and during crises. Continued support is needed until the client has learned and mastered more effective ways to handle the illness situation. Providing relevant information and feedback about illness, the small gains that have been made, and responsibility for self-care enables clients to gain control over their situation and to participate actively in decision making about health care. Promoting realistic expectations about illness involves assisting clients to identify healthy behaviors, to deal with the present, and to anticipate the future, rather than deal with the past. It also enables them to identify appropriate and helpful adaptive tasks. Focusing on care rather than cure and on strengths rather than weaknesses promotes development of the client's self-concept, increases self-esteem, and encourages development of independent living skills and interpersonal relationships. Promoting development of effective coping skills such as problem solving, involvement in self-care, and social interaction enables clients to regain a sense of mastery and helps preserve a sense of hope. It may also help clients avoid potential crises and facilitate planning activities to reduce or negate the impact of the crisis event (see "Crisis State," p 8).

G. The goal of intervention is to help clients achieve a quality of life that is compatible with their chronic illness. Continued monitoring and evaluation are essential in order to anticipate and avoid potential crises or exacerbations of illness.

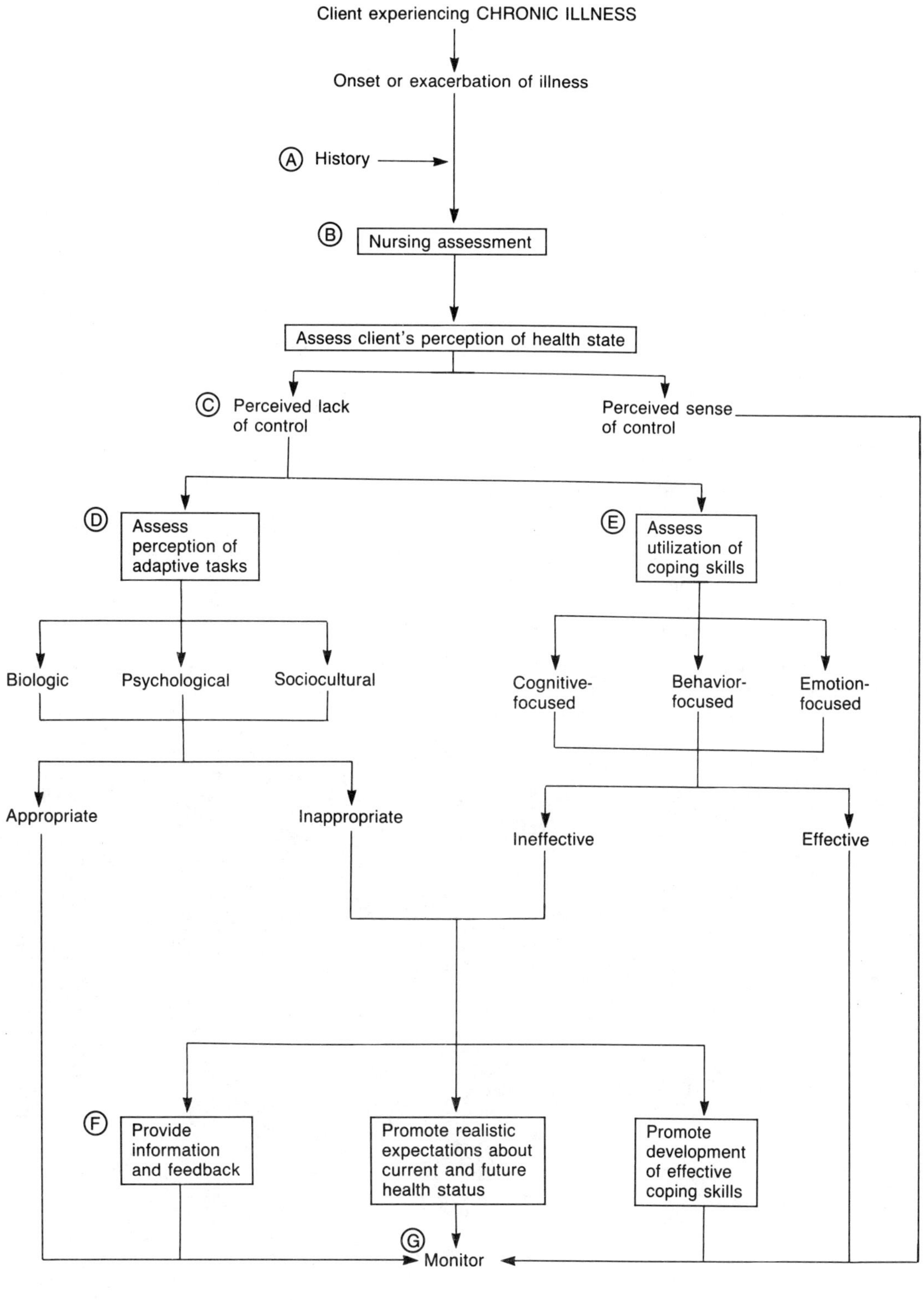

References

Bell RW. Care of the chronically mentally ill patient. In: Stuart GW, Sundeen SJ, eds. Principles and practice of psychiatric nursing. 3rd ed. St. Louis: CV Mosby, 1987:1011–1036.

Craig HM, Edwards JE. Adaptation in chronic illness: an eclectic model for nurses. J Adv Nurs 1983; 8:397–404.

Moos RH, Schaefer JA. The crisis of physical illness. In: Moos RH, ed. Coping with physical illness 2: new perspectives. New York: Plenum, 1984:3–25.

Munjas BA. Care of the chronically mentally ill: a continuing challenge to nursing. Iss Mental Health Nurs 1986; 8:203–212.

Strauss AL, Corbin J, Fagerhaugh S, Glaser BG, Mines D, Suczek B, Wiener CL. Chronic illness and the quality of life. 2nd ed. St. Louis: CV Mosby, 1984.

HOMELESSNESS

Deborah Antai-Otong

There are approximately 300,000 to 500,000 individuals classified as homeless in the United States. Factors that have contributed to this surge of homeless people include the uncertain national economy, cutbacks in local, state, and federal support, insufficient low-cost housing, unemployment, and the influx of psychiatric clients into the community over the past two decades, without adequate resources.

A. The nursing assessment includes assessing the client's physical, psychological, and sociological needs. Several studies of the homeless indicate a high prevalence of physical problems and substance abuse among this population. Many of them have chronic substance abuse problems, primarily alcoholism, with related chronic physical illness, i.e., heart and liver problems. Many of these clients are seriously ill, and the nurse must assess their symptoms and refer them to appropriate health-care centers. For further discussion of the nursing assessment, refer to chapters on depression (p 46), schizophrenia (pp 72–75), and substance abuse (pp 30–41).

B. Determine the availability of community resources through community meetings, resource centers, and agencies. The client's social support systems should be evaluated during this initial assessment and continuously assessed throughout contact.

C. Document clinical signs and symptoms of psychological distress and current and past psychiatric treatment. The literature suggests that large numbers of the homeless population have histories of schizophrenia, affective disorders, and substance abuse or dependence. Some of these individuals have dual diagnoses.

References

Bassak EL. The homeless problem. Sci Amer 1984; 241:40–45.

Koegel P, Burman A, Farr RK. The prevalence of specific psychiatric disorders among homeless individuals in the inner city of Los Angeles. Arch Gen Psychiatry 1988; 45:1085–1092.

Lipton FR, Sabitini A, Katz SE. Down and out in the city: the homeless mentally ill. Hosp Commun Psychiatry 1983; 34:817–821.

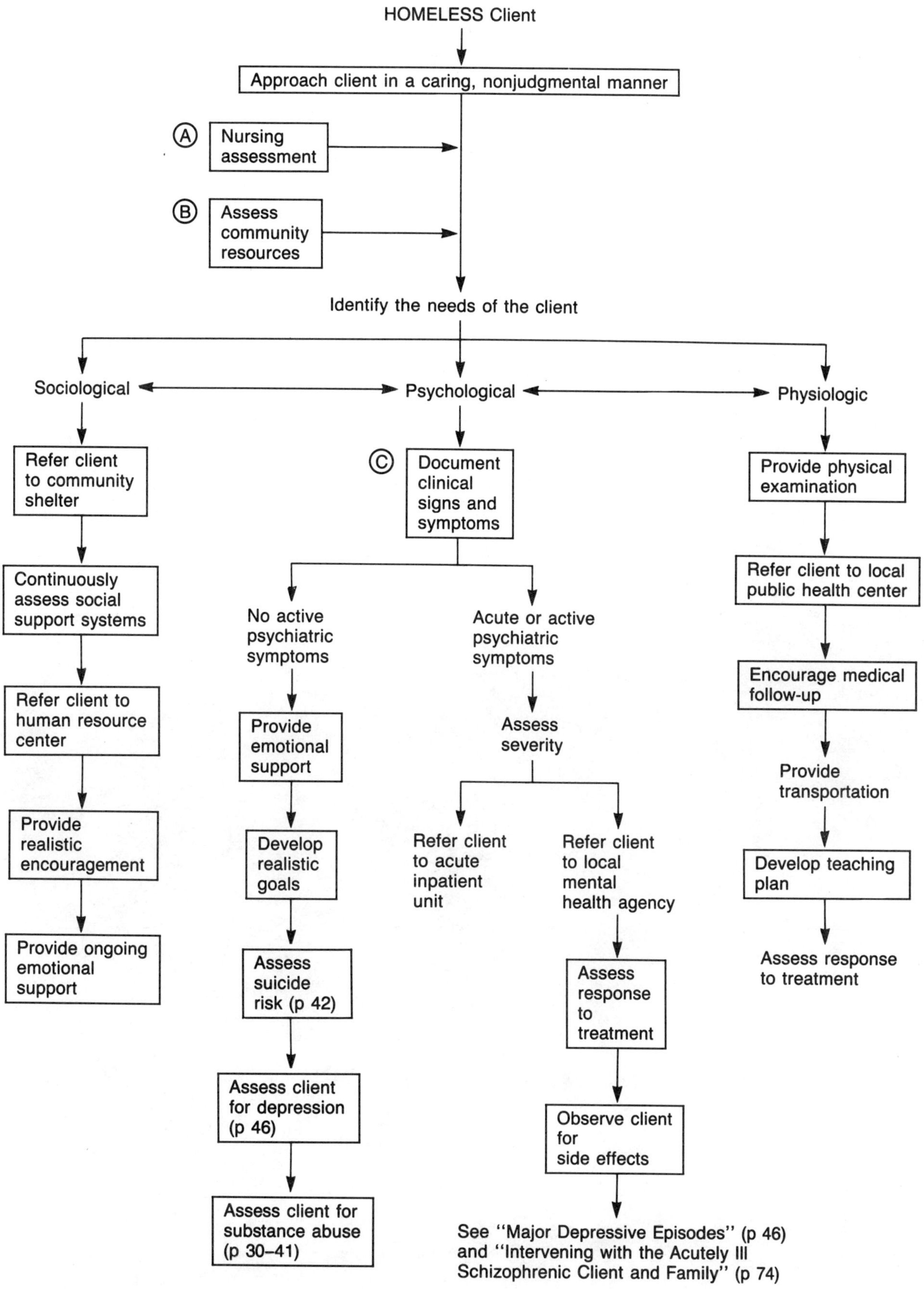
HOMELESS Client
Approach client in a caring, nonjudgmental manner
Ⓐ Nursing assessment
Ⓑ Assess community resources
Identify the needs of the client
Sociological
Psychological
Physiologic
Refer client to community shelter
Continuously assess social support systems
Refer client to human resource center
Provide realistic encouragement
Provide ongoing emotional support
Ⓒ Document clinical signs and symptoms
No active psychiatric symptoms
Provide emotional support
Develop realistic goals
Assess suicide risk (p 42)
Assess client for depression (p 46)
Assess client for substance abuse (p 30–41)
Acute or active psychiatric symptoms
Assess severity
Refer client to acute inpatient unit
Refer client to local mental health agency
Assess response to treatment
Observe client for side effects
See "Major Depressive Episodes" (p 46) and "Intervening with the Acutely Ill Schizophrenic Client and Family" (p 74)
Provide physical examination
Refer client to local public health center
Encourage medical follow-up
Provide transportation
Develop teaching plan
Assess response to treatment

VI SEXUALITY

CLIENT AT RISK FOR SEXUAL CONCERNS AND PROBLEMS

Marilyn E. Dewis

A. Sexual concerns and problems may be caused by a variety of factors. The client may perceive his or her own behaviors (such as vaginismus or orgasmic difficulties) as problematic. Changes in structural integrity (such as those caused by spinal cord injury) or physiologic alterations (diabetes, cardiac disease) may result in sexual dysfunction. Drugs such as oral contraceptives, tranquilizers, and antihypertensives may interfere with neurologic and circulatory mechanisms. Alterations in body image, as may occur with obesity and mastectomy, can influence sexual response, as may environmental influences such as hospitalization. Certain life-cycle events (menarche, pregnancy, menopause) may also influence sexual response. Negative emotional states (anxiety, depression) can adversely affect libido and interfere with the ability to form relationships.

B. Although dealing with sexual health is a relatively new domain for nursing, nurses can be involved in sexual health concerns of the well population as well as those for whom sexual dysfunction is associated with chronic illness or disability. Sex plays an important part in adjustment to chronic illness (see "Altered Body Image" [p 200] and "Chronic Illness" [p 212]), and it has been suggested that better sexual adjustment is related to better physical, social, and psychological functioning that is necessary for successful rehabilitation. The nurse's ability to deal with a client's sexuality depends on awareness and acceptance of her or his own sexuality as well as that of the client. He or she must have accurate, in-depth information about human sexuality and human dysfunction. The nurse should also have sufficient communication and interpersonal skills to relate easily to clients and to develop helping relationships. Preparation offered in the basic nursing education program should enable the nurse to intervene at the first three levels of the PLISSIT model.

C. When clients have sexual concerns, they want to discuss them, and they want direction and support in reestablishing sexual functioning or relationships. Many clients spontaneously identify their sexual concerns or problems; however, many do not. They expect the health-care provider to initiate the discussion. Sensitivity to potential problem areas can facilitate case finding and anticipatory guidance. Clients usually want their sexual partner included in the counseling.

D. The PLISSIT model is a useful format for direction of nursing intervention in helping client and family cope with sexual health problems. This hierarchical model moves in accordance with the nurse's skills and the setting in which treatment is to occur. The first step is simply to give **p**ermission for certain behaviors such as masturbation, fantasies, or feelings. The second step is to give **l**imited **i**nformation related to the problem, such as telling a cardiac patient that sudden death during intercourse almost never occurs. Step three involves **s**pecific **s**uggestions regarding a problem that has been clarified by comprehensive sexual health history taking, so that suggestions are relevant and appropriate to the client's specific concerns. The fourth step, **i**ntensive **t**herapy, may occur after the nurse's initial assessment of client need and his or her own competence, or after unsuccessful intervention at the first three levels. At this level of intervention the nurse refers the individual or couple to a professional with more advanced training.

References

Annon JS. The behavioral treatment of sexual problems. Vol 1. Brief therapy. Honolulu: Enabling Systems, 1974.

Annon JS. The PLISSIT model: a proposed conceptual scheme for the behavioral treatment of sexual problems. J Sex Educ Ther 1975; 2:1–15.

Fogel CI. Sexual dysfunction. In: Fogel CI, Woods NF, eds. Health care of women: a nursing perspective. St. Louis: CV Mosby, 1981:146–170.

Lubkin IL. Chronic illness: impact and interventions. Boston: Jones & Bartlett, 1986; 180–208.

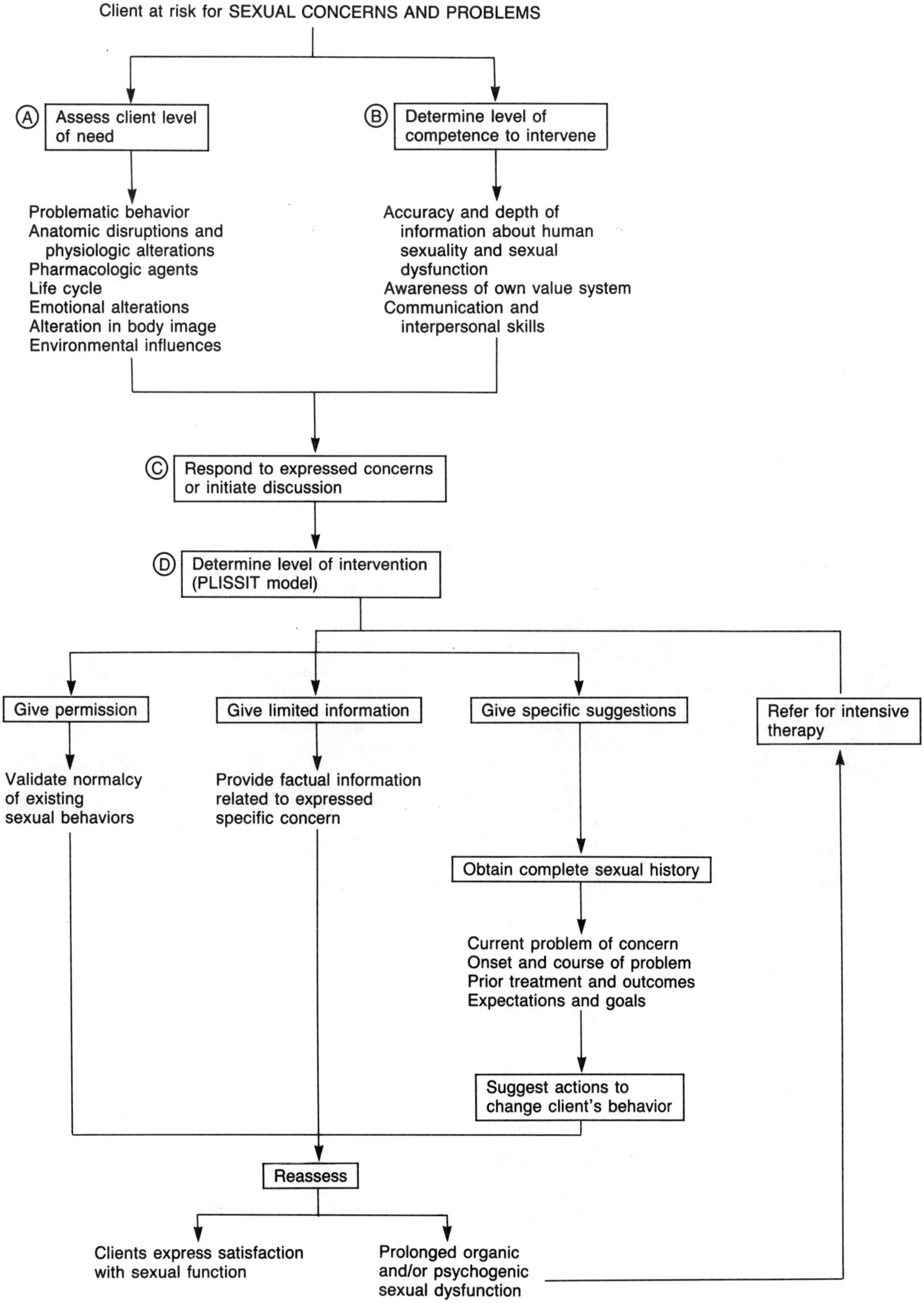
Client at risk for SEXUAL CONCERNS AND PROBLEMS
(A) Assess client level of need
(B) Determine level of competence to intervene
Problematic behavior
Anatomic disruptions and physiologic alterations
Pharmacologic agents
Life cycle
Emotional alterations
Alteration in body image
Environmental influences
Accuracy and depth of information about human sexuality and sexual dysfunction
Awareness of own value system
Communication and interpersonal skills
(C) Respond to expressed concerns or initiate discussion
(D) Determine level of intervention (PLISSIT model)
Give permission
Give limited information
Give specific suggestions
Refer for intensive therapy
Validate normalcy of existing sexual behaviors
Provide factual information related to expressed specific concern
Obtain complete sexual history
Current problem of concern
Onset and course of problem
Prior treatment and outcomes
Expectations and goals
Suggest actions to change client's behavior
Reassess
Clients express satisfaction with sexual function
Prolonged organic and/or psychogenic sexual dysfunction

THE INFERTILE COUPLE

Marilyn E. Dewis

It is estimated that one of every six couples of childbearing age in North America is involuntarily infertile. It is also estimated that only one-half of those couples who are evaluated and treated in major infertility clinics are likely to become pregnant. For those who wish to achieve pregnancy and cannot, infertility represents a major life crisis.

A. Identifying and treating the causes of infertility in a couple is often a long and discouraging ordeal that does not necessarily reach a satisfactory conclusion. The diagnostic tests are complex, repetitive and, for some people, acutely embarrassing. To enhance the chances of achieving pregnancy and to minimize individual or couple feelings of inadequacy and anxiety, the nurse can provide accurate and detailed information about specific procedures as they occur. She can also prepare the couple for each phase of the investigation and treatment by providing anticipatory counseling. Since high levels of anxiety may interfere with retaining important information, written instructions should follow verbal messages so that they can be reviewed at a later time.

B. The meaning of a diagnosis of infertility to the couple is likely to reflect their motivations for parenthood. They may wish to conform to societal pressures, to experience the rites of passage to adulthood, to relive their own childhood, to fulfill sex role expectations, or simply to experience the joys of childbearing and childrearing. Responses to infertility will vary: surprise, denial, anger, guilt and unworthiness, depression and grief. Because many persons perceive their infertility as stigmatizing, they isolate themselves from others who might be able to support or allow them to share their feelings. Surrender of control to health workers who conduct the infertility assessment often provokes feelings of helplessness and anger. The nurse has the opportunity to help the individual to link these feelings to the present circumstances, and to realize that they are normal, understandable reactions. The nurse may encourage participation in existing support groups.

C. The grief that ensues from the knowledge of sterility as a permanent condition comes as the response to losses—the loss of life goals, of the ability to give new life, and of the ability to transmit a familial genetic heritage. Although the losses are potential rather than actual, they are very real. They may, however, go unrecognized as such by the couple and even more so by others in their lives. Grieving is, therefore, to be recognized, encouraged, and assisted by the nurse (see "Grief" [p 192] and "Loss" [p 198]).

D. As the couple accepts the permanence of their sterility, they face further decisions. They may choose to continue as a family without children. They may choose adoption, which can be as difficult and frustrating a process as that of infertility diagnosis and treatment. The ability to proceed to these decisions is an indicator that progression to a stable existence is being made. Regardless of which option is chosen, the nurse can offer validation and support of the couple's mutual choices.

References

Kjeruik D, Martinson I. Women in health and illness. Life experiences and crises. Philadelphia: WB Saunders, 1986:167–174.

Wells MP. The infertile couple. In: Knor ER, ed. Decision making in obstetric nursing. Toronto: BC Decker, 1987:256–257.

Williamson M. Infertility. In: Griffith-Kenney J, ed. Contemporary women's health: a nursing advocacy approach. Menlo Park, CA: Addison-Wesley, 1986; 480–496.

Woods NF. Infertility. In: Fogel CI, Woods NV, eds. Health care of women: a nursing perspective. St. Louis: CV Mosby, 1981:257–284.

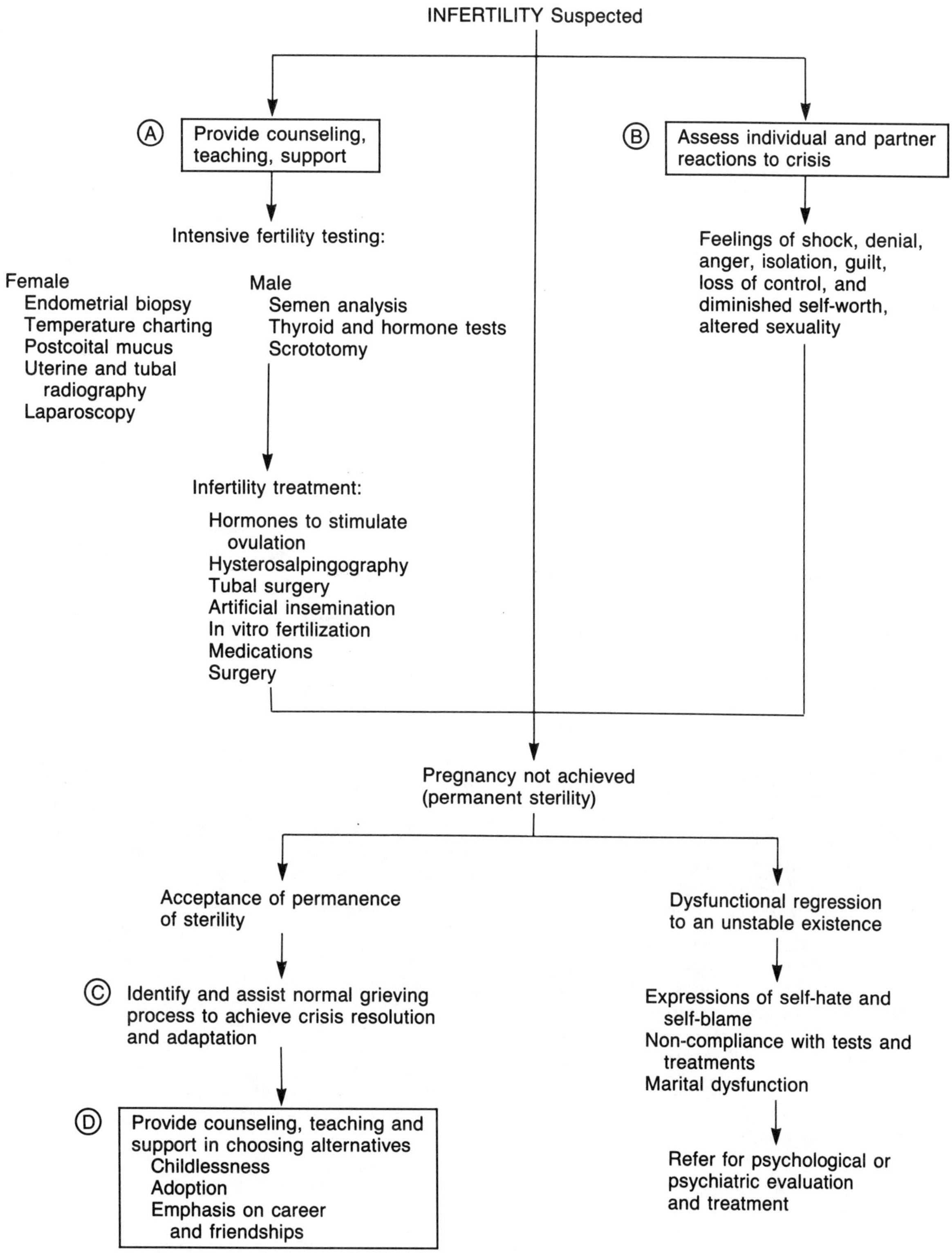
INFERTILITY Suspected
A
Provide counseling, teaching, support
Intensive fertility testing:
Female
Endometrial biopsy
Temperature charting
Postcoital mucus
Uterine and tubal radiography
Laparoscopy
Male
Semen analysis
Thyroid and hormone tests
Scrototomy
Infertility treatment:
Hormones to stimulate ovulation
Hysterosalpingography
Tubal surgery
Artificial insemination
In vitro fertilization
Medications
Surgery
B
Assess individual and partner reactions to crisis
Feelings of shock, denial, anger, isolation, guilt, loss of control, and diminished self-worth, altered sexuality
Pregnancy not achieved (permanent sterility)
Acceptance of permanence of sterility
C
Identify and assist normal grieving process to achieve crisis resolution and adaptation
D
Provide counseling, teaching and support in choosing alternatives
Childlessness
Adoption
Emphasis on career and friendships
Dysfunctional regression to an unstable existence
Expressions of self-hate and self-blame
Non-compliance with tests and treatments
Marital dysfunction
Refer for psychological or psychiatric evaluation and treatment

SEXUAL DYSFUNCTION

Deborah Antai-Otong

A. Couples complaining of sexual dysfunction must be approached in a calm, reassuring manner. The nurse must be aware of his or her own sexuality, take into consideration the couple's age and cultural and religious background, and have knowledge of the "norm" societal sexual issues. The couple must have a complete medical evaluation to rule out underlying organic dysfunction. Explore the use of medications such as antihypertensive and psychotropic agents or the presence of physical problems such as diabetes and chronic alcoholism, which may cause sexual dysfunction. Psychosocial issues include major depression, numerous situational stressors, and altered body image. Most sexual dysfunctions have a psychological basis, especially erectile and orgasmic disorders.

B. Gathering of information about sexual issues must include a thorough assessment of the dyad and include marital issues such as intimacy, communication patterns, and conflict resolution. Other issues that may contribute to sexual dysfunction are significant recent changes such as childbirth, unemployment, and role changes. Assess whether the presenting problem is new and, if not, how the problem has been resolved in the past. The couple's level of comfort when discussing sexual issues and their sexual language must be established in order to work more effectively with them. Psychosocial issues that may contribute to sexual dysfunction include psychiatric illnesses. Treatment for psychiatric disorders must begin as soon as possible, and the couple should be reassured that once these symptoms have abated, sexual function will return (if there are no organic or psychological issues involved and if there has been a "normal" sexual relationship prior to psychiatric episode).

C. Determine the couple's and individual needs from treatment by asking the couple to list their reasons for seeking treatment and determining what each wants from the relationship. These needs may range from improving their self-esteem and confidence to becoming more assertive in the relationship. These unmet needs may also contribute to feelings of powerlessness and spill over into the sexual relationship.

D. Assist the couple to look at options to enhance the sexual relationship such as trying different positions and longer foreplay, encouraging couples to ask what is stimulating and exciting to each other, and experimenting with new ideas. Encourage them to engage in these new activities in a relaxed and comfortable atmosphere rather than a mechanical and task-oriented one.

E. Medications such as beta blockers (antihypertensive agents, cardiovascular agents, and psychotropic agents), stimulants, and other psychoactive agents may or may not inhibit sexual arousal or cause anorgasm. Alcohol may also contribute to sexual dysfunction.

F. Patients who experience altered body-image problems often develop sexual dysfunction. Clients who have had recent heart attacks or who have longstanding heart conditions often experience sexual dysfunction because of fears of having another heart attack and underlying feelings of inadequacy. The spouse may reinforce these feelings by being hesitant or reluctant to participate in sexual relations. Explain that initially there may be temporary impotence, but with several attempts normal sexual function will return. (Patients are encouraged by their physician to resume "normal" activities with modification prior to discharge and during cardiac rehabilitation following an acute myocardial infarction.) Other conditions that may alter body image include surgical procedures such as hysterectomies and mastectomies. Often women and their husbands feel they are less feminine and thus less sexually attractive after these operations. These issues and associated fallacies must be discussed with the couple, and referrals should be made to community support groups. The last group of conditions that may contribute to altered body image include colostomies, ileostomies, and prostatectomies (see p 218). There are many hospital- and community-based support groups that assist individuals and couples to deal with sexually related issues that result from disfiguring surgical procedures. Older couples may experience physiologic changes that decrease their sexual functioning. Inform these clients that changes such as less firmness of the male erection and decreased vaginal lubrication with resulting dyspareunia are normal. The older couple should be encouraged to look at options and alternatives to deal with these changes.

G. A penile implant should be considered when the primary cause of impotence is considered irreversible or neurologic by a urologist. These devices are usually inflatable. Initially, some patients and their spouses may be embarrassed to discuss the prospect of a prosthesis, but the nurse can provide a calm, reassuring approach and refer the patient to a urologist or surgeon when appropriate. The spouse may also express feelings of anxiety, and she should be encouraged to discuss her feelings and thoughts about a penile prosthesis.

References

Byers S. Sexuality and sexual concerns. In: Johnson BS, ed. Psychiatric mental health nursing: adaptation and growth. Philadelphia: JB Lippincott, 1989:311–331.

Elster S, Zarling K. Coronary artery disease and congestive heart failure. In: Lewis SM, Collier IC, eds. Medical-surgical nursing: assessment and management of clinical problems. New York: McGraw-Hill, 1983:710–738.

May JL, Bobele M. Sexual dysfunction and the unemployed male professional. J Sex Marital Ther 1988; 14:253–261.

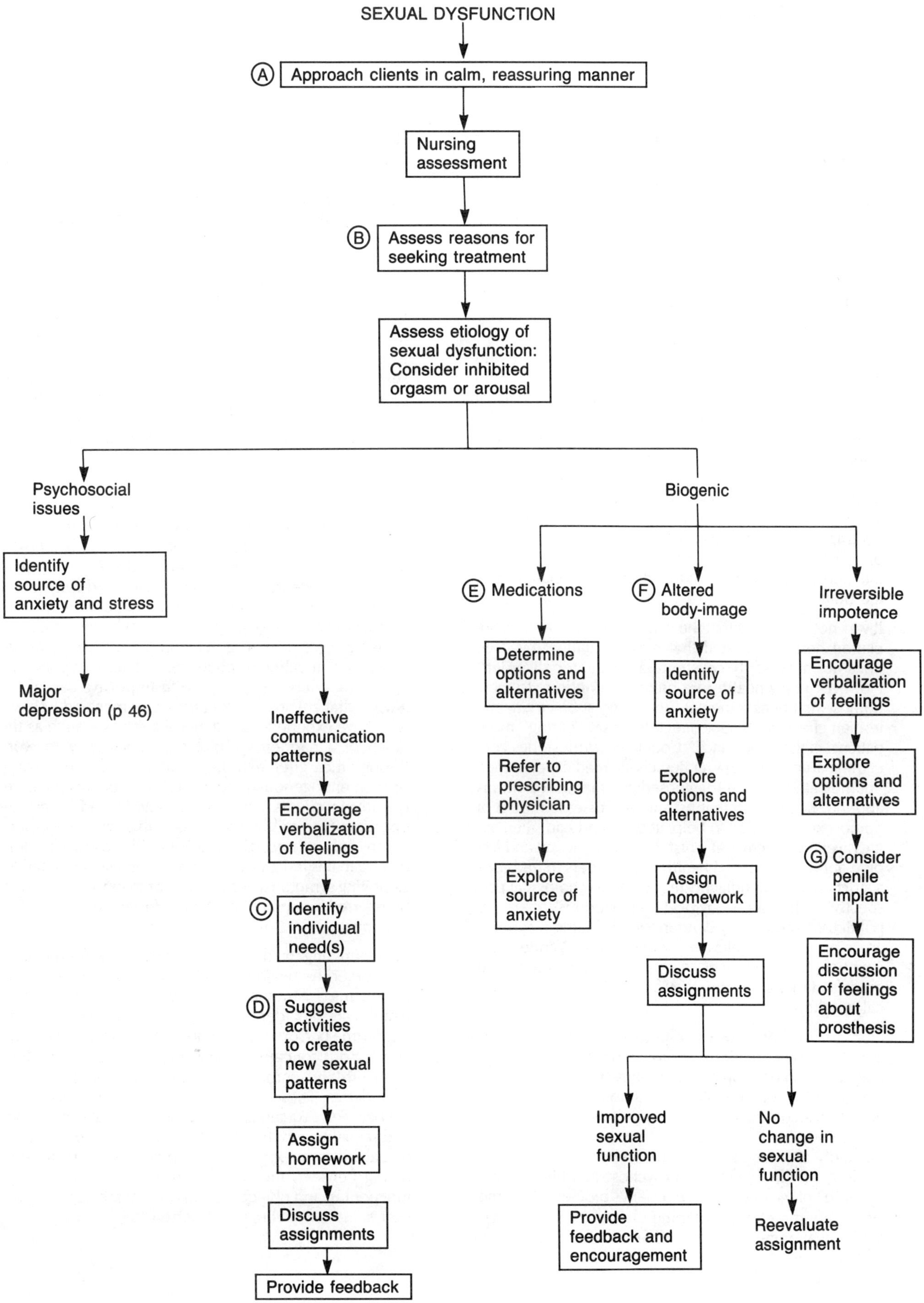
SEXUAL DYSFUNCTION
A
Approach clients in calm, reassuring manner
Nursing assessment
B
Assess reasons for seeking treatment
Assess etiology of sexual dysfunction: Consider inhibited orgasm or arousal
Psychosocial issues
Identify source of anxiety and stress
Major depression (p 46)
Ineffective communication patterns
Encourage verbalization of feelings
C
Identify individual need(s)
D
Suggest activities to create new sexual patterns
Assign homework
Discuss assignments
Provide feedback
Biogenic
E
Medications
Determine options and alternatives
Refer to prescribing physician
Explore source of anxiety
F
Altered body-image
Identify source of anxiety
Explore options and alternatives
Assign homework
Discuss assignments
Improved sexual function
Provide feedback and encouragement
No change in sexual function
Reevaluate assignment
Irreversible impotence
Encourage verbalization of feelings
Explore options and alternatives
G
Consider penile implant
Encourage discussion of feelings about prosthesis

HOMOPHOBIA

Karen Perkins

A. Sex sells everything in this country from toothpaste to cars. However, most people (including health care professionals) experience marked difficulty in talking about or dealing with issues even peripherally related to sexuality. If a client's sexual orientation lies outside the boundaries of mainstream heterosexual thought and behavior, he or she may be understandably unwilling to disclose information that might well affect the quality of his or her health care. Health care providers often unwittingly enter into collusion with the client in avoiding addressing pertinent sexuality concerns.

This mutual avoidance stems from a pervasive and generalized societal (external) as well as personal (internal) homophobia (the extreme, irrational fear of homosexuality and homosexuals). Those mental health care providers who believe that a client's sexual or affectional orientation does not matter when it comes to providing mental health care often do a grave disservice to the client. Comfort with one's own sexuality and a genuine willingness to develop a constructive and accepting attitude in working with clients whose sexual or affectional orientation may differ from one's own is the foundation upon which true therapeutic relationships are built.

B. It was not until 1973 that the American Psychiatric Association hesitantly stated that homosexuality "by itself does not necessarily constitute a psychiatric disorder." However, many health care providers continue to view homosexuality as a mental illness and subject gay and lesbian clients to therapy directed toward "curing" these patients of their "deviance." Countless horror stories concerning aversive therapy, antipsychotic medication (when not indicated), and misdiagnosed psychiatric conditions abound. Realization that psychiatry's disease model of homosexuality failed to help, at best, and had been aggressively destructive, at worst, has led many gay and lesbian affirmative mental health practitioners to embrace a strict antitrait, antidiagnostic, social-psychological perspective of human behavior. This position is inherently politicized and usually denounces psychiatric diagnoses as being invalid, irrelevant, or destructive. While there is much to recommend gay and lesbian affirmative models of mental health, they are not useful in all clinical conditions.

C. Homosexual concerns or behaviors are seen in a number of clinical conditions. In order to make a differential diagnosis and develop a comprehensive treatment plan, one must be able to distinguish among behaviors suggestive of a coming-out crisis, serious psychopathology, and a combination of both.

Only after a careful and comprehensive history, including a skillfully extracted psychosexual history, will a "sense" of the origins of the patient's problems become clear. The three most common clusters of symptomatology that require careful, differential diagnosis are schizophrenia (paranoid), affective disorders, and borderline personality disorder.

D. Recognition of symptoms suggestive of schizophrenia, most commonly of the paranoid type, must be clearly differentiated by means of a thorough history, and the clinician must be aware that *any* major threat to one's sexual identity may elicit paranoid defenses. In those clients who show no evidence of homosexual desire, either present or past (as determined by history), the thoughts are characteristically delusional: cerebral and ruminative ideas with little basis in homosexual actions. In a delusional-appearing, genuinely homosexual individual, a paranoid reaction may well be reality-based as a result of severe interpersonal rejection, physical or sexual assault, or a loss of livelihood as a result of being "found out" to be homosexual. The mental health care provider must be ever cognizant that a coming-out crisis may be the stressor which triggers an underlying schizophrenic process.

E. A careful history is the foundation for determining earlier affective problems and previous same-sex interests. Denial in true hypomania has a rigid, brittle quality which, when confronted, is met with irritability, hostility, and a possible flight into euphoria. A person with a true sexual identity crisis, when confronted with it, may become more anxious to the point of *appearing* hypomanic (without developing a full-blown hypomanic state) as he or she comes to grips with the fact of his or her sexual or affectional preference. These hypomanic-appearing clients may engage in impulsive sexual behaviors that are atypical for *them*. Gay men and lesbians who have experienced a major life stressor, such as the death of a partner, without the opportunity to work through their grief, may appear at first to be chronically or even endogenously depressed. This occurs most frequently in clients who are "closeted" and have little opportunity to talk of their loss with supportive others. Again, only a thorough history will disclose a symptom picture that is indicative of a major depression. A patient exhibiting symptoms of a major depression should always be referred to a psychiatrist for definitive diagnosis and treatment.

F. In determining the difference between a client experiencing borderline personality disorder and one who is experiencing a genuine sexual identity crisis, the mental health care provider must keep in mind that those with borderline personality disorder, while appearing to have coming-out concerns, have as their real issue a relatively severe and chronic lack of ego differentiation and boundaries. These individuals are unable to differentiate between acquaintanceship, friendship, affection, love, and sexuality and may, in fact, have both chaotic heterosexual and homosexual relationships. The key to differentiating between the two lies in a careful look at ego functioning and object relations *before* the current crisis over same-sex feelings and behavior.

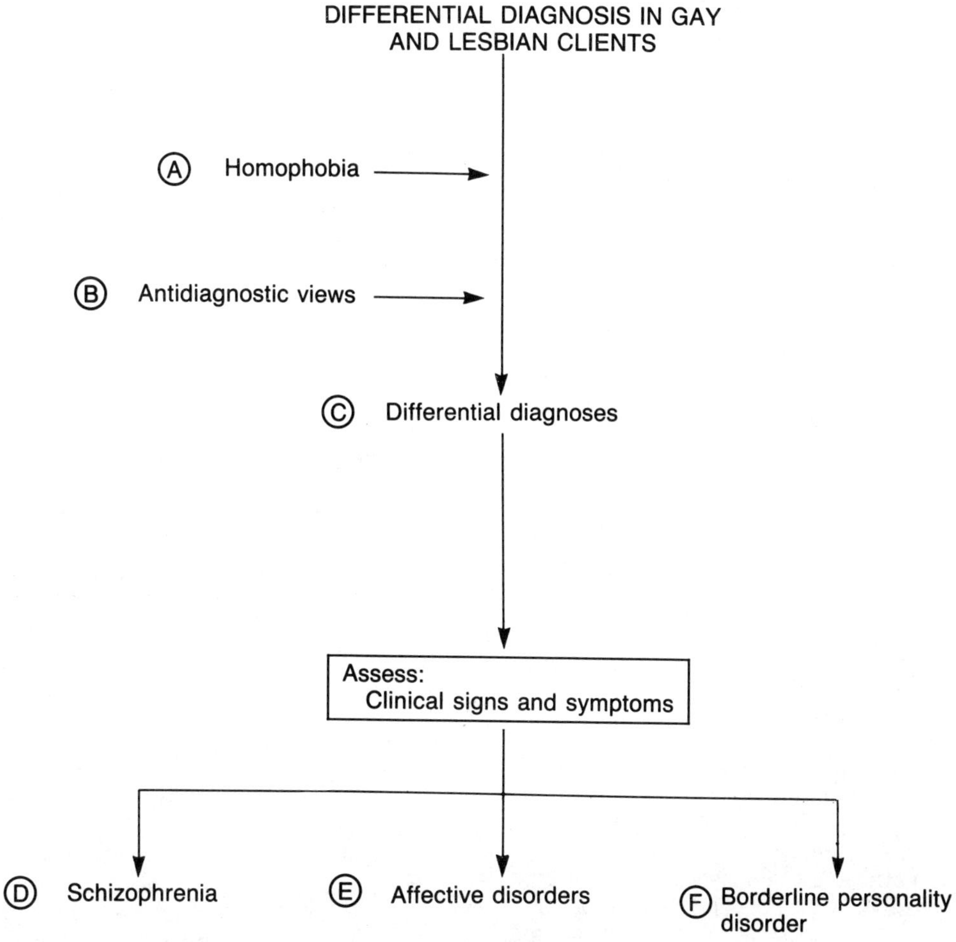

References

Finnegan DG, McNally EB. Dual identities. Center City, MN: Hazelden, 1987.

Gonsiorek JC, ed. A guide to psychotherapy with gay and lesbian clients. New York: Harrington Park Press, 1985.

The Boston Lesbian Psychologies Collective. Lesbian psychologies. Urbana and Chicago: University of Illinois Press, 1987.

SEXUALLY ASSAULTED CLIENT

Rosa Belgard

A. It is estimated that 40 to 50 percent of all women are victims of an actual or attempted sexual assault; approximately one-third of these cases go unreported. Therefore, there is a high probability of unresolved sexual trauma in any population. A recommended routine assessment question is: "Have you ever been pressured or forced to have sexual activity of any kind?" Predisposing variables that are associated with poor postassault adjustment include prior physical or sexual victimization, previous psychiatric diagnosis for the victim or immediate family, suicide ideation or attempts, or substance abuse.

B. Initial assessment for clients seeking assistance related to sexual assault or rape (A/R) should include when, where, the nature of the sexual act, and how long the assault occurred. Did the victim know the assailant? Were there threats (verbal or physical), a struggle, or conversation before, during, or after the assault? Was it the victim's first sexual experience, and had the victim been sexually assaulted before? Assess previous and present coping behavior.

C. Victims of a recent sexual A/R are likely to be in the disorganization phase of the rape trauma syndrome. Predominant feelings observed in this stage include fear, anger, humiliation, and self-blame. Incessant thoughts, nightmares, and flashbacks of the event are common. Emotional responses indicative of coping styles may be either expressive—anxiety, fear, and anger expressed by talking, crying, shaking, smiling—or controlled—masking of feelings with a subdued, calm, or composed affect. Proceed with a calm, directive, incident-oriented approach. Explore with the client options regarding physical care, legal action, and counseling. The response of significant others to the victim strongly influences resolution of the crisis. Encourage significant others to approach the client in a supportive, nonjudgmental manner.

D. Nurses are frequently called as witnesses in A/R trials; their documentation is a major source of evidence. A complete accurate account of physical findings and signs of mental and emotional trauma with exact quotes from victim should be recorded. Pictures of injuries should be taken with the client's permission.

E. Delayed treatment seekers are victims who never reported their assault or received only a medical rape examination. These clients often enter treatment following some precipitating event such as an anniversary date of the assault, impaired interpersonal relationships, or because of an unfulfilling and unsatisfying life.

F. Indicators of unresolved rape trauma syndrome include sudden onset of phobic symptoms regarding being alone, avoidance of relationships with members of the opposite sex, a marked change in sexual behavior, negative shifts in relationships with significant others, loss of self-esteem and confidence, and feelings of guilt, self-blame, or paranoia. During the interview, sudden increased anxiety, long periods of silence, blocking, stuttering, or physical distress may indicate unresolved assault issues.

G. The overall goal of counseling is for the client to regain control over physical, psychological, social, and sexual life-style disruptions. Therapeutic tasks include: (1) discussion of the assault in detail, with the full range of feelings; (2) questioning motives if a previous assault was unreported; (3) assisting the client to regain a feeling of physical well-being and safety; (4) working through fears or phobias and anger; (5) reestablishing self-esteem and trust; (6) gaining a realistic perception of the event; and (7) assimilating the event into the sense of self.

References

Burgess AW. Psychiatric nursing in the hospital and community. 4th ed. Englewood Cliffs, NJ: Prentice-Hall, 1985.

Burgess AW, Holmstrom LL. Rape: victims of crisis. Bowie, MD: Robert J Brady, 1974.

Foley T, Davies M. Rape: nursing care of victims. St. Louis: CV Mosby, 1983.

Jaber J, Hoskins P, Leach A, Sideleau B. Comprehensive psychiatric nursing. New York: McGraw-Hill, 1987.

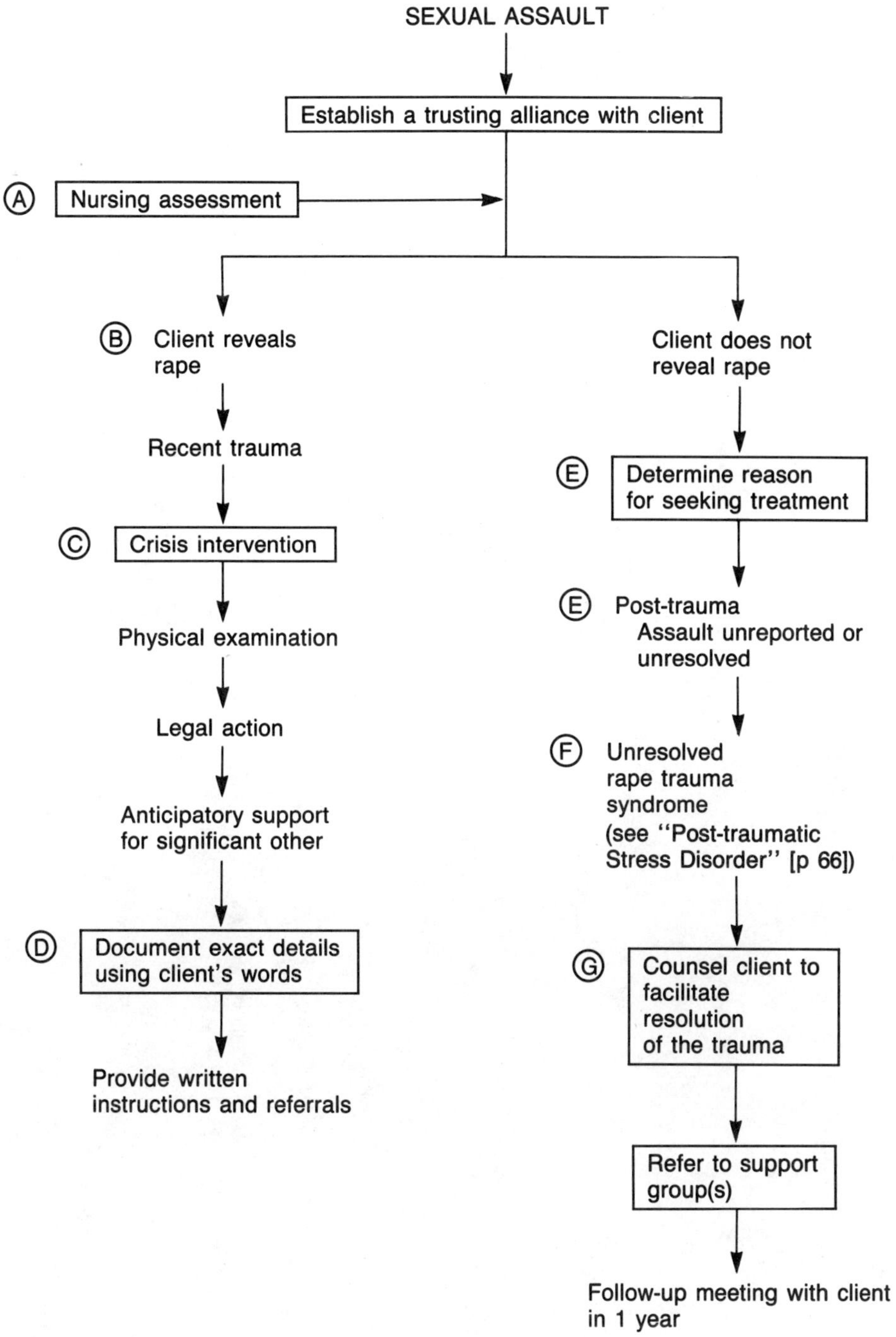
SEXUAL ASSAULT
Establish a trusting alliance with client
Ⓐ Nursing assessment
Ⓑ Client reveals rape
Recent trauma
Ⓒ Crisis intervention
Physical examination
Legal action
Anticipatory support for significant other
Ⓓ Document exact details using client's words
Provide written instructions and referrals
Client does not reveal rape
Ⓔ Determine reason for seeking treatment
Ⓔ Post-trauma Assault unreported or unresolved
Ⓕ Unresolved rape trauma syndrome (see "Post-traumatic Stress Disorder" [p 66])
Ⓖ Counsel client to facilitate resolution of the trauma
Refer to support group(s)
Follow-up meeting with client in 1 year

VII MISCELLANEOUS

THE LAW AND INFORMED CONSENT

Deborah Antai-Otong

Informed consent is an active process that involves the client, physician, and nurse. The ultimate responsibility lies with the physician, but the nurse is actively involved in presenting the consent form and carrying out the process of explanation and obtaining the client's signature. Signed consent forms are required by law before routine and nonroutine treatment and procedures are performed.

A. The nursing assessment should focus on assessing the client and family members' knowledge about the prospective treatment or procedures. A history of past and present psychiatric treatment will assist the nurse to develop an individualized teaching plan. The client's previous response to treatment also provides valuable information. A thorough physical examination and assessment are essential, including current medical problems and medications. A current mental status is also essential in assessing the client's ability to give informed consent and make a sound decision. Psychiatric admission does not mean that clients give up their rights to consent for treatment. Factors that influence an individual's capacity to give informed consent are age and competence. Each state has a mental health code which defines age of consent. The nurse must recognize that the informed consent is voluntary and can be revoked at any time. Informed consent is an ongoing process and must be evaluated continuously. The client must not be coerced into signing this form. The purpose of the consent form is to protect not only the client, but also the physician and other hospital personnel. The nurse must be available for clarification and answer questions that may be generated by the proposed procedures. The client must be allowed to read the informed consent at his own pace, in his own language and in terms that are familiar to him.

B. The informed consent form assures the following client rights:
   1. The right not to consent to treatment or procedures
   2. Freedom to revoke the form at any time
   3. Protection of the client's privacy
   4. Freedom to ask questions and clarify terms and treatment

C. Knowledge deficit issues must be addressed with an individualized teaching plan.

References

Antai-Otong DJ. Psychopharmacology. In: Johnson BS, ed. Psychiatric nursing: adaptation and growth. 2nd ed. Philadelphia: JB Lippincott, 1989:268–294.

Munetz MR, Roth LH, Cornes CL. Tardive dyskineasia and informed consent: Myths and realities. Am Acad Psychiatry Law 1982; 10:77–82.

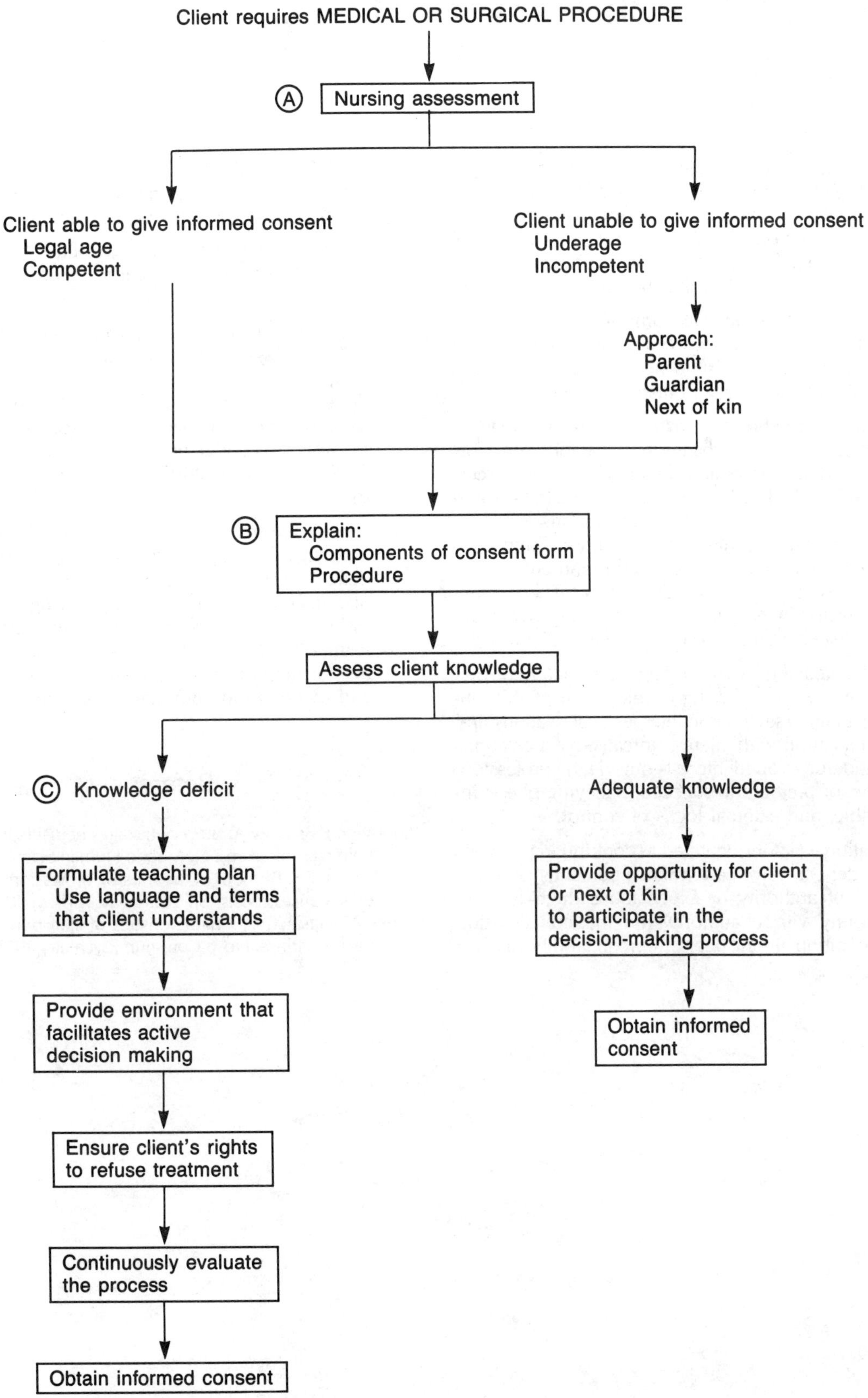
Client requires MEDICAL OR SURGICAL PROCEDURE
A Nursing assessment
Client able to give informed consent
Legal age
Competent
Client unable to give informed consent
Underage
Incompetent
Approach:
Parent
Guardian
Next of kin
B Explain:
Components of consent form
Procedure
Assess client knowledge
C Knowledge deficit
Adequate knowledge
Formulate teaching plan
Use language and terms that client understands
Provide environment that facilitates active decision making
Ensure client's rights to refuse treatment
Continuously evaluate the process
Obtain informed consent
Provide opportunity for client or next of kin to participate in the decision-making process
Obtain informed consent

PROFESSIONAL BURNOUT SYNDROME

Rosa Belgard

Burnout syndrome is characterized by the progressive stages of disillusionment observed in individuals involved in various human services and helping professions. Attitudinal and behavioral manifestations that may be precursors or indicators of dysfunctional job performance are associated with staff turnover, absenteeism, and less than optimal client services.

A. Somatic signs observable in burnout syndrome (BOS) include fatigue, headaches, low resistance to colds and viruses, gastrointestinal disturbances, weight loss or gain, insomnia, and shortness of breath.

B. Personality and behavioral manifestations that may be observed as a significant change from previous behaviors include: working harder and accomplishing less, excessive attention to details, low levels of frustration and enthusiasm, heightened sense of responsibility for clients, increased absenteeism, difficulty making decisions, and increased feelings of disillusionment, futility, guilt, confusion, resentment, defensiveness, boredom, anger, suspicion in work-related matters, and detachment from, or negative attitudes toward, clients.

C. Personal characteristics of individuals that may predispose or contribute to the development of BOS include: inability to set limits in interpersonal relationships, overidentification with clients, unrealistic expectations of job, underdeveloped interests outside the profession, high drive or pressure to succeed, believing one is indispensable, and external locus of control.

D. Organizational factors identified as contributing to burnout include: excessive performance demands, ambiguous lines of authority or expectations, high level of responsibility without authority, minimal collaboration and cooperation among peers, unpredictability, unclear goals or philosophy, pertinent information withheld, differences of opinion denied or ignored, and change introduced without thorough planning.

E. Identifying the beginning stages of disillusionment in self or employees facilitates earlier, more successful intervention.

F. Personal interventions involve: (1) providing necessary skills, i.e., assertiveness training, conflict management, bargaining skills; (2) assisting with realistic goal setting; (3) encouraging physical or relaxation exercises; (4) assisting the professional to expand nonjob-related interests; (5) conducting rational emotive therapy to confront cognitive distortions, and (6) promoting reality therapy.

G. Organizational interventions for staff include: (1) team building exercises, (2) addressing coping and knowledge deficits, (3) providing support groups, (4) utilizing planned change strategies, (5) clarifying expectations, (6) assigning responsibility congruent with authority, (7) adjusting the staff-client ratio, and (8) offering opportunities for time out and detachment from clients (retreats and planned time off), and continuing education.

References

Edelwich J, Brodsky A. Burn-out: stages of disillusionment in the helping professions. New York: Human Sciences Press, 1980.

McConnell EA. Burnout in the nursing profession: coping strategies, causes, costs. St. Louis: CV Mosby, 1982.

Pines A, Maslach C. Characteristics of staff burnout in mental health settings. Hosp Commun Psychiatry 1978; 29:233–237.

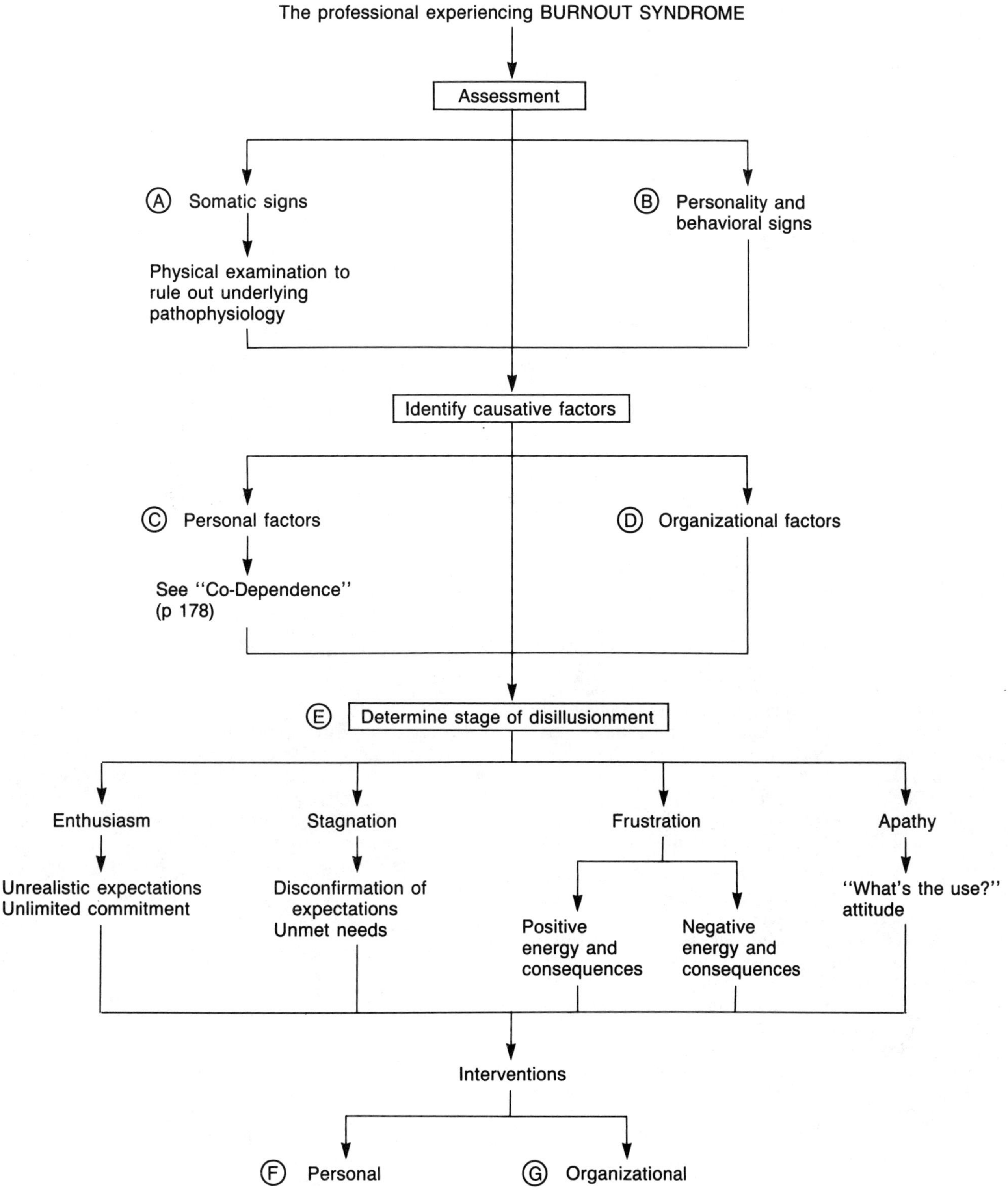
The professional experiencing BURNOUT SYNDROME
Assessment
Ⓐ Somatic signs
Physical examination to rule out underlying pathophysiology
Ⓑ Personality and behavioral signs
Identify causative factors
Ⓒ Personal factors
See "Co-Dependence" (p 178)
Ⓓ Organizational factors
Ⓔ Determine stage of disillusionment
Enthusiasm
Unrealistic expectations
Unlimited commitment
Stagnation
Disconfirmation of expectations
Unmet needs
Frustration
Positive energy and consequences
Negative energy and consequences
Apathy
"What's the use?" attitude
Interventions
Ⓕ Personal
Ⓖ Organizational

ACQUIRED IMMUNODEFICIENCY SYNDROME: PHYSIOLOGIC AND PSYCHOLOGICAL CONSIDERATIONS

Irene L. Goldstone
Rosemarie Riddell

Acquired immunodeficiency syndrome (AIDS) was identified in 1981, and defined by the Centers for Disease Control (CDC) as the presence of specific opportunistic infections and cancers, resulting from an unexplained defect in cell-mediated immunity. In 1984, with the discovery of the causative organism, human immunodeficiency virus (HIV), it was established that transmission occurred during intimate sexual contact, through parenteral exposure to blood and blood products, and from mother to infant during the perinatal period. For the protection of health-care workers, universal precautions must be instituted. The CDC developed a classification system to describe the spectrum of HIV infection, ranging from the initial exposure, through the latency period and other infections, to the end stage, which is AIDS. In North America, the majority of individuals with AIDS are homosexual and bisexual men. The proportion of women contracting AIDS from infected male partners is increasing.

A. Serologic tests are used to detect antibodies to HIV. Confirmatory testing indicating that seroconversion has occurred means that the individual is infected with HIV and is infectious to others, probably for life. Because HIV testing precipitates an emotional crisis, counseling must occur in order to ensure awareness of the implications of the test results, reduce anxiety, and promote changes in behavior. Seropositive individuals are counseled to inform their sexual partners of their HIV status and to seek out early medical assessment of their health status for possible treatment with zidovudine.

B. Nursing assessment of the person with HIV-related disease requires an understanding of his psychosocial make-up, current crisis, and stage of HIV-related disease. Psychological responses may include anxiety, anger, depression, somatization, and denial. Commonly occurring at specific crisis points (e.g., HIV testing, diagnosis of AIDS, impending death), these responses are reactions to a life-threatening and stigmatizing illness. Treatment includes participating in support groups, counseling, psychotherapy, pharmacotherapy, and education about the nature of the disease.

C. Bacterial and viral pneumonias and tuberculosis occur in HIV-infected persons, but the opportunistic infection *Pneumocystis carinii* pneumonia (PCP), which is diagnostic of AIDS, occurs in about 60 percent of patients as the index diagnosis. Although fatal if untreated, PCP responds to therapy in most cases if treated early. The nurse must be alert for acute respiratory failure requiring ventilatory support.

D. Bacterial infections of the gastrointestinal tract may precede the numerous AIDS-related opportunistic infections and malignancies. The AIDS diagnosis also includes the wasting syndrome: severe weight loss and diarrhea without superimposed opportunistic infection. Successful management of symptoms to maintain the patient's well-being is a nursing care challenge.

E. Two-thirds of AIDS patients experience neurologic complications related to opportunistic infections, lymphoma, or HIV, which result in a variety of symptoms ranging from mild to severe. Nursing assessment is complicated since behavioral changes may be caused by organic disease or may be functional, caused by the stress of living with a life-threatening disease.

F. Herpes zoster, herpes simplex, and oral candidiasis are common, and prognostic of AIDS. Kaposi's sarcoma of the skin and mouth is diagnostic of AIDS and represents 20 percent of primary diagnoses. These lesions are not usually fatal, but are visible and carry with them social stigma.

G. AIDS is a chronic and, at this time, a universally fatal disease. The percentage of HIV-infected individuals who will develop AIDS is unknown. To promote hope for these patients, the distinction must be made between being HIV infected and carrying the diagnosis of AIDS. The ordering of one's life affairs and decision making about the treatment desired (e.g., ventilation, code status) must be undertaken when AIDS is diagnosed. Internal conflicts about life-style, pressure to reveal life-style, guilt about transmission of the virus, acute anxiety attacks, depression, and suicidal ideation are common. The goal of treatment is to provide acute, aggressive therapy and support for both psychosocial and physiologic distress to maximize the quality of life. Palliative care is appropriate when the disease process becomes overwhelming.

References

Beaufoy A, Goldstone I, Riddell R. AIDS: what nurses need to know. Can Nurse 1988; 7:16–27.

Canada Diseases Weekly Report. Update universal precautions. 1988; 14(27):117–124.

Flaskerud JH. AIDS: psychosocial aspects. J Psychosoc Nurs 1987; 12:9–16.

Morbidity and Mortality Weekly Report. Revision of the CDC surveillance case definition for acquired immunodeficiency syndrome. 1987; 36(1S):3S–15S.

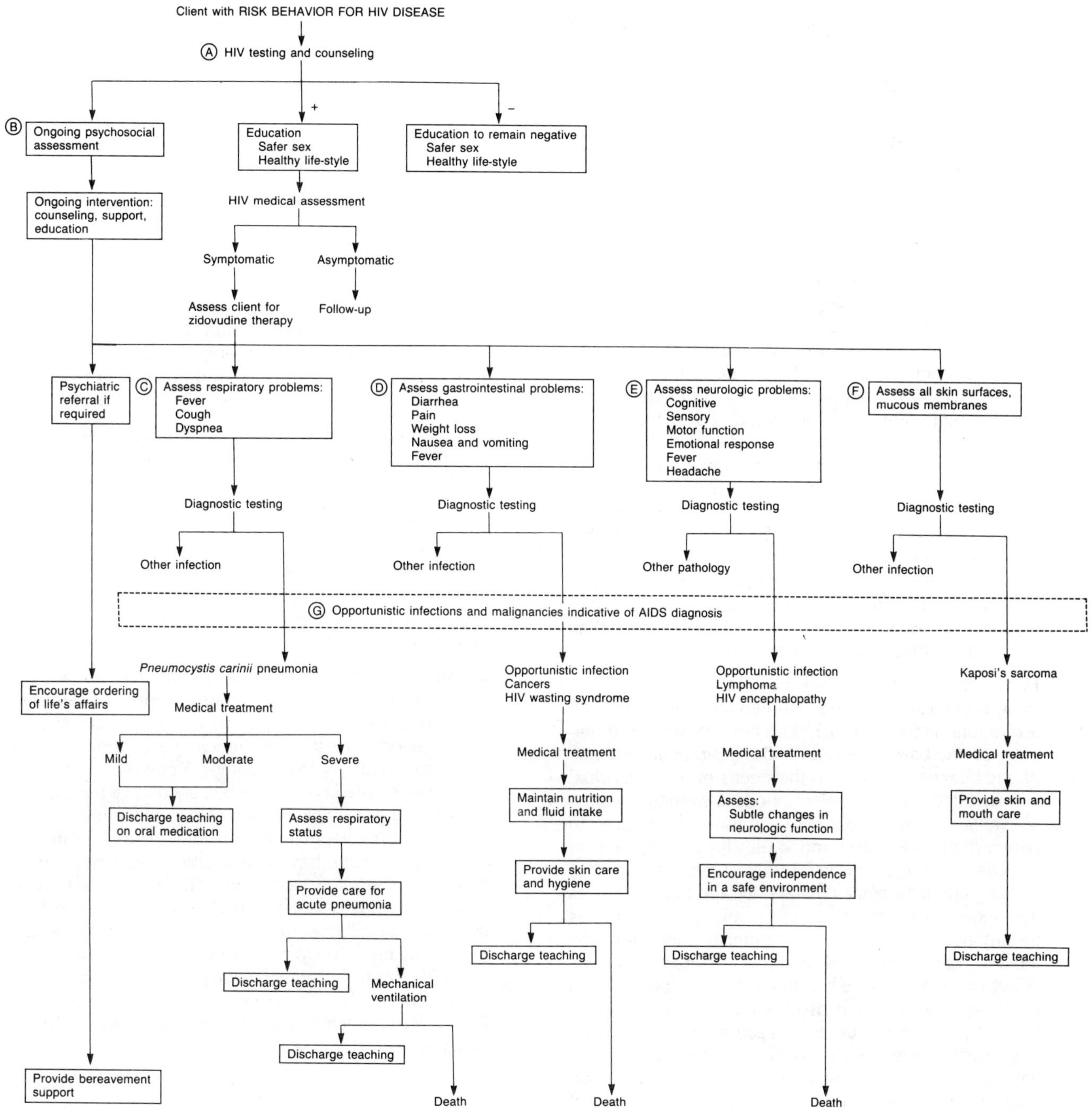
Client with RISK BEHAVIOR FOR HIV DISEASE
(A) HIV testing and counseling
+
−
(B) Ongoing psychosocial assessment
Education
Safer sex
Healthy life-style
Education to remain negative
Safer sex
Healthy life-style
Ongoing intervention: counseling, support, education
HIV medical assessment
Symptomatic
Asymptomatic
Assess client for zidovudine therapy
Follow-up
Psychiatric referral if required
(C) Assess respiratory problems:
Fever
Cough
Dyspnea
(D) Assess gastrointestinal problems:
Diarrhea
Pain
Weight loss
Nausea and vomiting
Fever
(E) Assess neurologic problems:
Cognitive
Sensory
Motor function
Emotional response
Fever
Headache
(F) Assess all skin surfaces, mucous membranes
Diagnostic testing
Diagnostic testing
Diagnostic testing
Diagnostic testing
Other infection
Other infection
Other pathology
Other infection
(G) Opportunistic infections and malignancies indicative of AIDS diagnosis
Pneumocystis carinii pneumonia
Opportunistic infection
Cancers
HIV wasting syndrome
Opportunistic infection
Lymphoma
HIV encephalopathy
Kaposi's sarcoma
Encourage ordering of life's affairs
Medical treatment
Mild
Moderate
Severe
Medical treatment
Medical treatment
Medical treatment
Discharge teaching on oral medication
Assess respiratory status
Maintain nutrition and fluid intake
Assess:
Subtle changes in neurologic function
Provide skin and mouth care
Provide skin care and hygiene
Encourage independence in a safe environment
Provide care for acute pneumonia
Discharge teaching
Discharge teaching
Discharge teaching
Discharge teaching
Mechanical ventilation
Discharge teaching
Provide bereavement support
Death
Death
Death

FEMINISM: A META-FRAMEWORK FOR PSYCHOTHERAPY WITH WOMEN

Patricia A. Gervaize
Alison Lee

A. Feminist psychotherapy can be defined as an approach to working with women which recognizes that many problems experienced by women are external and societally imposed rather than internal and a reflection of an individual's personality, psychopathology, maladaptive behavioral repertoire, diagnostic category, or any other description that places the locus of the precipitating problem within the woman rather than the society at large. Adult victims of childhood sexual abuse, battered women, women in power imbalance relationships, women caught in binds between work and family, and women discriminated against on the basis of sexual choice or life-style choice can all be viewed as candidates for feminist therapy, irrespective of the presenting complaint. For example, self-blame, depression, guilt, self-mutilation, and rage are viewed as an individual's response to societally imposed problems, rather than problems originating from within an individual.

B. Feminism is the meta-framework of the therapist. Thus, many approaches can be subsumed under feminist therapy as long as the approach does not treat women differently on the basis of gender and the direction of therapeutic change is based on the needs of the individual woman rather than role expectations of women in general. Therapists must continuously assess the degree to which their own biases and values have an impact on the client and must also scrutinize even the most discrete components of their therapeutic approach for biases that reflect or serve to reinforce misogynist attitudes toward women. For example, feminists reject not only the body of psychoanalytic and psychodynamic theories about women, but also practices that are derived from them, such as standard psychodiagnostic assessment. Similarly, therapists must guard against directing women toward political feminism, a position that is usually compatible with the value system of the therapist but has explicit role expectations of how women ought to be and limits the degree of individual choice as much as other, more traditional approaches.

C. The therapeutic relationship is a mainstay of feminist therapy, emphasizing support from an egalitarian position, teaching about the externally imposed event that has precipitated the client's problem, and granting permission to explore the client's idiosyncratic reactions, feelings, and alternatives through the use of therapeutic techniques. Control and choice about whether to proceed and what to explore rest with the client. The client utilizes the therapist's technical competence from within the safety of the relationship, but maintains control over what is addressed in each session and what changes will or will not occur. From the therapist's point of view, the goal of the relationship is to support the client's proactive behavior, rather than to encourage dependence.

D. Very often, women face practical problems that can be solved by resources available within the community. There are also support groups available for many aspects of women's experience. To refer women to these services and/or support groups reinforces the social basis of the problems they experience, provides a framework for support in a nonmedical, nontreatment setting, and provides guidance for women by women who have dealt with the same problems. This is a valuable adjunct to individual psychotherapy.

E. Therapeutic work focuses on the problem as it is defined by the woman. There is no labeling or formal diagnosis, no effort to discover the "real" meaning of what she says, and no effort to restructure the client's experience into one theoretical system or another. A common feature of therapy is the use of techniques to encourage the expression of strong feelings. This emphasis on feeling expression gives the client the opportunity of saying directly and fully what she has been unable to express, and to do it from the safety of therapy. The result is a clearer understanding of personal boundaries and behaviors that would enforce those limits in the client's extratherapy world. The final step in every session is detailed description and rehearsal of actual behaviors the client can carry out in the real-life situations she is apt to encounter. The choice of whether to carry them out always rests with the client.

References

Gartner A, Gartner AJ, Ouellette-Kobasa SC. Self-help. In: Blechman EA, Brownell KD, eds. Handbook of behavioral health for women. New York: Pergamon, 1988:330–342.

Lerman H. From Freud to feminist personality theory: getting here from there. In: Walsh MR, ed. The psychology of women: ongoing debates. New Haven: Yale University Press, 1987:39–58.

Mahrer AR, Gervaize PA. Impossible roles therapists must play. Can Psych 1983; 24:81–87.

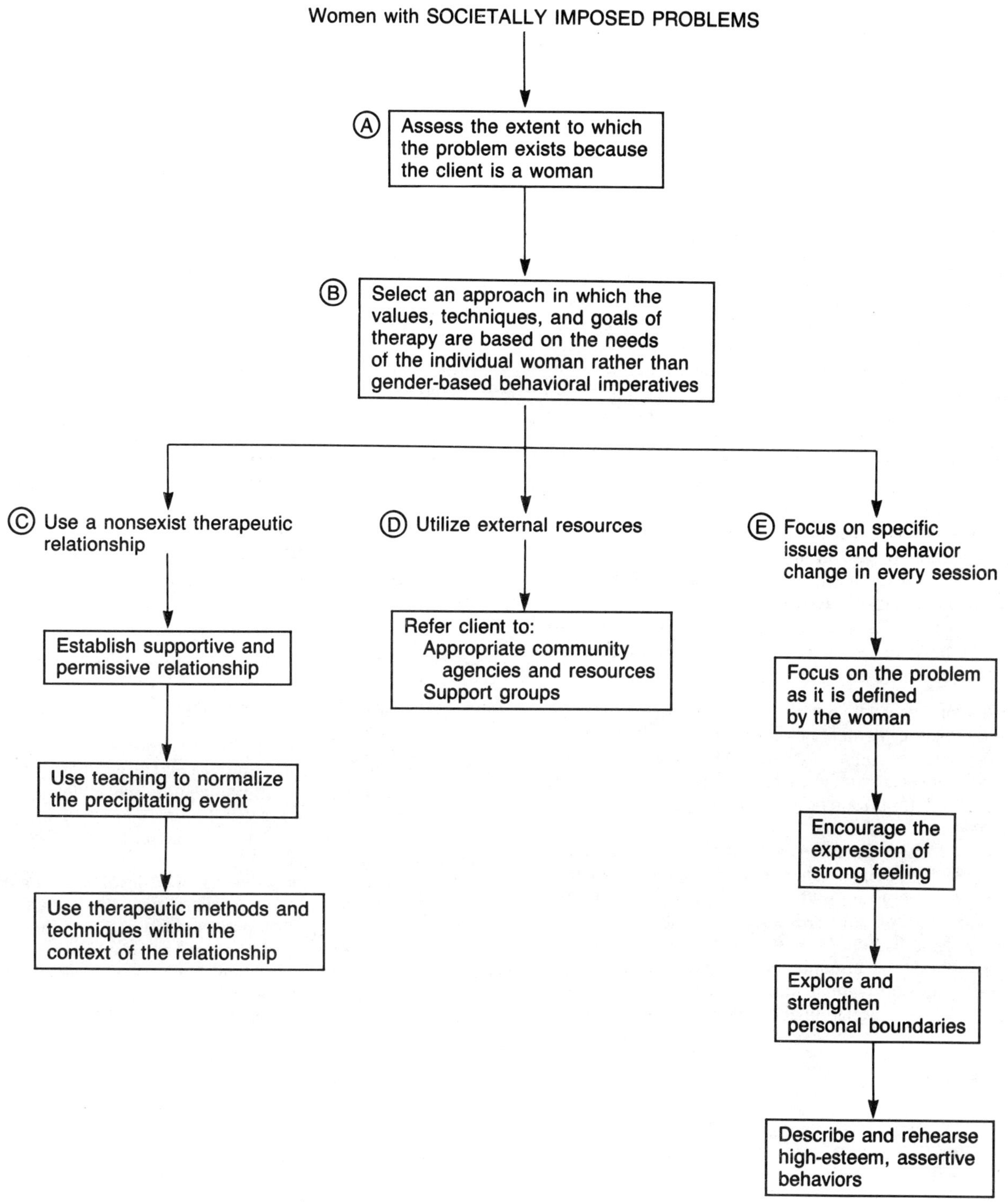
Women with SOCIETALLY IMPOSED PROBLEMS
A
Assess the extent to which the problem exists because the client is a woman
B
Select an approach in which the values, techniques, and goals of therapy are based on the needs of the individual woman rather than gender-based behavioral imperatives
C
Use a nonsexist therapeutic relationship
Establish supportive and permissive relationship
Use teaching to normalize the precipitating event
Use therapeutic methods and techniques within the context of the relationship
D
Utilize external resources
Refer client to:
Appropriate community agencies and resources
Support groups
E
Focus on specific issues and behavior change in every session
Focus on the problem as it is defined by the woman
Encourage the expression of strong feeling
Explore and strengthen personal boundaries
Describe and rehearse high-esteem, assertive behaviors

CLIENT ADVOCACY

Andrea Baumann

The word "advocate" means to help or speak out on behalf of someone else. An advocate is in a position to speak out for vulnerable and powerless clients and to ensure the right to self-determination. The client is considered to be the central participant in the decision-making process; an advocate acts on behalf of a client, not a system. The issues may focus on social, custodial, therapeutic entitlement, discharge planning, or other quality-of-life issues. Advocacy in some hospitals may provide advice to clients about their rights while they are hospitalized. There can be many barriers to implementation of an effective advocacy program. Although institutions may espouse philosophical commitment to the principle of self-determination and client decision making, there may be resistance due to long established rules and regulations and lines of bureaucratic communication (see 'Powerlessness,'' p 184). An effective advocate needs to break down barriers to change and open avenues for increasing the client's input into decision making about their own health. Advocacy is only viable when societal and environmental attitudes create a climate open to change and support the protection of the rights and entitlements of the society's most vulnerable and disadvantaged members.

A. Issues for advocacy focus on human and legal rights for the psychiatric client. Legal rights are entrenched in legislation, whereas human rights may be more expansive and refer to universal human values and rights. The advocate may be a staff nurse, a lay person, or a person solely appointed for the advocate position in the institution. The latter is considered to be best, because he or she has no conflict of interest. Although the nurse may often function as a client advocate, nurses may have restricted autonomy in this role owing to divided loyalties to the institution and client. A person acting in the capacity of an advocate must communicate well and be able to retain highly confidential information. Communication skills such as negotiation and mediation are important.

B. Self or case advocacy is based on the individual client's need. It focuses on change to meet an individual's needs, not a system change.

C. Collective advocacy is effective for system and policy change because more people are involved. Self-help groups and volunteer advocate associations are examples of collective advocacy.

D. There are three main areas of advocacy: (1) the quality-of-life issues or social rights advocacy, which focuses on privileges, economics, and contact with religious or family support; (2) quality-of-care issues (therapeutic advocacy), which focuses on issues such as therapeutic alternatives, second opinion, and conflicts with caregivers; (3) the right to self-determination, which is legal advocacy. The client needs information about such issues as informed consent (p 230), access to clinical charts, and review of committal and compulsory versus voluntary treatment.

References

Annas G. The patient rights advocate: can nurses effectively fill the role? Supervisor Nurse 1974; 5:21–25.

Appalbaum P. The rising tide of patient rights advocacy. Hosp Commun Psychiatry 1981; 37:9–10.

Atkinson S, Modell D, Sollerg D, Turner T. Mental health advocacy: paradigm or panacea? Can Ment Health 1985; 33:3–7.

Curtin L. The nurse as an advocate: a philosophical foundation for nursing. In: Heim E, Nicholson M, eds. Contemporary leadership behaviour: selected readings. Boston: Little, Brown, 1985:129–136.

Kohnke M. The nurse as an advocate: a philosophical foundation for nursing. In: Heim E, Nicholson M, eds. Contemporary leadership behaviour: selected readings. Boston: Little, Brown, 1985:137–140.

Milner N. The symbols and means of advocacy intervention. J Law Psychiatry 1986; 8:1–17.

Nelson M. Advocacy in nursing. Nurs Outlook 1988; 36:136–141.

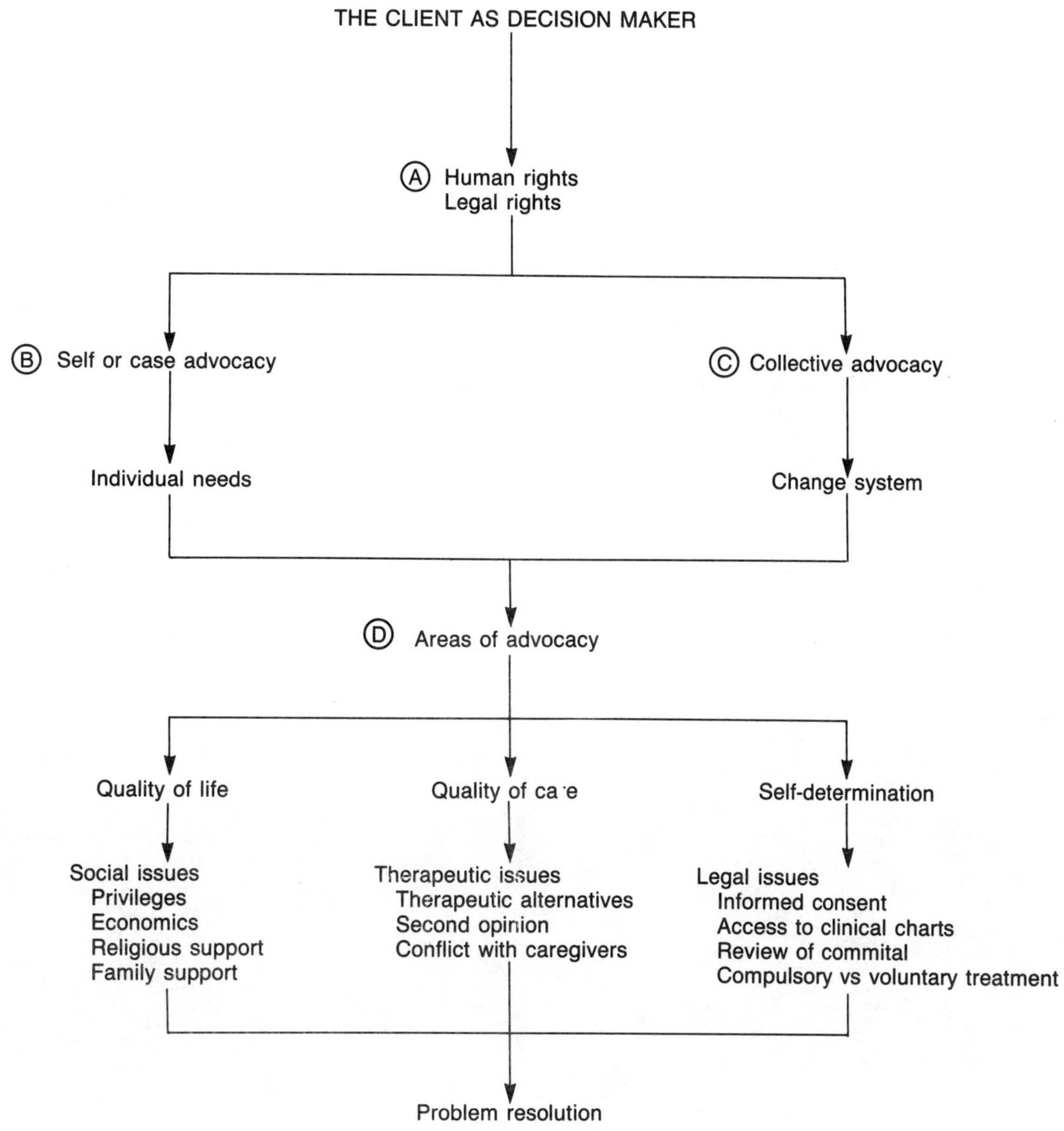
THE CLIENT AS DECISION MAKER
Ⓐ Human rights
Legal rights
Ⓑ Self or case advocacy
Ⓒ Collective advocacy
Individual needs
Change system
Ⓓ Areas of advocacy
Quality of life
Quality of care
Self-determination
Social issues
Privileges
Economics
Religious support
Family support
Therapeutic issues
Therapeutic alternatives
Second opinion
Conflict with caregivers
Legal issues
Informed consent
Access to clinical charts
Review of commital
Compulsory vs voluntary treatment
Problem resolution

INDEX

3168